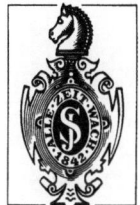

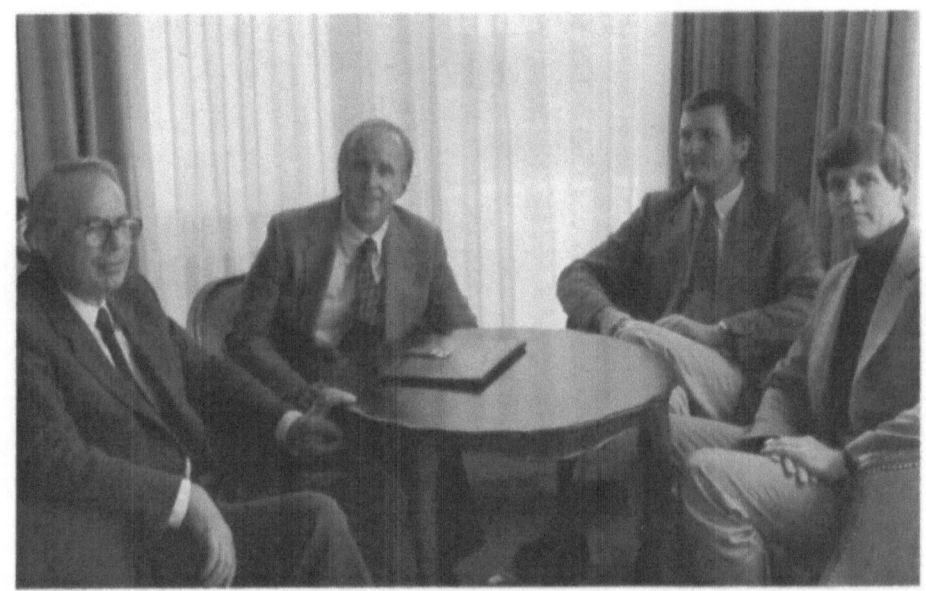

Editors (left to right): E. A. Quellhorst, M. J. Lysaght, C. A. Baldamus and L. W. Henderson

Hemofiltration

Edited by
L. W. Henderson   E. A. Quellhorst
C. A. Baldamus   M. J. Lysaght

With 121 Figures and 34 Tables

Springer-Verlag
Berlin Heidelberg New York Tokyo

Editors:

Professor Dr. med. Lee W. Henderson
Associate Chief of Staff for Research, VA Medical Center and Univ. of California
3350 La Jolla Village Dr., San Diego, CA 92161, USA

Professor Dr. med. Eduard A. Quellhorst
Nephrologisches Zentrum Niedersachsen, Abtl. Innere Medizin
– Nephrologie –, Vogelsang 105,
D-3510 Hann. Münden, West Germany

Professor Dr. med. Conrad A. Baldamus
Medizinische Klinik I – Nephrologie –, Universität zu Köln,
Josef-Stelzmann-Straße 9, D-5000 Köln 41, West Germany

Michael J. Lysaght
Director, Membrane Science, Travenol Laboratories, Inc.
Round Lake, Illinois IL 60073, USA

ISBN-13:978-3-642-69667-1   e-ISBN-13:978-3-642-68665-7
DOI: 10.1007/978-3-642-68665-7

Library of Congress Cataloging in Publication Data.
Hemofiltration. Bibliography: p. Includes index. 1. Blood-Filtration. I. Henderson, L.W. (Lee W.),
1930-RC901.7.H47H46   1986   615'.39   86-6435
ISBN-13:978-3-642-69667-1 (U.S.)

© Springer-Verlag Berlin Heidelberg 1986
Softcover reprint of the hardcover 1st edition 1986

2119/3145-543210

Preface

This book had its genesis in the spring of 1981 in Parma, Italy, where workers in the field of hemofiltration had assembled for an international symposium and for the organizational meeting of the International Society of Hemofiltration. The common wisdom held that the time was ripe for a comprehensive and archival volume on the subject. Dr. Stanley Shaldon convened the present authors and suggested that they work as a team to provide the proper balance of investigative, clinical, and scientific interests, as well as an appropriate degree of geographical dispersion.

The editors would like to thank the participating authors for the effort and scholarship underlying their contributions. It proved especially satisfying to assemble so many of the pioneers and champions of hemofiltration into one volume. Dr. Peter Kramer, one of the most prolific and innovative workers in this field, had agreed to prepare a chapter on continuous arteriovenous hemofiltration; his untimely death unfortunately precluded his participation.

For most contributing authors, as well as for the editors, hemofiltration represents not just a principal investigative enthusiasm but also the most important formative element in their career paths over the past decade. We hope that this volume serves hemofiltration well, both in recording its present status and defining its future directions.

June 1986

L. W. HENDERSON
E. A. QUELLHORST
C. A. BALDAMUS
M. J. LYSAGHT

Table of Contents

List of Contributors

B. VON ALBERTINI
Division of Renal Diseases
George Washington University Medical Center
2150 Pennsylvania Ave. N.W.
Washington, D.C. 20037, USA

C. A. BALDAMUS
Med. Klinik I – Nephrologie –
Universität zu Köln
Josef-Stelzmann-Str. 9
D-5000 Köln 41, West Germany

R. H. BARTLETT
Dept. of Surgery
University of Michigan
Ann Arbor, Michigan 48109, USA

V. BEHNCKE
Nephrologisches Zentrum Niedersachsen
Vogelsang 105
D-3510 Hann. Münden, West Germany

J. P. BOSCH
The George Washington University Medical Center
H. B. Burns Memorial Building
2150 Pennsylvania Avenue, N.W.
Washington, D.C. 20037, USA

C. K. COLTON
Dept. of Chemical Engineering
Massachusetts Institute of Technology
Cambridge, MA 02139, USA

G. M. EISENBACH
Medizinische Hochschule Hannover
D-3000 Hannover, West Germany

A.J.FÜRSCH
Z.I.M., Abtl. Nephrologie
Universitätsklinik
Theodor Stern Kai 7
D-6000 Frankfurt/M., West Germany

S.GLABMAN
The Mount Sinai School of Medicine
The Mount Sinai Medical Center
New York, N.Y. 10029, USA

H.GÖHL
Gambro Dialysatoren KG
Postfach 1323
D-7450 Hechingen, West Germany

L.W.HENDERSON
VA Medical Center and Univ. of California
3350 La Jolla Village Dr.
San Diego, CA 92161, USA

D.VON HERRATH
St.Joseph-Krankenhaus I
Med. Abt.II
Bäumerplan 24
D-1000 Berlin 42, West Germany

P.KONSTANTIN
Gambro Inc. American Membrane Div.
1450 Industrial Park Street
Covina, CA 91722, USA

A.LAUER
Long Island College Hospital
Brooklyn, N.Y., USA

J.K.LEYPOLDT
VA Medical Center
3350 La Jolla Drive
San Diego, CA 92161, USA

M.J.LYSAGHT
Travenol Laboratories
Round Lake, IL 60073, USA

J. R. MAULT
Dept. of Surgery University of Michigan
Ann Arbor, Michigan 48 109, USA

N. J. OFSTHUN
Dept. of Chemical Engineering
Massachusetts Institute of Technology
Cambridge, MA 02 139, USA

E. A. QUELLHORST
Nephrologisches Zentrum Niedersachsen
Innere Medizin – Nephrologie –
Vogelsang 105
D-3510 Hann. Münden, West Germany

K. SCHAEFER
St. Joseph-Krankenhaus I
Med. Abt. II
Bäumerplan 24
D-1000 Berlin 42, West Germany

M. SCHMIDT
Z. I. M., Abtl. Nephrologie
Johann-Wolfgang-Goethe-Universität
Theodor Stern Kai 7
D-6000 Frankfurt 70, West Germany

B. SCHÜNEMANN
Nephrologisches Zentrum Niedersachsen
Vogelsang 105
D-3510 Hann. Münden, West Germany

S. SHALDON
Dept. of Nephrology
University Hospital
Nimes, France

The History of Hemofiltration

M. J. LYSAGHT

Table of Contents

Introduction: Historical Overview

Writers in scientific and medical journals are fond of such sentences as "Polyvorpal Trans-jabberition, first introduced by SMITH in 1958[195-203]" or "Polyvorpal Trans-jabberitation was developed by SMITH[204-221] and JONES[222-250] in the late 50s." Such statements are rarely false, but are often oversimplified, inaccurate, and misleading. Scientific developments do not typically enjoy a discreet birthing, but instead emerge and take form rather like a major river gathering mass and momentum from disperse watersheds and from the confluence of many minor tributaries. Moreover, qualities such as perseverance, practicality, endurance, and exactitude are at least as important indices of a contributor's merit as is simple primacy. Accordingly, the purpose of this chapter is not to assign priority for the development of hemofiltration (HF), but rather to review the fascinating history of how and why this therapy came to be.

Early Stirrings (1928–1965)

FERRY's definitive 1936 review of ultrafiltration is 75 pages long, but devotes just the following seven lines to blood ultrafiltration [1]:

Ultrafiltration In Vivo. It is possible to lead the bloodstream of an animal through an ultrafilter, after injection of heparin to prevent clotting, and thus to obtain an ultrafiltrate of the blood in vivo. A convenient apparatus is described by GEIGER. BRULL performed this experiment, finding that chlorides, dextrose, and nonprotein nitrogen passed the filter in undiminished concentration, while phosphorus and calcium were partially retained, i.e., the results were similar to those of ultrafiltration in vitro.

Both BRULL [2] in France in 1928 and GEIGER [3] in Jerusalem in 1931 employed collodion membranes to obtain small samples of canine blood for analytical purposes; their principal interest appears to have been the relationship between electrolyte concentration in the filtrate and in what was retained. GEIGER was a peripatetic Hungarian doctor and his report is very impressive. His original cell design (Fig. 1) employs a spiral, thin-channel blood path; the same principle is employed in contemporary devices to minimize concentration polarization without turbulence. Moreover, he properly sorted out the role of protein volume (protocrit) in applying the Donnan correction to this system and in calculating what are now called sieving coefficients. Although GEIGER's first paper promised "a future communication" on this topic, none was forthcoming.

In 1947, MALINOW and KORZON [4] from Chicago described in the *Journal of Laboratory and Clinical Medicine* a technically successful canine HF. Their intent was clear. "Our purpose was to develop an ultrafilter which could duplicate glomerular function in a dog, both qualitatively and quantitatively, to be used in an attempt to prolong the life of uremic animals." Their ultrafilter contained 0.8 m^2 cellophane

A METHOD OF ULTRA-FILTRATION *IN VIVO.*

By ALEXANDER GEIGER, M.D.

(From the Department of Hygiene, Hebrew University, Jerusalem.)

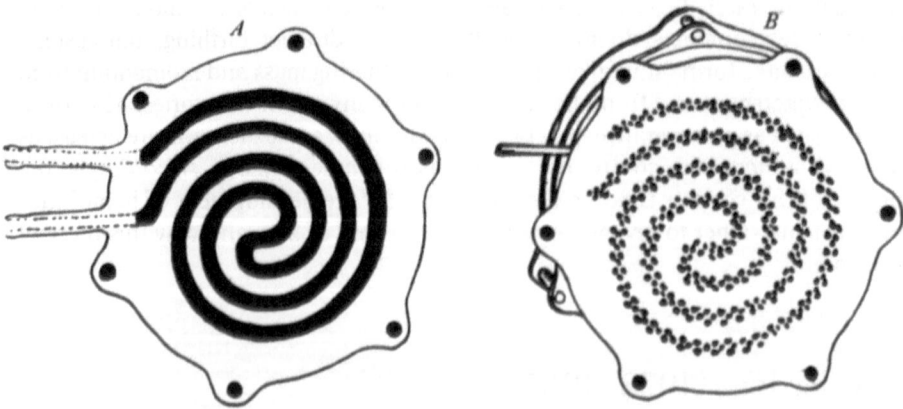

Fig. 1. Schematic drawing of ALEXANDER GEIGER's clinical ultrafilter, reprinted from [3]. GEIGER achieved thin-channel flow by cutting a spiral groove in a spacer and then sandwiching the spacer between the collodion membranes

468   MALINOW AND KORZON

TABLE I. OBSERVATIONS ON MALE DOG, WEIGHT 27 POUNDS, RENDERED ANEPHRIC AND CONNECTED TO ULTRAFILTER*

REMARKS		UREA N (MG./100 C.C.)	CREATININE (MG./100 C.C.)	PROTEIN (MG./100 C.C.)	CO_2 (VOL. %)	HEMATOCRIT (%)	Cl (MG./100 C.C.)
Preoperative	Blood	21		6.9	45	48	630
24 hr. after nephrectomy	Blood	65			32	47	680
48 hr. after nephrectomy	Blood	180		5.5	58	44	600
72 hr. after nephrectomy	Blood	175		5.4		38	540
After 1 hr. of filtration	Blood	135					590
	Plasma	145	8.6			42	590
After 8 hr. of filtration	Blood	75		3.9		39	640
	Plasma	83	6.0				600
Ultrafiltrate obtained at end of 1 hr.		160	7.2				660
Ultrafiltrate obtained at end of 8 hr.		80	5.0				660

	BEFORE FILTRATION	AFTER FILTRATION
Plasma volume	964 c.c.	1010 c.c.
Blood volume	1550 c.c.	1650 c.c.
Hematocrit	38%	39%

Total amount of filtrate, 7,200 c.c. collected in eight hr.
Total amount of urea N "excreted," 6.9 Gm.
Urea clearance (concentration in the blood assumed to be 125 mg./100 c.c., the mean between 175 and 75), 11.3 c.c./blood/minute.

*In this experiment the lag seen in Fig. 9 and explained in the text has not been taken into consideration. This lag explains the lack of parallelism between the plasma and ultrafiltrate concentrations of urea and creatinine.

Fig. 2. Table of results from MALINOW and KORZON's 1947 publication in Journal of Laboratory and Clinical Medicine [4]

arranged as parallel tubes. Blood flow rate (pumped) was ~100 ml/min. Filtration rate was 15–20 ml/min at 500 mmHg transmembrane pressure (TMP). Fluid balance was maintained by injecting Ringer-Krebs solution at 10-min intervals. In the course of an 8-h treatment, 7.2 liters was exchanged. Blood urea nitrogen in the nephrectomized test animal fell from 175 to 75 mg%. Other results are given in Fig. 2, which is a facsimile of Table 1 of the original article. Access was via the femoral artery and vein. In a footnote, the authors described a smaller version of their filter, one that functions without a blood pump. Three decades later, this version was to be called "spontaneous" or arteriovenous (AV) HF.

MALINOW and KORZON were rather deprecating of their results. ("A larger ultrafilter with more filtering surface, or one employing a much greater filtering pressure, may have sufficient clearance of urea for man, but the dialyzer described by KOLFF appears superior in simplicity and in obtainable results.") In retrospect, however, their accomplishment warranted greater enthusiasm.

In the late 1940s and early 1950s, ALWALL ([5], especially Chap. 6) in Stockholm experimented with dialyzer-ultrafilter designs with membrane support systems that produced rapid (by the standards of those days) ultrafiltration. In the main, ALWALL was treating the azotemia accompanying acute renal failure (ARF), and his protocols were simple variations on KOLFF's newly developed hemodialysis. Sometimes, however, ALWALL operated his devices as *isolated ultrafilters* with no dialysate, and documented substantial reductions in patient volume. These circuits often operated without blood or filtrate pumps and are the true clinical antecedents of continuous arteriovenous hemofiltration (CAVH), later developed by KRAMER. Interestingly, ALWALL's membranes had very low fluid permeability and, to generate the required transmembrane pressure, he sometimes hung his filtrate (siphon) line out the window. He notes, "In this case, the temperature of the air outside must not be below that of the fluid in the tube or it will freeze!!" (emphasis added). Although they were aggressive practitioners and promoters of blood ultrafiltration, ALWALL and his coworkers appeared primarily concerned with fluid removal. Urea was removed stoichiometrically with the excess fluid, and occasionally replacement fluid was given to correct imbalance. But this group did not embrace the blood-cleansing concept of HF, i.e., the reduction of urea concentration by plasma water exchange.

During the 1950s, LEONARDS, from the Cleveland Clinic, published two papers on the removal of edemic fluid, one with SKEGGS and KAHN in 1952 (canine) [6] and one with KOLFF in 1954 (human) [7]. In the early 1960s, NAKAMOTO [8] described the treatment of fluid overload with coil dialyzers. Again, this work focused on fluid removal, not on convective blood cleansing. In fact, there is nothing in the literature to suggest any recollection of MALINOW's original concept.

The Precommercial Decade (1966–1976)

The modern era of HF began in 1966. LEWIS BLUEMLE and LEE HENDERSON at the Medical School of the University of Pennsylvania were conducting a small National Institutes of Health (NIH) research program entitled "Evaluation of New Membranes for Hemodialysis." This group had been prevailed upon by ALAN MICHAELS, president of the just-founded Amicon Corporation, to include some of his firm's developmental membranes in their study. Their June 1966 letter report to the NIH read, in part, as follows [9]:

> Our attention has been directed to a new class of polyelectrolyte membranes produced by the Amicon Corporation . . . [Such] highly permeable membranes may be more useful in blood purification by ultrafiltration than by dialysis . . . Consequently, a method was conceived for continuous blood "diafiltration" in which neither the blood nor the patient becomes dehydrated, since reconstituting fluid is added as rapidly as ultrafiltrate is formed.

Additional information about their approach is given Fig. 3.

The process was described more fully in 1967 at an American Society for Artificial Internal Organs (ASAIO) meeting by HENDERSON and coworkers [10]. The National Institute of Arthritis and Metabolic Diseases (NIAMD), a division of the NIH, funded hemodiafiltration (as it was then called) in a major program that continued from 1968 through 1978. This program was directed by LEE HENDERSON with the support of Amicon Corporation (particularly CHERYL FORD), and also CLARK COLTON at the Massachusetts Institute of Technology (MIT). Their early activities

HOSPITAL OF THE UNIVERSITY OF PENNSYLVANIA
3400 SPRUCE STREET • PHILADELPHIA, PA. 19104

CLINICAL RESEARCH CENTER
SIXTH FLOOR • MALONEY BUILDING

June 2, 1966

LEWIS W. BLUEMLE, JR., M.D.
DIRECTOR

Dr. Irwin Siegel
Assistant Chief
Chronic Uremia/Dialysis Program
Institute of Arthritis and
Metabolic Diseases
Bethesda, Maryland 20014   Re: Contract No. PH-43-66-45

Dear Doctor Siegel:

This letter will serve as a brief interim report on the above contract entitled "Evaluation of New Membranes for Hemodialysis".

To state our tentative conclusion first, it would appear that highly permeable membranes which require reinforcement to avoid rupture may be more useful in blood purification by ultrafiltration rather than by dialysis.

Our attention has been directed to a new class of polyelectrolyte membranes produced by the Amicon Corporation under the trade name of Diaflo (formerly Diaplex). Briefly these membranes are composed of polymeric anions and cations (e.g. sodium polystyrene sulfonate and polyvinyl benzyl trimethyl ammonium chloride) in stoichiometric proportions, forming ionically-cross-linked structures with controllable permeability to solutes of varying molecular size. Void fractions of up to 8.0 have been reported.

Permeability studies were conducted in a batch dialyzer in which the effect of fluid films can be controlled by varying rotor speed. Sodium chloride, urea and glucose were the test solutes. Permeability was calculated as follows:

$$P = \frac{s}{A(1/V_L + 1/V_R)}$$

where s = slope of ln ΔC, or ln $(C_L - C_R)$, with
            time
        A = membrane area
        V_L = fluid volume in left chamber
        V_R = fluid volume in right chamber

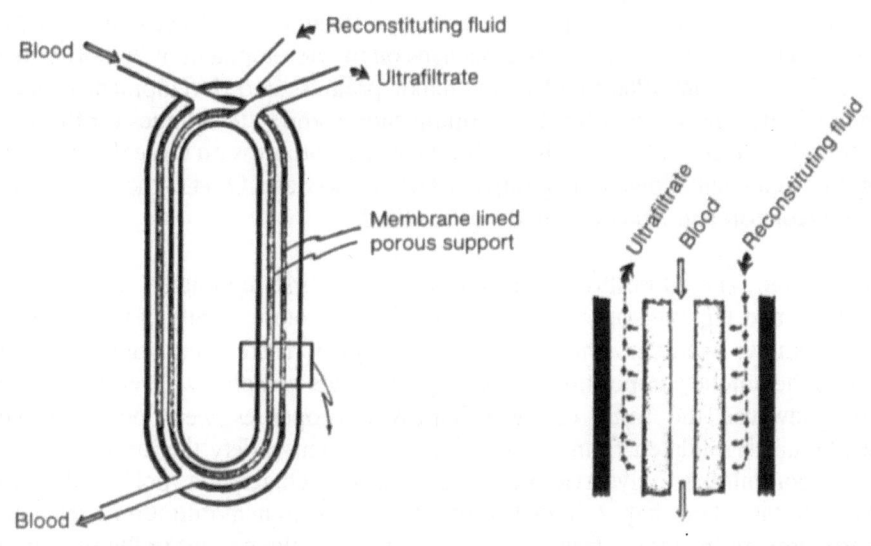

Fig. 3. The beginning of the modern era of hemofiltration: Letter and accompanying drawing for NIH contract PH 43-66-45

are chronicled in several reports presented at ASAIO meetings [11-15] and in the annual transactions of the NIAMD contractors conferences.

A second center of HF activity grew up in Göttingen, Federal Republic of Germany (FRG), under the leadership of EDWARD QUELLHORST. (Curiously, Göttingen had earlier housed R. ZSINGIMONDY's pioneering membrane laboratories during 1920s and 1930s.) Apparently, QUELLHORST's involvement with HF began in much the same way as that of HENDERSON and BLUEMLE when Sartorius, a Göttingen firm diversifying into membranes, asked him to evaluate some of their developmental membranes for hemodialysis. Filtration rates were too high, and QUELLHORST suggested that the filters be evaluated for hemofiltration instead. QUELLHORST's work was first described in 1971 [16]; subsequent progress was reported at several European Dialysis and Transplantation Association (EDTA) congresses [17-19].

DORSON and MARKOVITZ and their collaborators at Arizona State University also experimented with an "artificial glomerulus" [20] and then a "molecular separation artificial kidney" [21]. This group consistently incorporated reverse osmosis as a second stage in the circuit to purify the ultrafiltrate for eventual return to the donor. Ongoing developments were reported at ASAIO meetings [22, 23].

A review of references [9-23] reveals that each of the three groups whose work is included had its own character and a somewhat different sense of purpose. HENDERSON regarded HF primarily as a powerful means of exploring the role of middle molecules in uremia. He and his colleagues emphasized transport theory, the characterization and optimization of membranes and filters, and carefully structured clinical ABA cross-over protocols (A, hemodialysis; B, hemofiltration). QUELLHORST, in contrast, seems to have viewed HF as a method that should be adapted for clinical application. Accordingly, he worked at simplifying the process, at using commercially available products to provide reliable and reasonably economical treatment, and at building up a credibly large patient population at the earliest possible date. DORSON and his group believed that to be practical, HF required reprocessing of the spent filtrate. All of their studies embodied a second stage to remove the toxins from uremic plasma, allowing the useful portions to be returned to the patient. Both HENDERSON [24] and DORSON and PIZZICONI [25] have contributed review articles summarizing their perspectives on the development of hemofiltration.

The decade from 1966 to 1976 saw major progress and development in membranes, in transport theory for device optimization, and in techniques for fluid balance and management. It was, in the final analysis, progress on these three technological fronts that allowed the groups of HENDERSON and QUELLHORST to succeed where KORZON and MALINOW had earlier failed.

Membranes. The ultrafiltration membranes that first stimulated the work of BLUEMLE and HENDERSON were prepared from an esoteric family of inorganic hydrogels known as Ioplex. Their observed high transport rates were originally attributed to the unique composition of the polyelectrolyte complexes. Over the next decade, however, the same or even improved properties were obtained with membranes formulated from a wide range of garden variety thermoplastics [26]: dynel, polysulfone, polyacrylonitrile, polymethyl methacrylate, polyamides, and others discussed in Chap. 2. In fact, scientists working in hemofiltration were major contributors to the rationalization of membrane formulation and to the realization of techniques for prospectively designed ("tailored") membranes for molecular separation. Moreover, the development of hollow fibers for HF by FORD and PAULSEN [24] represented the first time that any asymmetric membrane had been achieved in hollow-fiber format for any purpose. This development has since been widely exploited in other commercial fields.

Transport Theory. By themselves, very permeable membranes did not guarantee rapid ultrafiltration rates; boundary layers of nonpermeated species could very rapidly accumulate at the membrane surface and eventually reduce the transmembrane flow to virtually nothing. Certain operating formats had been developed empirically that minimized this so-called "concentration polarization," but the relationships between filtration rate and conditions of geometry and flow were very complicated. This situation was sorted out in rather brilliant fashion, largely by COLTON, and the results were published in kinetics papers [27, 28] that have served as the foundation of mass transport in HF ever since. The early availability of a rational and comprehensive transport theory greatly facilitated the growth of HF; our current understanding is summarized in Chap. 3.

Fluid Balance and Management. HF requires some means of balancing the 8–12 liters of fluids being filtered and infused per hour. In the original, *volumetric* approach, fluid was pumped into and out of the patient by means of matched piston heads on a common reciprocating shaft. The problem with this circuit, aside from its intrinsic complexity, was the large surface area of hardware to which the parenteral fluid had to be exposed. This feature was almost certainly implicated in the on-again/off-again history of pyrogen responses in early HF attempts. In 1975 and 1976, the Hannovers-Münden group perfected a *gravimetric* approach to fluid balance that has since become standard [29]. The infusate and filtrate were combined onto a common scale and deployed in a fashion such that any change in their net weight (easily sensed by a transducer and acted upon by a microprocessor) was equal and opposite to that of the patient. As a side benefit, this approach prompted the supply of fluid in larger containers (3.5–5 liters), which were more economical than single-liter containers.

Medical attention during this period focused on patient tolerance of HF and other obvious and readily observable differences in outcome parameters. In 1973, HENDERSON et al. observed the improved symptomatic tolerance of the process. "If anything, it was felt that deliberate negative fluid balance was better tolerated (few, if any, leg cramps) with diafiltration than dialysis" [14]. HENDERSON did not dwell on this finding and instead pursued the general control of hypertension with HF. In 1976, QUELLHORST et al. [19] presented their first clinical experience with HF and heavily emphasized the putative advantages of the process with regard to both intratreatment hypotension and intertreatment hypertension. Virtually no attention was then paid to the improved biocompatibility of hemofilters relative to contemporary dialyzers. Of course, HF did not develop in a vacuum. Its theoretical progress was closely interwined with the achievements of FUNK-BRENTANO et al. in developing high-permeability membranes for dialysis [30] and of BERGSTROM et al. with isolated ultrafiltration [31].

So, a decade after BLUEMLE and HENDERSON began working on HF, the process had basic feasibility and was being separately pursued by different groups in different countries. The literature contained a total of about 30 publications, mostly from groups mentioned above. Perhaps a dozen German centers had begun to evaluate the process independently, but had not yet published their experiences. Commercial firms did not promote HF at exhibits and trade shows, and did not offer appropriate disposables and hardware. All this was about to change abruptly.

Growth and Maturation (1976–1985)

The emergence of HF as a commercial process, rather than as a scientific tool or development entity, can be pinpointed rather precisely. In September 1976, a German firm, Fresenius, convened a day-long workshop, inviting the various centers experimenting with HF to present their findings [32]. The meeting was organized by HANS RUDOLPH using the RP6 (which Fresenius distributed) for HF. BENJAMIN BURTON of the NIH attended as a special guest. The meeting was conducted entirely in German; a list of the speakers and their subjects is given in Table 1. Many of the participants are still active in the investigation and application of HF and many of the topics are still under discussion in contemporary workshops. Some of the papers were coordinated into proceedings and were later published (in 1977) in a special issue of *The Journal of Dialysis* [33].

In January 1977, four leading European investigators (QUELLHORST, MAN, FRANZ, and KRAMER) were invited, along with HENDERSON, to give short presentations on HF at the 10th Annual Contractors Conference. This occasion provided the first cross exposure of American and European investigators. Here, as detailed in the published synopsis [34], reduced symptomatic hypotension, which has proved to be the most enduring clinical advantage of HF, first received dominant emphasis. FRANZ wrote, "Even taking off 6 to 8 kg water in one treatment, filtration patients seem less zonked out than those on dialysis." QUELLHORST presented graphs demonstrating smaller decreases in mean arterial pressure for a given weight loss during HF than during a dialysis control. Then, as now, the exact mechanism of improved tolerance was only speculative.

The European and American efforts began to merge. Both QUELLHORST's and HENDERSON's groups presented papers at the Newcastle upon Tyne symposium "Technical Aspects of Renal Failure" [29, 35]. QUELLHORST was on the March 1977 ASAIO program [36]. Terminology became standardized, with the Americans adapting the European expression "hemofiltration" over their earlier term "hemodiafiltration." The frequent local meetings in Europe now all had at least one or two sessions devoted to HF, often with speakers from both sides of the Atlantic.

Also, in the spring of 1977, the NIH announced its intention to sponsor a multicenter, controlled study comparing HF with hemodialysis (HD). Four groups were selected (two from Europe and two from America) from the 15 or so centers that submitted proposals. This effort, which lasted 2 or 3 years, provided a skeletal continuity to research in HF during its rapid-growth phase. The participants were HEN-

Table 1. Program of the Braunlage Workshop on Hemofiltration, September 25, 1976

Introduction	F. Scheler, Göttingen
Principles of hemofiltration in comparison to hemodialysis	E. Quellhorst, Hannovers-Munden
Construction and special features of hemofiltration systems	J. Rieger, Göttingen; B. Doht, Hannovers-Munden
Predilution hemofiltration	H. Mann, Aachen
Variations in negative pressure during hemofiltration	M. Hueffler, D. V. Herrath, G. Asmus, K. Schaeffer, Berlin
Hemofiltration with hollow fibers	E. Streicher, H. Schneider, Stuttgart
Application of convective transport to artificial kidneys by means of hemofiltration	N. K. Man, A. Sausse, Paris
Hollow-fiber membranes	U. Mylius, Tuchingen
Cellulose-nitrate membranes	H. Perl, Göttingen
Lactate or acetate substitution fluid buffer	C-D. Seufert, H. D. Soling, Göttingen
Calcium balance in hemofiltration	Ch. Fuchs, Göttingen
Loss of amino acids in hemofiltration	H. Mann, Aachen
Role of clotting factors during hemofiltration	H. Koestering, Göttingen
Kinetics of leukocyte and colony-forming units in the blood of uremic patients on hemofiltration and hemodialysis	H. L. Franz, U/M
Clinical results of hemofiltration	B. Doht, Hannovers-Munden; D. V. Herrath, M. Hueffler, G. Asmos, K. Schaeffer, Berlin; H. Schneider, E. Streicher, Stuttgart
Control of dialysis-resistant hypertension with hemofiltration	B. Schunemann, Hannovers-Munden; J. Girnbdt, Göttingen
Changes in nerve-conduction velocities with long-term hemofiltration	H. Beckemen, Hannovers-Munden
Comparison of lipid changes in hemodialysis and hemofiltration	H. Henning, Göttingen
Elimination of drugs during hemofiltration	P. Kramer, K. W. Rumpf, Göttingen
Excursions in PTH, vitamin D, and digoxen during chronic hemofiltration	K. Schaeffer, G. Offerman, D. Herrath, G. Asmus, M. Huffler, Berlin

DERSON [37] (University of California), GLABMAN, BOSCH, ALBERTINI, and GERONO-MOS [38] (Mount Sinai Medical Center, New York), QUELLHORST [39] Munden (FRG), and KOCH and BALDAMUS [40] (University Hospital, Frankfurt, FRG).

Commercial interest heightened. At EDTA in Helsinki in June 1977, both Amicon and Sartorius introduced their hemofilters. Sartorius exhibited a fluid cycler, as well. The German firms of Braun and Schiwa began selling infusion fluid and Fresenius began marketing fluid of its own manufacture and also distributed the Sartorius filter and cycler. ASAHI introduced a hollow hemofilter in 1978. Gambro hardware and disposables were first displayed at EDTA in Istanbul in 1978 and entered the market shortly thereafter.

SCHELER's group at the University of Göttingen published a monograph containing their papers on HF in 1977 [41]; this was an early German-language primer in the field. The literature was expanding rapidly. In September 1978, Amicon issued a HF bibliography with over 250 entries [42].

In 1979 HENDERSON first described sterile fluid generation [43]. In the same year, the Mount Sinai group introduced high-clearance, postdilution HF, which for the first time allowed HF to provide the same urea clearance as HD [44]. In 1978, at EDTA, STANLEY SHALDON published the first of his many important contributions to this topic [45].

PETER KRAMER, of Göttingen, first described "spontaneous" or "continuous" arteriovenous HF in 1977 [46]. This highly cybernetic process proved enormously appealing to practitioners. By 1980, it was being widely utilized in intensive and critical care stations around Germany. In May 1981, KRAMER chaired a two-day workshop on this treatment in Göttingen; the proceedings of this workshop were published in German in 1982 [47]. An updated revision, in English, appeared late in 1985 [48]. CAVH was acclaimed even by those who were more restrained in their enthusiasm for continuous intermittent HF and was approved by the United States Food and Drug Administration (FDA) in March 1983.

Three workshops on HF were held in 1981-1982: "Symposium sur l'hemofiltration," September 24-26, 1981, La Grande Motte, France, organized by MION and SHALDON; "Hemofiltration: Present Status and Prospects," April 29-30, 1982, Durma, Italy, organized by MIGONE, MINETTI, CIVATI, and GUASTOMI; and, "Hemofiltration, II," December 4-5, 1981, Berlin, Germany, organized by SCHAEFFER, KOCH, and QUELLHORST. These meetings were supported by Gambro and were international in character; the proceedings of all three were published [49, 50, 51].

In 1982, the International Society for Hemofiltration was formed, with KOCH of Hannover as its first president. The society, which held annual meetings in 1983, 1984, and 1985, publishes its own journal, *Blood Purification,* edited by K. SCHAEFFER and published by Karger.

These meetings, colloquia, and literature provided a continuous appraisal of the medical performance and technical progress of HF. A degree of ebb and flow attended the common perception of the issues. HF was at first lauded as a long-awaited panacea, then revisionists began to view it as oversold, unduly complex, and hazardous. The current wisdom, which lies somewhere in between, is summarized throughout this book.

Figure 4 shows the growth in number of patients receiving chronic HF. At this writing (mid-1984), virtually all HF patients reside in Europe, since the process was not approved by the FDA for the USA until 1983 and economical replacement fluid is not yet available in Japan. The 2%-5% market penetration in various European countries has been achieved despite the fact hat HF therapy is more expensive than HD. Of course, further growth is likely to depend very much on process economics.

The primary indication for HF has been patient-specific vascular instability during HD (see the chapter by BALDAMUS). A very small fraction of patients (well under 1%, often acute or chronic cases with collateral complications) simply cannot tolerate the stresses of HD, are unsuited for continuous ambulatory peritoneal dialysis (CAPD), and thus need HF to survive. A second group, variously estimated at 1%-5% of end-stage renal disease (ESRD) patients, display sufficient intolerance to HD to require specially elongated treatment schedules or frequent staff intervention. This is the group for whom HF is prescribed in Europe and who might be reasonable candidates in the United States, despite higher disposable costs. A third subset (5%-40%) experience some intratreatment discomfort, but not enough for

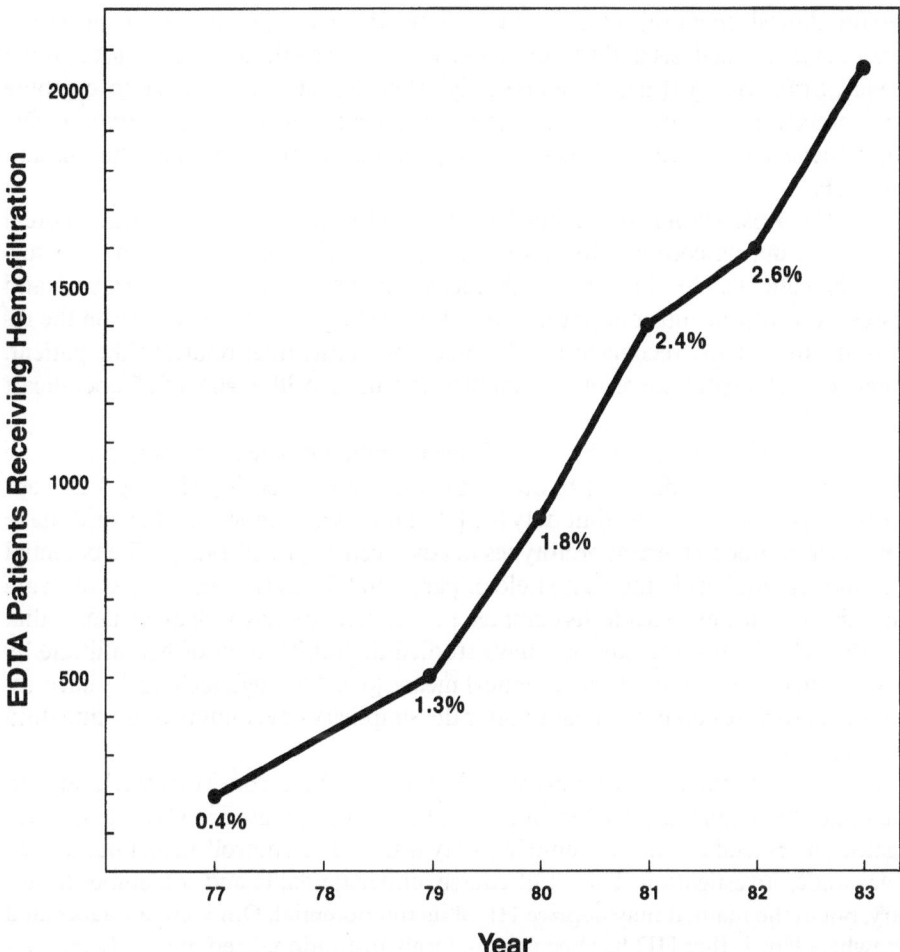

Fig. 4. Growth in the number of patients receiving hemofiltration. Percentages are based on total EDTA population from EDTA registry and industry sources

this to be regarded as a medical or economic issue. For HF to expand to this group, the treatment would have to be fully cost equivalent to alternative therapies. The goal of cost equivalency is not unrealistic. Some centers have reported that with fluid generation and device reuse, HF is no more expensive than comparable dialysis [52, 53, 54]. Patients in other than those groups detailed above would probably not shift to HF unless advantages other than symptomatic tolerance were identified. Such advantages could either be medical or dramatically reduced treatment times [55].

There have been several attempts to meld HF and HD into a single treatment modality. SHINABERGER [56] attempted this combination in 1969, but lacked suitable devices or hardware. In 1974, HENDERSON [57] described the conduct of both processes in series using separate filters for dialysis and fluid removal. In 1982, CHEUNG and HENDERSON [58] proposed a two-filter hybrid system capable of combining dialysis, HF, and in situ fluid generation. Von ALBERTINI [59] described successful clinical operation in 1984. LEBER [60] advanced the concept of using the same device for dialysis and filtration, but with separate fluid infusion distal to the device. STREICHER [61] has developed high-flux dialysis that appears to combine both processes in a single device with fluid replenishment by retrofiltration. The consequence of all such processes is a treatment midway between pure dialysis and pure HF.

In 1976, ROMAGNOLI first applied hemofiltration technology to extracorporeal circulation during coronary bypass surgery [62]. During oxygenation in such surgery, the patient's blood is often deliberately diluted to minimize both trauma and losses; ROMAGNOLI introduced the concept of placing a small hemofilter on the return line to partially reconcentrate the blood before its final return to the patient. Some form of membrane reconcentration is now used in 30%–40% of all open-heart surgery.

HENDERSON's technique for on-line fluid generation has been the subject of much research interest [43, 52, 53, 54], but is not yet widely used in HF. The FDA approved this process in 1983 (but only for HF) and both Gambro and Sartorius have a number of precommercial prototypes in advanced stages of testing. The potential for this methodology in the entire field of parenteral fluids is enormous; as this area unfolds over the next decade, its commercial significance may well overshadow that of HF itself. Several investigators have studied the purification of hemofiltrate by absorption [45, 63, 64] or electrochemical means [65]. Although technically successful, such processes do not appear to offer the simplicity or economy of on-line fluid generation.

With the encouraging exception of CAVH, HF has been consistently relegated to the same "three times a week for four-to-six hours" format used in HD. Most investigators, in fact, take pains to maintain parity with a "HD control" in all but the variables under investigation. This is, of course, understandable and sometimes necessary, but in the main, it may deprive HF of its full potential. Our view, as elaborated elsewhere [66], is that HD has been prematurely institutionalized in a far from optimal format, a format that traps patients in a marathon dance of endless tedium where survival alone is the operative index of merit and where quality of life is far too often ignored. HF should strive to avoid the same mistake. It is to be hoped that future investigative efforts will be directed toward

a) simple at-home overnight treatments as envisioned by KRAMER [67],

b) further pursuit of NEFF's [68] and SHALDON's [69] concepts for continuous ambulatory HF, and

c) reduction to practice of the proposals of KRAMER [70] and BLACKSHEAR [71] for wearable or implantable devices capable of reprocessing or reabsorbing the primary filtrate. Such approaches bring us closer to the ultimate endpoint of returning the patient to true health instead of simply prolonging life. That is the challenge of the future and the goal toward which the considerable promise of hemofiltration should be directed.

Acknowledgments

Dr. LEE HENDERSON provided the letter which is reproduced, in part, in Fig. 3. I am indebted to Ms. CAROL WORSTER for considerable research assistance and to Mr. BRUCE DAVIS for editing the manuscript.

References

1. Ferry JD (1936) Ultrafilter membranes and ultrafiltration. Chem Rev 18: 373–455
2. Brull L (1928) Realisation de l'ultrafiltration in vivo. Biol C R 99: 105–107
3. Geiger A (1931) A method of ultra-filtration in vivo. J Physiol 71: 111–120
4. Malinow MR, Korzon W (1947) An experimental method for obtaining an ultrafiltrate of the blood. J Lab Clin Med 32: 461–471
5. Alwall N (1963) Therapeutic and diagnostic problems in severe renal failure. Scandinavian University books (Munksgaard), Copenhagen
6. Skeggs LT, Leonards JR, Kahn JR (1952) Removal of the fluid from normal and edematous dogs by continuous ultrafiltration of blood. Lab Invest 1: 488–494
7. Kolff WJ, Leonards JR (1954) Reduction of otherwise intractable edema by dialysis or filtration. Cleveland Clin Quat 21: 61–71
8. Nakamoto S (1961) Removal of edema fluid by ultrafiltration with the disposable twin coil artificial kidney. Clev Clin Q 28: 10–15
9. Bluemle LW (1966) Evaluation of new membranes for hemodialysis. Interim report on NIH contract PH-43-66-45
10. Henderson L, Besarb A, Michaels A, Bluemle LW (1967) Blood purification by ultrafiltration and fluid replacement (diafiltration). Trans Am Soc Artif Intern Organs 16: 216–222
11. Bixler HJ, Nelsen LM, Bluemle LW (1968) The development of a blood purification system for blood purification. Trans Am Soc Artif Intern Organs 14: 99–107
12. Henderson LW, Ford CA, Colton CK, Bluemle LW, Bixler HJ (1970) Uremic blood cleansing by diafiltration using a hollow fiber ultrafilter. Trans Am Soc Artif Intern Organs 16: 107–114
13. Hamilton R, Ford C, Colton C, Cross R, Steinmuller S, Henderson LW (1971) Blood cleansing by diafiltration in uremic dog and man. Trans Am Soc Artif Intern Organs 17: 259–265
14. Henderson LW, Livoti LG, Ford CA, Kelly AB, Lysaght MJ (1973) Clinical experience with intermittent hemofiltration. Trans Am Soc Artif Intern Organs 19: 119–123
15. Silverstein ME, Ford CA, Lysaght MJ, Henderson LW (1974) Response to rapid removal of intermediate molecular weight solutes in uremic man. Trans Am Soc Artif Intern Organs 20: 614–621
16. Quellhorst E, Plashues E (1971) Ultrafiltration: Elimination harnpflichtiger Substanzen mit Hilfe neuartiger Membranen. In: Ditrich P, Skabal F (eds) Aktuelle Probleme der Dialyseverfahren und der Niereninsuffizienz. Bindernagel, Friedberg, pp 216–226
17. Quellhorst E, Fernandez F, Scheler F (1972) Treatment of uremia using an ultrafiltration-filtration system. Proc Eur Dial Transplant Assoc 9: 584–587
18. Reiger J, Quellhorst E, Lowitz HD, Kong RG, Scheler F (1974) Ultrafiltration for middle molecules in uremia. Proc Eur Dial Transplant Assoc 11: 158–164
19. Quellhorst E, Rieger J, Doht B, Beckmann H, Jacob I, Kraft B, Mietzsch G, Scheler F (1976) Treatment of chronic uremia by an ultrafiltration kidney: first clinical experience. Proc Eur Dial Transplant Assoc 13: 314–321
20. Markovitz M (1968) An artificial glomerulus. Ariz Med 25: 35–37
21. Dorson W, Markovitz M (1968) A pulsating artificial kidney. Chem Eng Prog Symp Ser 84: 85–89
22. Dorson WJ, Markovitz M, Pizziconi VB, Walter JA (1970) Molecular separation as an artificial kidney technique. Trans Amer Soc Artif Intern Organs 16: 127–133
23. Dorson WJ, Pizziconi VB, Vorhees ME, Calkins R, Christianson HB, Cotter DJ, Fargotstein R, Markovitz M, Monty DE, Tomisaka DM (1973) Initial trials of a molecular separation artificial kidney. Trans Am Soc Artif Intern Organs 19: 109–118

24. Henderson LW (1982) The beginning of hemofiltration. Contrib Nephrol 32: 1-19
25. Dorson WJ, Pizziconi VB (1979) Present status of the hemofiltration molecular separation artificial kidney. Artif Organs 3 (1): 6-7
26. Lysaght MJ, Ford CA (1974) Biomedical applications of anisotropic membranes. In: Hopfenberg HB (ed) Permeability of plastic films and coating to gases, vapors, and liquids. Plenum, New York, pp 459-468
27. Colton CK, Henderson LW, Ford CA, Lysaght MJ (1975) Kinetics of hemodiafiltration: in vitro transport characteristics of a hollow fiber blood ultrafilter. J Lab Clin Med 85 (3): 355-371
28. Henderson LW, Colton CK, Ford CA (1975) Kinetics of hemodiafiltration II: clinical characterization of a new blood cleansing modality. J Lab Clin Med 85 (3): 372-391
29. Quellhorst E, Schuenemann B, Doht B (1978) Hemofiltration - a new method for the treatment of chronic renal insufficiency. In: Frost TH (ed) Technical aspects of renal dialysis. Pitman Medical, Kent, pp 96-106
30. Funk-Brentano JL, Man NK, Sausse A, Zingraff J, Boudet J, Becker A, Cueille GF (1976) Characterization of a 1100-1300 MW uremic neurotoxin. Trans Am Soc Artif Intern Organs 22: 163-167
31. Bergstrom J, Asaba H, Furst P, Oules R (1976) Dialysis, ultrafiltration and blood pressure. Proc Eur Dial Transplant Assoc 13: 293-305
32. Quellhorst E, Scheler F (1976) Arbeitstagung über Hämofiltration Braunlage/Harz 25. September 1976. Wissenschaftliche Information Aktuelle Nephrologie (Fresenius Stiftung) 4: 85-103
33. Journal of Dialysis 1 (6): 529-649
34. Mackey BB (ed) (1977) Proceedings tenth annual contractors conference of the artificial kidney program of the National Institute of Arthritis, Metabolism, and Digestive diseases. DHEW publication 77-1422: 130-157, 166-191
35. Lysaght MJ, Ford CA, Colton CK, Stone RA, Henderson LW (1978) Mass transfer in clinical blood ultrafiltration devices - a review. In: Frost TH (ed) Technical aspects of renal dialysis. Pitman Medical, Kent, pp 81-95
36. Quellhorst E, Schuenemann B, Doht B (1977) Hemofiltration - A new method for treatment of chronic renal insufficiency. Trans Am Soc Artif Intern Organs 23: 681-682
37. Henderson LW, San Felippo ML, Stone RA (1981) Comparison of hemodialysis and hemofiltration. Proc 12th Annu Contract Conf, Dept HEW Publ No. NIH 81-1979: 169
38. Bosch JP, Albertini B, Geronomos A, Glabman S (1981) Comparison of hemofiltration and ultrafiltration + hemodialysis to conventional hemodialysis. NIH Report AK-1-2228-F
39. Quellhorst E, Schuenemann B (1981) Controlled study to compare hemodialysis and hemofiltration treatment in patients with chronic renal insufficiency. NIH Report AK-1-8-2229-F
40. Koch K, Baldamus C (1981) Hemodialysis/hemofiltration: a comparison of medical, technical, and cost factors. NIH Report AK-1227-F
41. Scheler F, Von Henning H (1977) Hamofiltration. Dustri, Munich
42. Hemofiltration Bibliography (1978) Amicon Corporation, Lexington MA USA Publication # 1430
43. Henderson LW, Beans E (1978) Successful production of sterile pyrogen-free electrolyte solution by ultrafiltration. Kidney Int 14: 522-525
44. Bosch J, Geronomos R, Glabman S, Lysaght MJ, Kahn T, Von Albertini B (1978) High flux hemofiltration. Artif Organs 2 (4): 339-342
45. Shaldon S, Beau MC, Claret G, Deschodt G, Ramperez P, Mion C (1978) Haemofiltration with sorbent regeneration of ultrafiltrate: First clinical experience in end stage renal disease. Proc Eur Dial Transplant Assoc 15: 220-227
46. Kramer P, Wigger W, Rieger J, Matthaei D, Scheler F (1977) Arterovenous haemofiltration: a new simple method for treatment of overhydrated patients resistant to diuretics. Klin Wochenschr 55: 1121, 1122
47. Kramer P (1982) Arterio-venoese Haemofiltration - Nieren-(Ersatz)-Therapie im Intensivpflegebereich. Vandenhoeck and Ruprecht, Göttingen
48. Kramer P (1985) Arteriovenous hemofiltration: A kidney replacement therapy for the intensive care unit. Springer, New York Berlin Heidelberg
49. Mion C (1982) Symposium sur l'hémofiltration. Opuscula Medico-technica lundensia XXIV. Rahms, Lund
50. Schaeffer K, Koch K-M, Quellhorst E, Von Herrath D (1982) Hemofiltration. Contrib Nephrol 32

51. Intern J Artif Organs (1983) 6: 1
52. Luehman D, Hirsch D, Ebben J, Collins A, Shapiro F, Keshaviah P (1984) Central on-site preparation of substitution for hemofiltration. Trans Am Soc Artif Intern Organs 30: 195-198
53. Ramperez P, Beau MC, Deschodt G, Flavier JL, Nilsson L, Mion C, Shaldon S (1981) Economic preparation of sterile pyrogen free infusate for hemofiltration. Proc Eur Dial Transplant Assoc 18: 293-296
54. Rameoofsky JA, Prestidge H, Ford C, Sanfelippo ML, Henderson LW (1981) Novel applications for hemofiltration membranes. Trans Am Soc Artif Intern Organs 27: 613-617
55. Shaldon S, Beau MC, Deschodt G, Mion C (1981) Mixed hemofiltration: 18 months experience with ultrashort treatment time. Trans Am Soc Artif Intern Organs 27: 610-612
56. Shinaberger JH, Miller JH, Rubini ME, Gardner PW, Martin FE (1969) Initial clinical evaluation of "Diafiltration." Trans Am Soc Artif Intern Organs 15: 97-102
57. Silverstein ME, Ford CA, Lysaght MJ, Henderson LW (1974) The treatment of intractable fluid overload. N Engl J Med 291: 747-751
58. Cheung AC, Kato Y, Leypoldt JK, Henderson LW (1982) Hemodiafiltration using a hybrid membrane system for self-generation of diluting fluid. Trans Am Soc Artif Intern Organs 28: 61-65
59. von Albertini B, Miller J, Gardner P, Shinaberger J (1984) High flux hemofiltration: under 6 hrs/week treatment. Trans Am Soc Artif Intern Organs 30: 227-231
60. Leber HW, Wizeman V, Goubeaud G, Rawer P, Schuetterle G (1978) Simultaneous hemofiltration/hemodialysis: an effective alternative to hemofiltration and conventional hemodialysis in the treatment of uremic patients. Clin Nephrol 9: 115-121
61. Streicher E, Schneider H (1985) The next generation of dialysis membranes: barriers or pathways. Contr Nephrol 44: 125-136
62. Romagnoli A, Hacker J, Keats A, Milam J (1976) External hemoconcentration after deliberate hemodilution. (Abstr). Ann Meet Am Soc Anesthesiol
63. Shapiro WB, Faubert PF, Fein PA, Tzeng T, Porush JG (1978) Hemofiltration with sorbent recycling of ultrafiltrate in uremic dogs. Trans Am Soc Artif Intern Organs 24: 185-191
64. Shettigar UR, Kablitz C, Stephen R, Kolff WJ (1983) A portable hemodialysis/hemofiltration system independent of dialysate and infusion fluid. Artif Organs 7 (2): 254-256
65. Schueneman B, Nebendahl K, Schunk O, Quellhorst E, Mund K, Richter G (1982) Regeneration of hemofiltrate using an absorption and electrochemical oxidation scheme. Contrib Nephrol 32: 192-199
66. Lysaght MJ (1985) Contemporary ESRD therapy: quagmire or eschaton? Contrib Nephrol 44: 255-284
67. Kramer P, Wigger W, Matthaei D, Langenscheid C, Reiger J, Fuchs C, Rumpf KW, Scheler F (1978) Clinical experience with continuously monitored fluid balance in automatic hemofiltration. Artif Organs 2: 147-149
68. Neff MS, Sadjadi S, Slifkin R (1979) A wearable artificial glomerulus. Trans Am Soc Artif Intern Organs 25: 71-73
69. Shaldon S, Beau MC, Deschodt G, Lysaght MJ, Ramperez P, Beau MC (1980) Continuous ambulatory hemofiltration. Trans Am Soc Artif Intern Organs 26: 210-211
70. Trautmann M, Groene HJ, Heuer E, Kramer P (1982) Intestinale substitution bei arteriovenoeser haemofiltration. In: Kramer P (ed) Arterio-venoese Haemofiltration - Nieren-(Ersatz)-therapie im Intensivpflegebereich. Vandenhoeck and Ruprecht, Göttingen, pp 259-268
71. Blackshear PL (1978) Two new concepts that might lead to a wearable artificial kidney. Kidney Int [suppl] 13: S-133-137

Determinants of Fluid and Solute Removal Rates During Hemofiltration

N. J. OFSTHUN, C. K. COLTON and M. J. LYSAGHT

Table of Contents

The rates at which fluid and solutes are removed from blood during hemofiltration depend on device dimensions and operating conditions. The purpose of this chapter is to describe these factors qualitatively and quantitatively in order to give the reader both an understanding of the physical phenomena involved and a grounding in the mathematical models available to quantify such phenomena.

Introduction

Hemofilters replace the blood purification function of the normal kidney with a convective ultrafiltration process which removes waste products from the blood stream using the same principles that are employed in a common vacuum cleaner.

Nomenclature

A	Membrane surface area (cm^2)	Φ	Volume fraction of hydrated pro-
	CWhole-blood clearance (cm^3/min)		teins in plasma
D	Molecular diffusion coefficient	$\Delta\pi$	Osmotic pressure (mmHg)
	(cm^2/s)	σ	Staverman reflection coefficient
H	Hematocrit, or volume fraction of		
	red cells in blood		
J	Flux [cm^3/(min·cm^2) or cm/s]		
K	Partition coefficient, or equilibrium		**Subscripts**
	distribution coefficient		
L	Length of hemofilter (cm)	Aug	Shear-augmented
L_p	Permeability [cm^3/(s·cm^2·mmHg)]	B	Blood
M	Mass removal rate of solute by de-	D	Diluting fluid
	vice (g/min)	Eff	Effective
ΔP	Transmembrane pressure difference	F	Filtrate
	(mmHg)	M	Inside membrane
Q	Volumetric flow rate (cm^3/min)	O	Observed
R	Rejection coefficient	P	Plasma
S	Sieving coefficient	Part	Particle
a	Particle radius (cm)	RBC	Red blood cell
c	Concentration (g/100 cm^3)	S	Solute
h	Channel height of filter (cm)	W	Plasma water
k	Mass transfer coefficient (cm/s)		
n	Number of fibers in hemofiltration	a	Arterial
	device	b	Bulk
t	Membrane thickness (cm)	i	Filter inlet (before predilution)
x	Distance from inlet (cm)	m	Maximum
y	Distance from wall (cm)	o	Filter outlet (after postdilution)
		p	Protein
δ	Boundary layer thickness (cm)	v	Venous
γ	Shear rate (s^{-1})	w	Wall

In both devices, a pressure difference generates bulk fluid motion, which carries solutes to the filter surface. This process is called convection, from the Latin verb *convehere,* meaning "to carry together." Small solutes pass freely through the filter and very large solutes above a particular cut-off size are completely retained. While a vacuum cleaner filter retains dust particles and allows free passage of air and molecules dissolved in the air, a hemofiltration membrane retains macromolecules (e. g., proteins) and formed elements, and allows free passage of water and small solutes. A hemofilter differs from a vacuum cleaner in that it transports the undesired, rather than the desired, species through the membrane. Nevertheless, both processes use convection to achieve the intended mass transport and membrane filters to provide selectivity. Water and vital solutes are replenished in hemofiltration, either before (predilution) or after (postdilution) the ultrafiltration step.

Hemofiltration, with its convective filtration process, is distinctly different from hemodialysis, the commonly used technique for separating blood components. Hemodialysis relies on diffusion rather than convection to transport solute molecules through the membrane. Diffusion, from the latin verb *diffundere,* meaning "to pour or spread out in different directions," refers to the net movement of a species down a concentration gradient as a result of thermally driven random ("Brownian") motion of individual molecules. An example of diffusion at work is a tea bag resting in a quiescent cup of water. Molecules which give tea its flavor and color diffuse out of the highly concentrated environment in the tea bag to the less concentrated solution outside it. The tea bag membrane prevents particles above a certain "cut-off" size from escaping into the tea. Similarly, a hemodialysis membrane prevents molecules above a certain size from leaving the blood, while molecules below the cut-off size diffuse through the membrane to the dialysate. Large molecules diffuse more slowly than small molecules. Consequently, the removal rate of solutes during hemodialysis decreases with increasing molecular weight.

In hemofiltration, on the other hand, a solute which can pass freely through the membrane is removed at a rate proportional to its concentration in the blood and independent of its size. Consequently, so-called "middle molecules" of molecular weight 500–5000 are removed at higher rates in hemofiltration than in hemodialysis. It has been proposed that the improved removal rate of middle molecules may be the reason for better vascular stability (i.e., control of blood pressure) and better patient tolerance in hemofiltration than in equivalent hemodialysis [1]. An alternative explanation is that hemofiltration allows greater control of water volume and electrolyte balance, which leads to the improved vascular stability and patient tolerance [2]. Differences in blood membrane biocompatibility may also contribute to the effect [3].

The glomerular basement membrane of the human kidney functions by convective filtration. Additional renal control of the net removal rates of certain solutes is provided downstream of the glomerular membrane by reabsorption of the solute from the filtrate or by secretion of the solute from capillaries into the filtrate. A comparison of various filtration parameters for typical conventional hemofiltration devices, continuous arteriovenous hemofiltration (CAVH) devices, and a typical pair

Table 1. Comparison of typical hemofilters and a pair of human kidneys

	Conventional hemofilter [4]	CAVH hemofilter [5]	Human kidneys [6]
Membrane area (m^2)	0.5–1.5	0.2–0.5	1.5
Number of fibers/capillaries	4000–12000	2500	5×10^6
Inside diameter of fiber (cm)	0.02	0.02–0.11	8×10^{-4}
Transmembrane pressure difference (mmHg)	200–500	50–100	50
Maximum blood flow rate (cm^3/min)	200–400	100	1200
Wall shear rate (s^{-1})	2000	400	−[a]
Ultrafiltrate flux (10^{-4} cm/s)	0.7–2.3	0.8	1.3
Filtration fraction (filtration rate divided by inlet blood flow rate)	0.35/0.50[b]	0.1/0.4[c]	0.2

[a] The wall shear rate cannot be calculated using the formula for parabolic flow, because complicated flow patterns develop as red cells pass through capillaries which have diameters comparable to those of the cells.
[b] Values are for postdilution and predilution, respectively.
[c] Values are for CAVH, and CAVH with filtrate siphoning, respectively.

of human kidneys, is given in Table 1. Note that a hemofilter with approximately the same membrane area as a pair of human kidneys is limited to a lower blood flow rate than normal flow through the kidneys and requires a greater transmembrane pressure difference to produce a filtrate flux comparable to that of the kidneys.

Overview of the Hemofiltration Process

In this section we consider from a qualitative standpoint the factors which influence fluid and solute removal rates in hemofiltration. Each of these factors is then discussed, along with useful mathematical relationships, in the subsequent sections.

We begin be defining certain important quantities while at the same time ignoring spatial variations along the device. The volumetric flow rate of ultrafiltrate is denoted by Q_F. The ultrafiltrate flux, J_F, is the volumetric flow rate per unit membrane surface area, A, defined by

$$J_F = \frac{Q_F}{A} \tag{1}$$

which is equivalent to the superficial velocity of ultrafiltrate across the membrane. The rate of mass removal, M, of a particular solute is given by

$$M = Q_F c_F \tag{2}$$

where c_F is the solute concentration in the ultrafiltrate, which is related to the solute concentration in the bulk plasma water, c_{Wb}, by the observed sieving coefficient, S_O,

$$S_O = \frac{c_F}{c_{Wb}} \tag{3}$$

$S_O = 1$ if the solute is freely passed by the membrane, and $S_O = 0$ if it is completely retained. A related term which is often used in the literature is the observed rejection coefficient, R_O, defined by

$$R_O = 1 - S_O \tag{4}$$

From Eqs. 1-4, the solute flux is then defined by

$$J_S = \frac{M}{A} = J_F c_{Wb} S_O = J_F c_{Wb} (1 - R_O) \tag{5}$$

The solute flux is thus determined by both the ultrafiltrate flux and the observed sieving coefficient, each of which is discussed separately below.

Ultrafiltration Rate

Because the ultrafiltrate flux during hemofiltration is easily measured, the dependence of the flux on parameters such as device dimensions and operating conditions has been well studied. Under typical hemofiltration conditions, the flux depends primarily on five parameters, namely membrane hydraulic permeability, transmembrane pressure difference, blood flow rate, device geometry and dimensions, and blood protein concentration, and secondarily on protein composition, hematocrit, and temperature. The flux varies in a complicated but reproducible fashion with these parameters, and the relative importance of each parameter depends on the operating conditions.

The transmembrane pressure difference, ΔP, is defined as the hydrostatic pressure on the upstream side of the membrane minus the pressure downstream of the membrane. A typical plot of ultrafiltrate flux vs transmembrane pressure difference for hemofiltration, ignoring the effects of osmotic pressure, is shown in Fig. 1. Examination of this flux behavior reveals two distinct hemofiltration operating regimes: a pressure-dependent region and a pressure-independent region. At low applied pressures, the flux is linearly dependent on pressure. In this region, transmembrane pressure difference and membrane hydraulic permeability completely determine the flux; increasing either parameter increases the ultrafiltration rate. Therefore the pressure-dependent region is said to be "membrane-limited." At high applied pressures, the flux is independent of transmembrane pressure difference and membrane permeability. In this region, blood flow rate, device geometry, and protein concentration primarily influence the flux. For example, increasing the blood flow rate, decreasing the channel height, and decreasing the protein concentration all increase the flux. Since these factors affect the buildup of cells and proteins in the concentration boundary layer near the membrane surface, such a boundary layer is believed to be responsible for constraining the flux in this region. Therefore, the pressure-independent region is said to be "boundary layer-limited." At low pressures where the flux is small, boundary layer formation does not signifi-

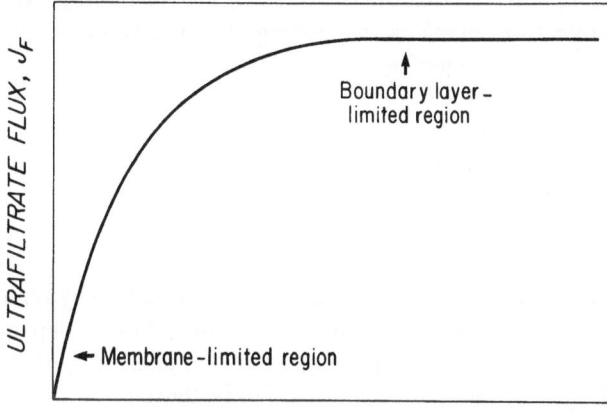

Fig. 1. Typical curve for ultrafiltrate flux vs transmembrane pressure difference in hemofiltration

cantly affect the membrane-determined flux. Between these two extremes, all of the aforementioned parameters can influence the flux.

Both membrane-limited behavior and boundary layer-limited behavior are seen clinically and will be discussed later in this chapter in terms of the effects of the individual parameters.

Membrane Sieving Coefficient

Observed sieving coefficients depend upon the nature of the membrane and the solute and on the conditions of use [7], which may affect solute transport in a variety of ways. First, adsorbed protein molecules may reduce the effective pore size of the membrane, thereby increasing the rejection of some species [8–10]. Adsorption occurs almost instantaneously, but surface-bound proteins may adjust their composition, packing density, and thus their pore occlusion over several hours [11]. Second, the concentrated boundary layer of cells and proteins which forms at the membrane surface may itself act as a dynamically formed secondary membrane, with sieving properties for smaller proteins different from those of the underlying hemofiltration membrane [12–14]. Since boundary layer formation depends on operating conditions, solute clearance may also depend on such variables as blood flow rate, device geometry, protein concentration, and cell concentration. Finally, even in the absence of protein adsorption and secondary membranes, sieving coefficients between 0.0 and 1.0 do not depend solely on the nature of the membrane and permeating solute; they also vary slightly with ultrafiltration velocity and retentate flow conditions. These effects, which arise from concentration polarization of partially rejected solutes and from the interaction of convection and diffusion within the membrane pores, are of largely theoretical interest, because the magnitude of such effects is usually small over the range of ultrafiltration velocities encountered clinically. Recently, experimental evidence of this has been presented. NAKAO et al. [15] found that both apparent and true solute rejection coefficients depended on bulk flow rate, transmembrane pressure difference, and filtrate velocity. HENDERSON et al. [16] observed that the clearance of intermediate-sized molecules decreases as the filtrate flux increases, suggesting that increasing concentration polarization increases solute rejection.

Compartmentalization Effect

Since hemofiltration removes solutes from blood by removing the plasma water in which they are dissolved, the rate of solute removal depends on solute compartmentalization between the plasma water, the plasma proteins, and the red blood cells. These effects have been observed to be more pronounced than in hemodialysis, especially in postdilution.

Whole-blood clearance, C, is used as a measure of the effectiveness of both natural and artificial kidneys. It is defined as the removal rate of a solute divided by its initial concentration in whole blood, c_B,

$$C = \frac{M}{c_B} \tag{6}$$

and can be thought of as the equivalent volume of whole blood, per unit time, from which solute is completely "cleared" (i.e., removed) by the kidneys. Since the solute removal rate, M, in a hemofilter is equal to the ultrafiltration rate, Q_F, times the solute concentration in the plasma water filtrate, c_F, clearance will exceed Q_F if the solute concentration in plasma water, $c_{W,}$ is greater than its concentration in whole blood, c_B. This requirement is met by all solutes which are partially or totally excluded from the red cells and are not bound to plasma proteins. However, clearance can never exceed the blood flow rate through the device.

Prediction and measurement of clearance in hemofiltration is complicated by solute compartmentalization for several reasons. Any solute which remains bound to plasma proteins or enclosed in red cells as the blood passes through the hemofilter cannot be cleared. Dilution reduces the solute concentration in the plasma water and leads to movement of solute from the proteins and/or red cells to the plasma water. Predilution therefore makes some of the previously bound or sequestered solute available for removal. However, since the filtrate concentration of the solute to be removed is also reduced, more filtrate must be produced in predilution than in postdilution to remove a given amount of solute. In postdilution hemofiltration, the volume fractions of red cells and protein, and thus the ratio of c_W to c_B, increase along the length of the filter and there is a corresponding increase in the magnitude of the compartmentalization effects. Partition coefficients (i.e., equilibrium distribution constants) have been measured for only a few solutes, and rates of attaining equilibrium are unknown. If it is assumed that equilibrium between compartments is reached instantaneously, then equilibrium among compartments is maintained throughout the length of the hemofilter. To determine the solute removal rate, either the filtrate volume and solute concentration are measured, or blood (plasma water) solute concentrations are measured as the blood leaves and enters the body, before predilution and after postdilution.

Solute compartmentalization within the body may also be important. Recent work by HAAS et al. [17] indicates that equilibration of solute compartments in the body tissue is not achieved during hemofiltration. Consequently, rebound of solute concentrations occurs after hemofiltration is completed.

Analysis of Ultrafiltration Rate

In the quantitative approach that follows, a distinction will be made between local values for ultrafiltrate and solute transport rates and average values for an entire hemofiltration device. This is necessary because these rates may depend on the composition and thickness of the boundary layer formed at the membrane surface and on hematocrit and protein concentration, all of which vary along the length of the device. The usual approach, which we shall follow here, is to develop approximate equations to describe local rates and then to integrate them along the length of the device in order to predict device-averaged values, making simplifying assumptions as needed in order to carry out the integration. Some of these techniques will be discussed in this section. Alternatively, if the appropriate constitutive relationships can be obtained, a more rigorous and detailed system of partial differential equations for the entire device may be set up and solved. Such a model can provide both local and device-averaged filtration and solute removal rates.

Membrane-Limited Region

A more detailed description of the relationship between flux and transmembrane pressure difference for hemofiltration is shown in Fig. 2. All three curves are representative of data obtained with a membrane that does not compress under the applied transmembrane pressure difference. The dashed line applies to filtration of distilled water or saline through the membrane prior to its exposure to blood or plasma. The flux increases linearly with ΔP. The membrane hydraulic permeability, L_p, which is defined as the slope of this flux vs pressure relation, does not change with pressure. The dotted line is the result of saline perfusion through the same membrane after the membrane has been exposed to blood or plasma and then thoroughly rinsed. The flux again increases linearly with ΔP, but the permeability is typically lower than it was prior to exposure to the protein-containing solution [18]. This decrease results from adsorption of proteins onto the surface or into the pores of the synthetic membrane. The magnitude of the decrease depends on the nature of the adsorbed proteins and the composition of the membrane; for example, aromatic polymers adsorb more than olefinic or hydrophilic structures. The adsorption is virtually instantaneous, although the adsorbed proteins slowly rearrange to form a

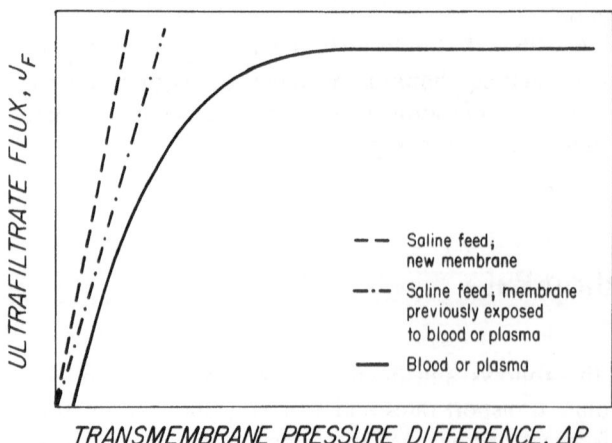

Legend:
- - - Saline feed; new membrane
- ·- Saline feed; membrane previously exposed to blood or plasma
— Blood or plasma

ULTRAFILTRATE FLUX, J_F

TRANSMEMBRANE PRESSURE DIFFERENCE, ΔP

Fig. 2. Various forms of ultrafiltration behavior in hemofiltration

more tightly packed configuration [11]. Thus the dotted line, here shown after in-stantaneous exposure, might shift slightly clockwise during prolonged exposure to plasma.

The solid curve in Fig. 2 applies to ultrafiltration of plasma or blood through the same membrane [5]. A finite applied pressure is required in order to produce an in-finitesimally small flux. This pressure, represented by the non-zero intercept of the curve on the ΔP axis, is that which is required to overcome the osmotic pressure dif-ference ($\Delta\pi$) across the membrane, essentially equal to the colloid osmotic pressure of the proteins in the blood. At applied pressures below this osmotic pressure, any fluid present on the filtrate side will flow "backward" into the plasma or blood com-partment. The colloid osmotic pressure of the proteins in whole plasma is normally about 28 mmHg and varies with protein composition and concentration [19]. (The colloid osmotic pressure should not be confused with the much larger total osmotic pressure of plasma, which includes the osmotic pressure resulting from small ions which pass through both capillary walls and hemofiltration membranes.) Above this level, the flux begins to rise linearly with the net driving force for flow, which is the difference between the applied (hydrostatic) transmembrane pressure differ-ence, ΔP, and the colloid osmotic pressure of the plasma or blood, $\Delta\pi$. The hydrau-lic permeability is usually slightly lower than the water permeability of the same membrane following exposure to plasma.

To summarize the observed flux behavior in the membrane-limited region, we can write the following expression for the local filtrate flux $J_F(x)$:

$$J_F(x) = L_p [\Delta P(x) - \Delta\pi(x)] \tag{7}$$

where x is the axial distance from the inlet of the device. This expression can be in-tegrated to give the device-averaged flux, provided any variation of L_p, ΔP, and $\Delta\pi$ with position is known. If we assume that the hemofiltration membrane is incom-pressible, so that its hydraulic permeability will not depend on the transmembrane pressure, then L_p will be independent of position. The transmembrane pressure dif-ference decreases along the length of the filter by an amount which depends on the pressure drop of the channel. The device-averaged transmembrane pressure, $\overline{\Delta P}$, may be approximated as the arithmetic average of the inlet and outlet values. As-suming that the fraction of fluid which is removed as filtrate is small, $\Delta\pi$ will be ap-proximately constant along the length of the device. Therefore the device-averaged flux, $\overline{J_F}$, in the membrane-limited region is given by

$$\overline{J_F} = \frac{1}{L} \int_0^L J_{F_0}(x)\, dx \approx L_p (\overline{\Delta P} - \Delta\pi) \tag{8}$$

This expression has been shown to be valid in describing the flux behavior observed in high-flow-rate arteriovenous or "spontaneous" hemofiltration devices [5]. (It is not valid in low-flow-rate arteriovenous hemofilters, in which filtration fractions greater than 20% result in significant nonlinear increases in the osmotic pressure along the device [20]. Arteriovenous hemofilters operate in the membrane-limited region because the arterial and venous pressures, which provide the driving force for ultrafiltration (in combination with any vacuum applied to the filtrate compartment), generally result in a transmembrane pressure difference of less than 100 mmHg.

Two implications for device design arise from Eq. 8 and our understanding of membrane-limited filter operation with arteriovenous hemofiltration [5]. First, excessive filtration fractions, which may occur with large membrane area, too high a rate of ultrafiltrate pumping, and low blood flow rates, must be avoided, since they can lead to very high blood viscosity and flow stasis. This is less of a problem in conventional hemofilters, in which the concentration polarization phenomenon (described in "Plateau Region") limits the filtration fraction, because

a) the asymptotic flux is insensitive to the transmembrane pressure difference, and
b) the flux decreases as the blood flow rate is reduced.

Second, the importance of the membrane hydraulic permeability in setting the flux implies that the membrane permeability should be the focus of both quality control and product development for membrane-limited hemofilters.

Plateau Region

At higher pressures, typically 250–300 mmHg, the ultrafiltration rate approaches an upper limit or plateau beyond which further increases in pressure do not lead to further increases in flux. This pressure-independent flux cannot be increased by substitution of a more permeable membrane. Thus, the two factors which had controlled the filtration rate at low pressures – membrane permeability and transmembrane pressure difference – have no effect at high pressures. The principal factors which influence the flux in the pressure-independent region are blood flow rate, device geometry, and blood protein concentration. The effect of hematocrit, which becomes significant only at concentrations far removed from the normal range of operation, will be discussed later.

Numerous experimental observations show that increasing the blood flow rate or decreasing the channel height (i.e., the diameter of a hollow fiber or the gap width in a parallel-plate device) increases the flux. The wall shear rate (i.e., the velocity gradient at the membrane surface), which is proportional to the ratio of mean velocity to channel height, provides a convenient measure of these two effects. As illustrated in Fig. 3a, the logarithm of the filtrate flux has been observed to be linearly proportional to the logarithm of the wall shear rate. Therefore the flux is proportional to the shear rate raised to a power which is given by the slope of that log-log plot. The flux is inversely proportional to the log of the blood protein concentration, as shown in Fig. 3b. Both of these observations are consistent with the theoretical models discussed later.

Any satisfactory explanation for hemofiltration flux behavior must provide plausible reasons for

a) the existence of two distinct flux regimes (the pressure-dependent linear region and the pressure-independent plateau region), and

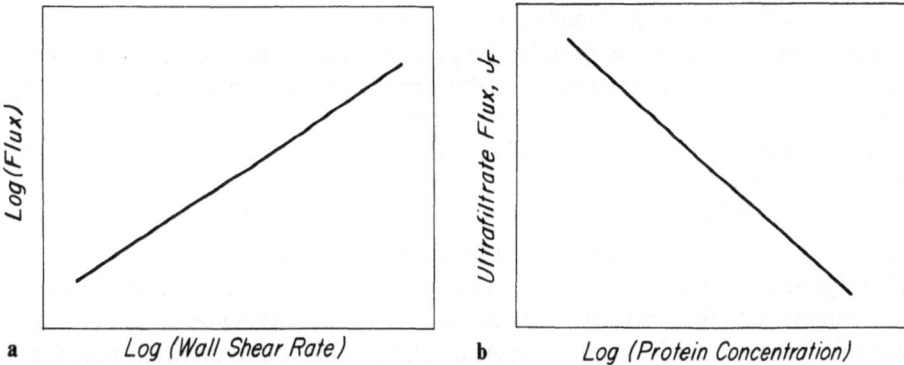

Fig. 3a, b. Experimental observations of the dependence of hemofiltration flux on design and operating parameters. **a** wall shear rate; **b** protein concentration

b) the lack of influence of either membrane hydraulic permeability or transmembrane pressure difference on the flux in the plateau region.

One theory which can explain these observations (and consequently has received considerable attention) is the thin-film concentration polarization boundary layer model [21]. The essence of this theory is that at sufficiently high transmembrane pressure differences the ultrafiltrate flux is limited by the formation of a concentration polarization boundary layer near the membrane, consisting of a high concentration of cells and/or proteins which do not pass through the membrane.

The extent of concentration polarization of any species depends on the relative rates of convection toward the membrane and diffusive transport away from it. At steady state the boundary layer is in dynamic equilibrium; the rate of convection of each species to the membrane is balanced by diffusion back into the bulk. Although the rate of convective transport of all species to the membrane surface (and therefore the ultrafiltrate flux) is determined by the rate of back-diffusion, the concentration polarization boundary layer of cells and/or proteins reduces the ultrafiltrate flux either

a) by providing a hydraulic resistance in addition to that of the membrane [22, 23] or
b) by increasing the osmotic pressure at the membrane surface, which reduces the driving force for ultrafiltrate flow [24, 25].

The available evidence suggests that osmotic pressure is important with proteins of low molecular weight, especially highly charged molecules such as albumin, but that it cannot be the dominant mechanism with much larger proteins and particles [25]. At this time, it is unclear whether increased hydraulic resistance, osmotic pressure, or some combination of the two is responsible for the reduction in the convective flux of various protein solutions during ultrafiltration [26]. This is especially true in hemofiltration because of the complex composition of blood. However, the mechanism of flux reduction is not crucial to understanding of steady-state flux behavior, and will not be discussed further.

At low transmembrane pressure differences, the convective flux is sufficiently small that no significant concentration polarization boundary layer can form, and the observed flux is approximately the same as that which is obtained when membranes previously exposed to proteins are perfused with saline, corrected for colloid osmotic pressure according to Eq. 8. At these pressures, the convective flux is set by the membrane permeability and the applied pressure; the concentration profile of each polarizable species adjusts itself so that its diffusive flux away from the membrane equals its convective flux toward the membrane.

The transition from the pressure-dependent region to the pressure-independent region may most easily be understood in terms of the transient response to an increased transmembrane pressure difference. At higher transmembrane pressure the flux increases and the convective flux toward the membrane is greater than the diffusive flux away from the membrane. As a result, species build up (i.e., "polarize") at the membrane surface. The rising concentration of the species at the membrane increases its rate of back-diffusion. Adjustment of the polarization boundary layer continues until diffusion balances convection, and no additional material collects in the boundary layer. Thus, increasing the transmembrane pressure raises the concentration at the membrane, which increases the rate of back-diffusion and increases the steady-state flux. At sufficiently high transmembrane pressures, further increases in pressure cannot effect further increases in the rate of back-diffusion because the concentration at the membrane surface reaches or approaches a constant value limited, for example, by solubility or osmotic pressure constraints. The result is a pressure-independent maximum hemofiltration flux, seen as a plateau in flux vs pressure curves. When the ultrafiltrate flux is limited by boundary layer phenomena, the flux can be influenced by the shear rate. For example, increasing the wall shear rate (by increasing the blood velocity or decreasing the channel height) reduces the boundary layer thickness, making the concentration gradient steeper. This increases the back-diffusion rate, thereby increasing ultrafiltrate flux.

As whole blood contains a complex mixture of proteins and cells, all of which can contribute to the concentration polarization phenomenon, satisfactory theoretical models have not yet been developed to describe hemofiltration. By way of introducing the available data and correlations, we first consider two simpler limiting cases:

a) ultrafiltration of protein solutions (containing no cells), and
b) microfiltration of blood or red cell suspensions, as in membrane plasmapheresis, in which only the cells are retained by the membrane.

Ultrafiltration of Protein Solutions

To develop the flux expressions for the plateau region, consider a differential (i.e., vanishingly small) element, dx, along the length of a membrane. The steady-state equality between the convective ultrafiltrate flux of proteins toward the membrane and the diffusive flux away from the membrane may be written as

$$J_F(x)\, c_p = -D\frac{dc_p}{dy} \tag{9}$$

where $J_F(x)$ is the flux at a distance x from the inlet, y is the distance from the membrane surface (wall), and c_p is the protein concentration. Integration across the thickness, $\delta(x)$, of the boundary layer, assuming constant D, yields

$$J_F(x) \int_0^{\delta(x)} dy = D \int_{c_{pb}}^{c_{pw}} \frac{dc_p}{c_p} = D\ln\left(\frac{c_{pw}}{c_{pb}}\right) \tag{10}$$

where c_{pw} and c_{pb} are the protein concentrations at the wall and in the bulk, respectively. If the boundary layer is approximated by an equivalent stagnant film, the ratio $D/\delta(x)$ may be equated to the local convective mass transfer coefficient, $k(x)$, giving

$$J_F(x) = k(x)\ln\left(\frac{c_{pw}}{c_{pb}}\right) \tag{11}$$

where $k(x)$ is a function of the velocity profile. Using the classical solution of Leveque [27] for the case of constant c_{pw} and a linear velocity gradient across the boundary layer, which is applicable to proteins which have a small diffusion coefficient and form a thin boundary layer, one obtains

$$k(x) = 0.538\left(\frac{D^2\gamma_w}{x}\right)^{1/3} \tag{12}$$

Combination of Eqs. 11 and 12 leads to the following expression for the local flux:

$$J_F(x) = 0.538\left(\frac{D^2\gamma_w}{x}\right)^{1/3}\ln\left(\frac{c_{pw}}{c_{pb}}\right) \tag{13}$$

The device-averaged flux, J_F, is obtained by integrating the local expression over the length of the channel. It is assumed that c_{pw} is constant, and the numerically small differences between inlet and outlet bulk concentrations are neglected; therefore the ratio of wall to bulk concentration remains constant from device inlet to outlet, and

$$\overline{J_F} = \frac{1}{L}\int_0^L J_F(x)\,dx = 0.807\left(\frac{D^2\gamma_w}{L}\right)^{1/3}\ln\left(\frac{c_{pw}}{c_{pb}}\right) \tag{14}$$

The maximum flux, i.e., that obtained when operating in the plateau region, is given by the above expression with c_{pw} replaced by c_{pm}, the maximum value of the protein concentration at the wall, which is attained if the transmembrane pressure is sufficiently high. In general, c_{pm} is not directly measured but is obtained by extrapolation of a plot of J_F vs $\ln(c_{pb})$ (as in Fig. 3) to the intercept where $J_F=0$.

Data from several authors for the ultrafiltration of plasma [21–23, 28–29] and albumin solutions [23, 29–31] have been found to fit Eq. 8 quite well. For example,

COLTON et al. [21] developed the following semiempirical expression using data for ultrafiltration of 1:1 diluted plasma in hollow fibers:

$$\bar{J}_F = 3.40 \times 10^{-5} \left(\frac{\gamma_w}{L}\right)^{1/3} \ln\left(\frac{28.7}{c_{pb}}\right) \tag{15}$$

JAFFRIN et al. [32] and ISAACSON et al. [33] found that their data fit COLTON's expression quite well.

By comparing Eqs. 14 and 15, the diffusion coefficient implied by Eq. 15 may be back-calculated. The resulting value is $2.7 \times 10^{-7}\,cm^2/s$, which is less than the Brownian motion diffusion coefficient of albumin, $7 \times 10^{-7}\,cm^2/s$ [34]. This is probably due to the high concentration of plasma proteins near the wall and to the presence of larger proteins such as lipoproteins, whose average diffusion coefficient is $2.5 \times 10^{-7}\,cm^2/s$ [35].

Although the dependence on shear rate was consistent in all of the albumin and plasma ultrafiltration studies listed above, the value of c_{pm} obtained by extrapolation of J_F vs $\ln(c_{pb})$ data varied considerably. Values ranged from 17.4 wt% to 57.5 wt% for bovine serum albumin, from 28 wt% to 45 wt% for human albumin, and from 20 wt% to 60 wt% for human plasma. Most values of c_{pm} were far below the solubility limit of albumin, which is 58.5 wt% [24]. No satisfactory explanation for such variation in c_{pm} is currently available, suggesting the need for further refinement of the simple polarization model for protein ultrafiltration.

Microfiltration of Red Cell Suspensions

In microfiltration of whole blood, plasma proteins pass freely through the membrane; the red cells and other formed elements are retained by the membrane and form a concentration polarization boundary layer. Although the concentration polarization model described in the previous section has proven successful in the ultrafiltration of solutions of proteins and other macromolecules, quantitative agreement with experimental data for the cross-flow filtration of colloidal suspensions, including blood, has been poor. ZYDNEY and COLTON [36] showed that agreement could be improved by incorporation of an enhanced diffusive motion of the large colloidal particles as a result of lateral migrations arising from mutually induced velocity fields in shear flow. They used the correlation developed by ECKSTEIN et al. [37] for the shear-enhanced diffusion coefficient of the red blood cells:

$$D_{RBC} = 0.03\, a^2 \gamma_w \tag{16}$$

where a is the particle radius (4.2 μm for red blood cells). Incorporation of this expression into Eqs. 13 and 14 leads to

$$J_F(x) = 0.052 \left(\frac{a^4}{x}\right)^{1/3} \gamma_w \ln\left(\frac{c_w}{c_b}\right) \tag{17}$$

$$J_F = 0.078 \left(\frac{a^4}{L}\right)^{1/3} \gamma_w \ln\left(\frac{c_w}{c_b}\right) \tag{18}$$

These results differ from Eqs. 14 and 15 in that the filtrate flux is predicted to be dependent upon the first power, rather than the 1/3 power, of the wall shear rate. Experimental data support this prediction, although the exponent on γ_w is generally somewhat less than 1.

Ultrafiltration of Blood

Flux data from several authors for ultrafiltration of whole and diluted blood follow neither the 1/3 nor the 1.0-power dependence on wall shear rate predicted by Eqs. 14 and 18, respectively [12, 21, 28–30, 38]. The variation of hemofiltration flux with hematocrit, plasma protein concentration, and wall shear rate was thoroughly studied by OKAZAKI and YOSHIDA [28]. They studied shear rate dependence for red cell suspensions with hematocrit ranging from $H=0$ to $H=44.3$ and protein concentrations of $c_{pb}=0.9$ to $c_{pb}=7.0$. The exponent on wall shear rate varied from 0.33 to 0.82, in general increasing with increasing hematocrit and decreasing with increasing protein concentration for $H>20$. Exponents observed by the other authors listed above lie in the range 0.33–1.0. Most exponents observed in whole-blood experiments were between 0.4 and 0.5.

The higher shear rate dependence in the presence of cells may be attributed to shear enhancement of the protein diffusion coefficient. To a first approximation, the effective diffusivity, D_{Eff}, of a solute (e. g., protein) can be expressed as the sum of the Brownian motion (D) and shear-augmented (D_{Aug}) contributions:

$$D_{Eff} = D + D_{Aug} \tag{19}$$

ZYDNEY [39] used a model analogous to eddy diffusivity in turbulent flow to show that the shear-augmented diffusivity term for a solute in a suspension of particles undergoing shear flow can be approximated by the augmented diffusion coefficient, D_{Part}, of the particles themselves, yielding

$$D_{Eff} = D + D_{Part} \tag{20}$$

Using Eq. 16 for D_{Part}, ZYDNEY obtained an expression for the effective diffusion coefficient of solutes in shear flow of a particle suspension:

$$D_{Eff} = D + 0.03\ a^2\gamma_w \tag{21}$$

and found that it satisfactorily correlated experimental data for a wide variety of experimental systems. If Eq. 21 is incorporated into the simple protein polarization model, i. e., Eq. 14, then the apparent dependence of flux on shear rate will depend on the relative magnitude of the Brownian motion and shear-augmented terms, which will in turn depend on the magnitude of the wall shear rate. For $\gamma_w=100$, the apparent exponent on shear rate using ECKSTEIN's correlation is 0.67, which is higher than that observed in the whole-blood ultrafiltration experiments. For higher shear rates, such as those normally encountered in hemofiltration, the apparent exponent is even larger. Therefore, the simple protein polarization model, modified to include a shear-enhanced albumin diffusivity, is not able to completely account for hemofiltration flux behavior. More sophisticated models, which have yet to be developed, may be more successful in predicting hemofiltration flux behavior.

While the simple protein concentration polarization model discussed above does not provide a complete explanation of hemofiltration flux behavior, it is sufficient to yield useful implications for design and operation of conventional (i.e., non-arteriovenous) hemofilters. For example, according to the concentration polarization model, increasing the number of fibers will increase the membrane area, but if the total blood flow rate is constant, it will also reduce the blood velocity through each fiber; this, in turn, will reduce the shear rate and thereby reduce the ultrafiltrate flux. Reducing the fiber diameter decreases the area per fiber, but increases the shear rate, which increases the flux. Because the local flux (i.e., the flux through a differential section of the membrane) decreases as the distance from the inlet increases, increasing membrane area by increasing the device length leads to a higher total ultrafiltration rate, but to a lower device-averaged flux or filtration rate per unit membrane area [40].

Because of these competing effects of varying fiber dimensions, it is necessary to consider the total ultrafiltration rate, non just the membrane area and flux separately, in choosing the optimal design. It is also necessary to realize which operating parameters can be varied independently in order to achieve the desired ultrafiltration rate in the device. For example, in determining the optimal hemofiltration fiber diameter, LYSAGHT et al. [41] found differing results for

a) conventional hemofiltration, in which blood flow rate is chosen independently from fiber diameter, and
b) arteriovenous hemofiltration, in which blood flow rate is dependent on both the fiber diameter (because it determines the hydraulic resistance) and the arteriovenous pressure drop, which is fixed at the physiologic value for each particular patient.

Using the semiempirical concentration polarization flux correlation of COLTON et al. [21], which corresponds to predilution hemofiltration, LYSAGHT found that in hemofilters of fixed membrane area hollow fibers should be as small as possible for conventional hemofiltration and as large as possible for arteriovenous hemofiltration, at least until blood flow reaches an asymptote dependent upon access and physiologic limits. In the actual choice of fiber dimensions, constraints related to preventing hemolysis, minimizing priming volume, avoiding coagulation problems, and changing the sieving properties of the membrane/boundary layer combination will usually limit the range of possible variation in design and operating parameters.

The simple protein polarization model also has implications for the operation of hemofilters after the design has been finalized. For example, the concentration polarization theory predicts that the ultrafiltration rate will decrease throughout patient treatment because of an increasing blood protein concentration. This agrees with clinical observations.

The reason why the simple concentration polarization model is so useful in qualitatively explaining flux behavior is probably that the basic physical picture of polarization is correct: there is physical evidence that plasma proteins do form concentration polarization boundary layers. NAKAO et al. [42] determined the density and permeability of a gel formed on an ultrafiltration membrane. VILKER et al. [43] used a shadowgraphic technique to determine the concentration profile of albumin in the boundary layer of an unstirred batch ultrafiltration system. Observed profiles fit the concentration polarization model quite well. IORIO et al. [44] used a scintigraphic technique to observe plasma protein buildup on both flat-plate and hollow-fiber cross-flow hemofiltration membranes. This technique could not measure concentration profiles, but did show an increase in the amount of polarized and/or adsorbed protein with increasing distance from the inlet, as predicted by concentration polarization theory.

Thus far, the five parameters which are primarily responsible for hemofiltration flux behavior – membrane hydraulic permeability, transmembrane pressure difference, blood flow rate, device geometry, and blood protein concentration – have been discussed. Other hemofiltration parameters – hematocrit, temperature, and protein composition – may also play a role in determining the steady-state ultrafiltrate flux and deserve mention here. OKAZAKI and YOSHIDA [28] studied the effect of hematocrit and found a complicated dependence in which variations from normal hematocrit led to variation in the flux. In particular, they noted that the shear-augmenting effect of the red blood cells was most prominent at low hematocrits and appeared to be damped out as the hematocrit was increased to normal or above-normal values. ISAACSON et al. [33] demonstrated that the effect of temperature is large enough that data taken at room temperature (22 °C) are not representative of data at body temperature (37 °C). Values of the flux at 37 °C are about 34% higher than those at 22 °C. While no quantitative studies have been carried out to date, the protein composition of plasma is also believed to have an effect on the hemofiltration flux. In the clinical setting, some patients have been identified as "slow" and others as "fast" compared with the norm, at equivalent blood flow rates and hematocrits, regardless of the hemofilter employed. It has been speculated that variation in protein composition – with higher concentrations of larger proteins, especially lipoproteins, in the "slow" patients – is the reason for such differences. On the basis of the concentration polarization model, one would expect that the presence of more large proteins might lower the effective protein diffusion coefficient and also, therefore, the plateau filtration rate.

Analysis of Solute Transport

Since the primary purpose of hemofiltration is solute removal, it is important to understand the factors which affect observed membrane sieving characteristics. Some of these factors are discussed in this section; in addition, equations which relate solute clearances to membrane properties and ultrafiltrate flow rates are summarized and problems with such predictions identified.

Observed Sieving Coefficients

The ability of a membrane to reject a solute is usually measured in terms of an observed sieving coefficient, S_O. At any point along the membrane, the observed sieving coefficient is the ratio of the solute concentration in the filtrate, c_F, to the concentration in the bulk plasma water, c_{Wb}, as defined by Eq. 3. The true sieving coefficient, S_T, a more accurate measure of the ability of a membrane to reject a solute, is the ratio of c_F to the concentration of solute in the plasma water at the membrane surface, c_{Wm}:

$$S_T = \frac{c_F}{c_{Wm}} \tag{22}$$

The limits on S_T are the same as those on S_O. A true membrane rejection, R_T, may be defined analogously to Eq. 4.

The observed sieving coefficient is equal to the true sieving coefficient times the polarization modulus, c_{Wm}/c_{Wb}. Estimating the polarization modulus from the mass transfer coefficient yields the following relationship [13]:

$$S_O = \frac{S_T \exp (J_F/k)}{1 - S_T + S_T \exp (J_F/k)} \tag{23}$$

Equation 23 predicts that the observed sieving coefficient is always greater than or equal to the true sieving coefficient; i.e., that the effect of polarization is to raise the observed sieving coefficient above the true sieving coefficient because the solute concentration at the membrane surface is greater than that in the bulk as a result of concentration polarization.

The true sieving coefficient, S_T, is not constant, but depends on filtration conditions. It may be related to the Staverman reflection coefficient, σ, which is an intrinsic property of the membrane for each solute and which was originally derived from the theory of irreversible thermodynamics. SPIEGLER and KEDEM [45] developed the following expression, which demonstrates the dependence of S_T on ultrafiltrate flux and membrane transport properties:

$$S_T = \frac{1 - \sigma}{1 - \sigma F} \tag{24}$$

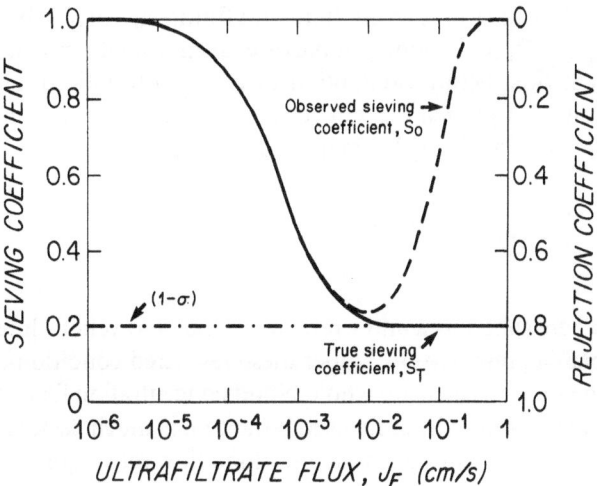

ULTRAFILTRATE FLUX, J_F (cm/s)

Fig. 4. Dependence of true and observed sieving coefficients on σ and J_F. Calculated from Eqs. 23 and 24 with $\sigma = 0.8$ (for inulin[14]), $D_M = 2 \times 10^{-6} \text{ cm}^2/\text{s}$, $t = 4 \times 10^{-3}$ cm and $k = 5 \times 10^{-2}$ cm/s. Note that J_F is expressed in units of cm/s

where $F = \exp [J_F (1 - \sigma) t / D_M]$, t is the membrane thickness in cm, and D_M is the effective solute diffusion coefficient in the membrane. S_T varies from 1 (as J_F approaches zero) to its minimum asymptotic value, $1 - \sigma$, at sufficiently high values of J_F.

A typical plot relating S_O and S_T to σ and J_F is given in Fig. 4. At low flux, S_O and S_T are equal, and both decrease from 1.0 toward $(1 - \sigma)$ as the flux is increased. At higher flux, the true sieving coefficient approaches its minimum value of $(1 - \sigma)$ asymptotically, while the observed sieving coefficient passes through a minimum and rises back to one. Thus at high flux the membrane appears to be losing its ability to reject the solute as the flux is increased, when in fact its rejection ability is not changing.

Because of the difficulty in measuring the concentration of a solute at the membrane surface, the true sieving coefficient must be calculated from a rearranged form of Eq. 23. Often, only the observed sieving coefficient is reported, in which case its variation with ultrafiltrate flux must be considered.

Clearance as a Measure of Solute Removal and Its Prediction from Operating Parameters

Whole-blood clearance, C, the equivalent volume of whole blood per unit time from which a particular solute is completely removed by an artificial kidney device, was defined by Eq. 6. The rate of solute removal is most easily determined from measurements with the ultrafiltrate, as given by Eq. 2. Measurements can also be made with the blood entering and leaving the hemofilter:

$$M = Q_{Bi} c_{Bi} - Q_{Bo} c_{Bo} \qquad (25)$$

If flow rates of diluting fluid and filtrate are precisely balances (i.e., $Q_D = Q_F$, and $Q_{Bi} = Q_{Bo}$), all blood samples are taken from the streams entering or leaving the patient (i.e., before predilution or after postdilution), and equilibrium between red cells and plasma is attained, then the ratio $c_B : c_P$ is the same for all samples, and Eqs. 6 and 25 may be combined to yield

$$C = Q_B \left(\frac{c_{Pa} - c_{Pv}}{c_{Pa}} \right) \tag{26}$$

where subcripts a and v refer to arterial and venous lines leaving and reentering the patient, respectively. Under these restricted conditions, Eq. 26 can be used without the need to calculate whole-blood concentration from plasma concentration. However, this form is rarely used because it is much easier to measure the filtration rate, Q_F, required in Eq. 2, than the blood flow rate required in Eq. 26, under clinical conditions.

One goal in hemofiltration design is to be able to relate clearance to measurable membrane properties (e.g., sieving coefficients), and thus to predict hemofilter performance *a priori*. The first step is to convert the whole-blood solute concentration used in the clearance expressions to the solute concentration in plasma water, c_W. The solute concentration in whole blood, c_B, may be calculated from the solute concentration in plasma, c_P, using a solute mass balance:

$$c_B = c_P (1 - H) + K c_P H = c_P (1 - H + HK) \tag{27}$$

where H is hematocrit and K is the equilibrium solute distribution (partition) coefficient between red cells and plasma. It is most convenient to assume here that no solute crosses the red cell membrane during passage through the device. $K = 1$ if the solute concentration is the same inside the red cells as in plasma, and $K = 0$ (the most common case for solutes larger than sucrose) if the red cell membrane is impermeable to the solute. The maximum possible value of K, which is attained if no protein binding occurs and the equilibrium concentrations of the solute in the red cell interior and in the plasma water are equal, is $1/(1 - \Phi)$, where Φ is the volume fraction of hydrated proteins in plasma (Φ can be calculated as 0.0107 times the concentration of proteins in plasma [21]). Failure to correct for the difference between c_B and c_P will lead to an erroneously low value for clearance.

In the absence of protein binding, c_W is related to the measured concentration in plasma by

$$\frac{c_P}{c_W} = 1 - \Phi \tag{28}$$

Using Eqs. 27 and 28 to relate solute concentrations in whole blood, plasma, and plasma water, it is possible to then formulate complete equations for predicting whole-blood clearance from the observed sieving coefficient and other specified operating conditions. By assuming a power law dependence of flux on axial position [18], the following equations [4] were developed:

for predilution

$$C = Q_B \left(\frac{1-H}{1-H+HK} \right) \left\{ 1 - \left[\frac{(1-\Phi)(1-H) + \dfrac{Q_D}{Q_B}(1 - \dfrac{Q_F}{Q_D})}{(1-\Phi)(1-H) + \dfrac{Q_D}{Q_B}} \right] S_O \right\} \qquad (29)$$

and for postdilution,

$$C = Q_B \left(\frac{1-H}{1-H+HK} \right) \left\{ 1 - \left[\frac{(1-\Phi)(1-H) - \dfrac{Q_F}{Q_B}}{(1-\Phi)(1-H)} \right] S_O \right\} \qquad (30)$$

where S_O is the device-averaged observed sieving coefficient, and Q_D is the diluting fluid flow rate in predilution.

In developing these equations, it was assumed that the solute concentration varies axially but not radially in the hollow fibers, and that solute transport out of red cells following dilution is sufficiently slow that no significant rebound of the solute concentration can occur while the blood flows through the hemofilter. In the case of very fast equilibration between red cells and plasma, Eq. 29 may still be used if H is taken to be the hematocrit at the filter inlet *after* predilution.

For the case of $S_O = 1$, i. e., no rejection of solute, maximum whole-blood clearance for specified operating conditions is achieved. Eqs. 29 and 30 may be simplified as follows:

for predilution

$$C = \frac{Q_F(1-H)}{[1-H+HK][(1-\Phi)(1-H) + \dfrac{Q_D}{Q_B}]} \qquad (31)$$

and for postdilution

$$C = \frac{Q_F}{(1-H+HK)(1-\Phi)} \qquad (32)$$

Since these simplified equations no longer contain S_O, they can be used to compare maximum performance of different devices or operating regimes for which only Q_F, Q_D, and Q_B are known.

References

1. Shaldon S, Beau MC, Deschodt G, Ramperez P, Mion C (1980) Vascular stability during hemofiltration. Trans Am Soc Artif Intern Organs 26: 391–393
2. Gotch FA (1983) Sodium-volume modelling of hemodialysis and hemofiltration therapy. Proc Clin Dial Transplant Forum 10 (6): 27
3. Shaldon S, Deschodt G, Branger B, Oules R, Granolleras C, Baldamus CA, Koch KM, Lysaght MJ, Dinarello CA (1985) Hemodialysis hypotension: the interleukin hypothesis restated. Proc Eur Dial Transplant Assoc 22: 229–243

4. Lysaght MJ, Ford CA, Colton CK, Stone RA, Henderson LW (1978) Mass Transfer in clinical blood ultrafiltration devices. In: Frost TH (ed) Technical aspects of renal dialysis. Pitman Medical, Kent, pp 81-95

5. Lysaght MJ, Schmidt B, Gurland HJ (1983) Filtration rates and pressure driving force in AV hemofiltration. Blood Purif 1: 178-183

6. Brenner BM, Rector FC Jr (1976) The kidney. Saunders, Philadelphia

7. Feldhof P, Turnham T, Klein E (1984) Effect of plasma proteins on the sieving spectra of hemofilters. Artif Organs 8 (2): 186-192

8. Matthiasson E (1983) The role of macromolecular adsorption in fouling of ultrafiltration membranes. J Membr Sci 16: 23-26

9. Reihanian H, Robertson CR, Michaels AS (1983) Mechanisms of polarization and fouling of ultrafiltration membranes by proteins. J Membr Sci 16: 237-258

10. Zeman LJ (1983) Adsorption effects in rejection of macromolecules by ultrafiltration membranes. J Membr Sci 15: 213-230

11. Horbett TA (1982) Protein adsorption on biomaterials. Adv Chem Ser 199: 233-244

12. Dorson WJ Jr, Pizziconi VB, Allen JM (1971) Transfer of chemical species through a protein gel. Trans Am Soc Artif Intern Organs 17: 287-292

13. Colton CK, Friedman S, Wilson DE, Lees RE (1972) Ultrafiltration of lipoproteins through a synthetic membrane. J Lab Clin Med 51: 2472-2481

14. Streicher E (1982) Transport properties in filtration and dialysis membranes. Contrib Nephrol 32: 31-39

15. Nakao S-I, Yumoto S, Kimura S (1982) Analysis of rejection characteristics of macromolecular gel layer for low molecular weight solutes in ultrafiltration. Jpn J Chem Eng 15 (6): 463-468

16. Henderson LW, Leypoldt JK, Frigon RP, Uyeji SN, Alford M (1984) Slow flow hemofiltration improves solute transport. Blood Purif 2: 9

17. Haas T, Dongradi G, Villeboeuf F, de Viel E, Fournier JF, Duruy D (1983) Plasma kinetics of small molecules during and after hemofiltration: decrease in hemofiltration efficiency related to increase in ultrafiltration rate. Clin Nephrol 19 (4): 193-200

18. Henderson LW, Colton CK, Ford CA (1975) Kinetics of hemodiafiltration. II Clinical characterization of a new blood modality. J Lab Clin Med 85 (3): 372-391

19. Guyton AC (1978) Textbook of medical physiology. Saunders, Philadelphia

20. Lauer A, Saccaggi A, Ronco C, Belledonne M, Glabman S, Bosch JP (1983) Continuous arteriovenous hemofiltration in the critically ill patient: clinical use and operational characteristics. Ann Intern Med 99 (4): 455-460

21. Colton CK, Henderson LW, Ford CA, Lysaght MJ (1975) Kinetics of hemodiafiltration. I In vitro transport characteristics of a hollow-fiber blood ultrafilter. J Lab Clin Med 85 (3): 355-371

22. Blatt WF, Dravid A, Michaels AS, Nelson L (1970) Solute polarization and cake formation in membrane ultrafiltration: causes consequences and control techniques. In: Flinn JE (ed) Membrane science and technology. Plenum, New York, pp 47-97

23. Probstein RF, Leung W-F, Alliance Y (1979) Determination of diffusivity and gel concentration in macromolecular solutions by ultrafiltration. J Phys Chem 83 (9): 1228-1232

24. Kozinski AA, Lightfoot EN (1972) Protein ultrafiltration: a general example of boundary layer filtration. A I Ch E Journal 18 (5): 1030-1040

25. Vilker VL, Colton CK, Smith KA, Green DL (1984) The osmotic pressure of concentrated protein and lipoprotein solutions and its significance to ultrafiltration. J Membr Sci 20: 63-77

26. Wijmans JG, Nakao S, Smolders CA (1984) Flux limitation in ultrafiltration: osmotic pressure model and gel layer model. J Membr Sci 20: 115-124

27. Leveque MA (1928) Les lois de la transmission de chaleur par convection. Ann Mines 13: 201

28. Okazaki M, Yoshida F (1976) Ultrafiltration of blood: effect of hematocrit on ultrafiltration rate. Ann Biomed Eng 4: 138-150

29. Kochinke F, Baeyer HV, Kiener St, Schnabel R, Marx M, Mohnhaupt R, Kessel M (1982) Formation of a hybrid membrane in porous glass capillaries during hemofiltration (HF). Trans Am Soc Artif Intern Organs 28: 488-493

30. Porter MC (1972) Concentration polarization with membrane ultrafiltration. Ind Eng Chem Prod Res Devel 11 (3): 234-248

31. Shen JJS, Probstein RF (1977) On the prediction of limiting flux in laminar ultrafiltration of macromolecular solutions. Ind Eng Chem Fundam 16 (4): 459-465

32. Jaffrin MY, Butruille Y, Granger A, Vantard G (1978) Factors governing hemofiltration (HF) in a parallel plate exchanger with highly permeable membranes. Trans Am Soc Artif Intern Organs 24: 448-453
33. Isaacson K, Duenas P, Ford C, Lysaght M (1980) Determination of graetz solution constants in the in vitro hemofiltration of albumin, plasma and blood. In: Cooper AR (ed) Ultrafiltration membranes and applications. Plenum, New York, pp 507-521
34. Keller KH, Canales ER, Yum SI (1971) Tracer and mutual diffusion coefficients of proteins. J Phys Chem 75 (3): 379-387
35. Schumaker VN (1973) Hydrodynamic analysis of human low density lipoproteins. Accts Chem Res 6 (12): 398-403
36. Zydney AL, Colton CK (1982) Cross-flow membrane plasmapheresis: theoretical models for flux and hemolysis prediction. Trans Am Soc Artif Intern Organs 28: 404-412
37. Eckstein EC, Bailey DG, Shapiro AH (1977) Self-diffusion of particles in shear flow of a suspension. J Fluid Mech 79: 191-208
38. Bixler HJ, Nelson LM, Besarab A (1968) The diaphron hemodiafilter: an alternative to dialysis for extracorporeal blood purification. Chem Eng Prog Symp Series 84 (64): 90-103
39. Zydney AL (1985) Cross-flow membrane plasmapheresis: an analysis of flux and hemolysis. Ph D Thesis, MIT, Cambridge, Mass
40. Lysaght MJ, von Albertini B, Bosch JP, Ford CA, Geronomus R (1978) Relationship between surface area and ultrafiltration rate in capillary hemofilters. Proc Eur Soc Artif Organs 5: 178-182
41. Lysaght MJ, Ford CA, Isaacson KA (1981) Selection of optimal capillary internal diameter in blood ultrafilters. Proc Eur Soc Artif Organs 8: 130-134
42. Nakao S-I, Nomura T, Kimura S (1979) Characteristics of macromolecular gel layer formed on ultrafiltration tubular membrane. A I Ch E Journal 25 (4): 615-622
43. Vilker VL, Colton CK, Smith KA (1981) Concentration polarization in protein ultrafiltration. Part II: theoretical and experimental study of albumin ultrafiltered in an unstirred cell. A I Ch E Journal 27 (4): 637-645
44. Iorio G, Drioli E, Memoli B, Andreucci V, Salvatore M, Alfano B (1984) Ultrafiltration processes in blood treatment. J Membr Sci 18: 297-311
45. Spiegler KS, Kedem O (1966) Thermodynamics of hyperfiltration (reverse osmosis): criteria for efficient membranes. Desalination 1: 311-326

Membranes and Filters for Hemofiltration

H. GÖHL and P. KONSTANTIN

Table of Contents

Nomenclature

c	Mean concentration of	n_h	Number of fibers
b	Width of effective membrane	D	Diffusion coefficient
C_{Bi}	Solute concentration in incoming blood	I	Solvent flux
		J	Volume flux
C_{Bo}	Solute concentration in outgoing blood	K_B	Whole blood clearance
		K_P	Plasma clearance
C_F	Solute concentration in filtrate	L_p	Hydraulic permeability
c_b	Protein concentration in blood	P	Solute permeability
c_g	Protein concentration on the membrane	P_m	Diffuse permeability
		Q_B	Mean blood flow
c_{Pi}	Solute concentration in incoming plasma	Q_F	Device filtration rate
		R	Rejection coefficient
d	Fiber diameter	S	Sieving coefficient
h	Height (thickness) of blood film	TMP	Transmembrane pressure
k	Solute coefficient $k = \dfrac{c_i}{c_o}$ of concentration inside (c_i) and outside (c_o) the membrane	γ_w	Shear rate
		ΔP	Pressure difference
		η	Blood viscosity
		π	Constant
k_{fs}	Constant for flat sheet	σ	Staverman coefficient
k_h	Constant for hollow fiber	$\Delta\pi$	Osmotiv pressure
l	length of effective membrane	Φ	Solute flux
n_{fs}	Number of layers flat sheet	Δc	Concentration difference

Membranes

Membranes from a wide variety of materials have been used as dialysis or filtration membranes for medical purposes. This goes back as far as 1913, when ABEL et al. [1] first demonstrated the feasibility of an artificial kidney by diffusively removing metabolites from animal blood by circulating the blood through cellulose tubing placed in saline. Also, the first human dialysis performed by HAAS in 1923 [35] utilized diffusion as the transport mechanism of the artificial kidney.

The first use of ultrafiltration by filtering of blood for the purpose of dehydration of patients was reported by BRULL in 1928 [14]. Twenty years later, ALWALL [3] wound cellophane tubing, normally used in the production of sausages, on a spiral and surrounded this by a second screen which provided a pressure-driven ultrafiltration. It was, however, not until the end of the 1960s that, with the development of new polymers, membranes suitable for hemofiltration (HF) were developed [72].

Various new concepts for water purification, such as reverse osmosis, ultrafiltration, and microfiltration, were a major impetus for these developments. The first clinical HF experiments, in today's sense, were carried out by HENDERSON et al. [40]. In those initial reports, the technique was named hemodiafiltration. Currently, hemodiafiltration (HDF) describes a separation process which uses filtration and diffusion simultaneously. For this purpose, membranes with thinner wall thickness and higher hydrophilicity than pure HF membranes are used. These so-called high flux membranes combine moderately high water flux and high diffusive transport properties.

A membrane can be used for clinical HF if it fulfills the following criteria:

a) good blood compatibility,
b) no passage of albumin, and
c) high plasma water flux.

Membrane Materials

Of the large number of polymeric materials suitable for HF membranes, some have become commercially available, while others are still under development for clinical application. Table 1 classifies these membranes according to polymerization methods. Cuprophan HDF and cellulose acetates, acetylated to varying degrees, are all derived from cellulose, a naturally occurring linear condensation-type polymer. The other materials, all of synthetic origin, include linear polycondensation polymers such as polyamides and polysulfones and linear addition polymers such as polyacrylonitrile. The list also includes an inorganic material, i.e., glass which has been evaluated as membrane material although it is not yet commercially available as such.

Table 1. Membrane materials

Polymer type	Polymer material	Clinical use	Commercial-ly available	Reference
Linear polycondensation (synthetic origin)	Polyamide (aromatic)	HF		64, 97
	Polyamide (aliphatic-aromatic)	HF	Yes	33, 73, 99
	Polycarbonate-polyether	HF, HDF		57, 58, 59, 93
	Polysulfone	HF	Yes	39
	Polyether sulfone	HF		38
	Sulfonated polysulfone	HF		17, 53
Linear polycondensation (cellulosic origin)	Cellulose, regenerated	HDF	Yes	42
	Cellulose acetate	HDF	Yes	22
	Cellulose diacetate	HF	Yes	54
	Cellulose triacetate	HF	Yes	74
Linear addition	Polyacrylonitrile	HF, HDF	Yes	6, 36, 37
	Polyacrylonitrile-Na methallyl sulfonate	HDF	Yes	18, 19
	Polyethylene-polyvinyl alcohol	HF, HDF	Yes	103
	Polymethyl methacrylate	HDF	Yes	76, 77, 91, 98
	Polyelectrolytes	HF		9
Inorganic	Glass	HF		7

HF, hemofiltration; HDF, hemodiafiltration

These polymers vary from low *hydrophilicity* such as polyacrylonitrile, poly-amide, or polymethyl methacrylate to hydrophilic compounds such as cellulose or polyethylene polyvinyl alcohol copolymer. A polymer is called hydrophilic if it has a strong interaction with water, i. e., it adsorbs water and its surface is easily wetted. A measure of wettability is the contact angle of a drop of water on the material surface. A material is called hydrophilic if the contact angle is below 90 degress. On a molecular basis, the responsible factor for hydrophilicity are end groups such as carboxyl, amino, or hydroxy groups which have an attraction to water by hydrogen bonding. Hydrophobic compounds are molecules which do not associate with water (e. g., hydrocarbons).

Surfaces of solids immersed in water can have an electric *charge* caused by groups which dissociate into ions. If the counter-ion dissociates, a fixed charge remains in its place. Negatively charged surfaces can be created by acidic groups incorporated into the polymeric structure (carboxyl or sulfonyl groups); positively charged surfaces can be made by quarternation of amino compounds. If an electrical charge is not evenly distributed throughout a molecule, polar centers arise. These can exist on solids as well as on solutes such as proteins.

In clinical application, hydrophilicity or hydrophobicity of a membrane material, as well as the interactions between charged surfaces and charged solutes, can play a major role influencing adsorption of solutes on membrane surfaces and thereby affect the transport characteristics of a membrane.

In what follows a description of some of the membrane materials for HF is given.

Cellulose Esters

Cellulose esters have the advantage of being soluble in a wide range of solvents. This facilitates variations in membrane properties and allows different manufacturing processes. Therefore, this is the most investigated material. Its hydrophilicity and hydrophobicity as well as moderate polarity make it suitable for water filtration processes. This was shown in 1962 by Loeb and Sourirajan who developed the first asymmetric cellulose diacetate membrane suitable for reverse osmosis [63]. The disadvantages are poor strength and poor chemical resistance; the mechanical weakness requires relatively high membrane thicknesses.

Among cellulose esters, cellulose diacetate with an acetylation range of 2.3 to 2.7 and cellulose triacetate have attracted most attention. Cellulose acetate membranes were first developed by Cordis Dow for use in hollow-fiber hemodialyzers. They were then modified for high-flux dialysis and can be used for HF with limited filtration capacity [22]. Flat-sheet membranes from cellulose triacetate manufactured by Sartorius [74] and cellulose diacetate manufactured by Daicel [54] followed.

Cellulose

Cellulose was the first membrane material used in hemodialysis (HD) and remains by far the most widely used membrane in this field (Cuprophan). Using a higher glycerin content, this material was modified (Cuprophan HDF) to achieve increased flux and higher solute transport characteristics [42]. Compared with the synthetic membranes, Cuprophan HDF has a relatively low water-filtration rate, but since it also exhibits high diffusive solute transport, it is mostly used in HDF.

Glass

The use of porous glass hollow fibers is reportedly the first use of an inorganic material for a HF membrane [7]. Glass provides higher dimensional and chemical stability than most polymeric materials, but has the disadvantages of high brittleness and low permeability. Glass is composed of the system $Na_2O-B_2O_3-SiO_2$. The manufacturing process involves an induced microphase separation resulting in alkali borate areas. Rinsing with mineral acids removes these areas leaving a porous silica matrix as the membrane wall. Then, with special treatment, the hydrophobic glass is rendered more hydrophilic to make it wettable. However, probably due to the brittleness of fragile glass hollow fibers (which poses a real problem during hemofilter manufacturing), no clinical use has been reported in the literature.

Polyacrylonitrile

Hollow-fiber and flat-sheet membranes are reportedly made from polyacrylonitrile (PAN) [36, 37] and PAN copolymers [18, 19], e.g., with sodium methallyl sulfonate [29, 69, 71]. These polymers dissolve well in water miscible solvents, such as dimethyl formamide and dimethyl sulfoxide, and their good wettability leads to high filtration rates combined with high diffusive permeability. They are, therefore, not only used for HF but also for HDF.

Polyamide

Out of the large number of polyamides (PA) which were evaluated for membrane formation, especially for reverse osmosis membranes, a few were described for use in HF. Careful selection of the material is necessary since some PA have a tendency to adsorb proteins. One aliphatic aromatic copolymer [33, 73, 99] and an aromatic PA [64, 97] are described extensively. PA have the advantage over cellulose acetates of possessing extremely asymmetric structures with high filtration rates. PA also have high mechanical strength and high flexibility allowing the fabrication of thin and pressure-resistant hollow fibers.

Polycarbonate Block Copolymer

Polycarbonate-polyether (PC-PE) block copolymer has been first described for use in a HD membrane [8, 43]. Modification of the manufacturing process reportedly increases the filtration rates and cut-off point of the membrane to make the membrane suitable for HDF [93] and HF [57, 59].

Polyelectrolytes

Early research in HF reported the use of membranes of the precipitated polyelectrolytes sodium polystyrene sulfonate and polyvinyl benzyl trimethyl ammonium chloride in stoichiometric proportions [9]. Hence, the membrane possesses a net neutral charge. The membrane itself was cast 20-50 µm thick and was quite fragile. For greater strength it was therefore cast on a stout backing of highly porous polyether felt.

Polyethylene-Polyvinyl-Copolymer

A modification of the dialysis membrane manufacturing process of polyethylene-polyvinyl-copolymer (EVAL) results in a typical HF membrane comprising a skin layer on its surface, supported by a porous layer [48, 103].

Polymethyl Methacrylate

A stereo complex of isotactic polymethyl methacrylate (PMMA) and syndiotactic PMMA results in a so-called hydrogel type semipermeable membrane having a high water content. Since the ultrafiltration rate of this membrane is lower than asymmetric membranes, it is better suited for HDF than for pure HF [76, 77, 91, 98].

Polysulfones

The first hemofilter which was clinically used was a polysulfone (PS) hollow-fiber device manufactured by Amicon [39]. A few years later, the copolymer polyether sulfone [38] was used because of better solubility than PS. Another modification resulting in a more hydrophilic negatively charged polymer is achieved by sulfonating polysulfone [17, 53]. However, clinical use of a sulfonated polysulfone membrane has not yet been reported and is so far restricted to technical ultrafiltration. Using blending of poly(vinylpyrrolidone) instead of chemical modification is another way to increase the hydrophilicity of PS [15]. According to Walch [100], this increases the diffusive solute transport, which enables the use of this normally hydrophobic membrane material to be also used in HDF. A device manufactured in this manner has been introduced recently [28].

Principles of Membrane Formation

The manufacture of HF membranes from the above-mentioned polymer materials is done by the so-called phase inversion technique, whereby a solution of the polymer is solvent cast via a doctor blade, extruded or spun through a spinnerette. The obtained film or hollow fiber is then brought into contact with a nonsolvent which replaces the solvent and causes the polymer to gel and be converted into the solid phase.

A single-step phase inversion takes place when the polymer solution is solidified immediately after passing the casting knife, the spinnerette, or the extruder, resulting in the final membrane. In some cases, however, before the membrane is obtained in its final structure, it may be desirable to alter its structure by one or more steps preceding the final formation of the membrane. This is accomplished by processes such as:

1) Partial evaporation of the solvent to form a skin on the membrane
2) Lowering the temperature to a temperature sufficient for the system to be transformed into a gel
3) Passing the polymer solution through a gelling medium having the capability of only gradually transferring the membrane into its solid state

These processes, one or more used consecutively, will influence the membrane formation and can be used to optimize the membrane structure and thereby the membrane properties for its intended purpose.

The manufacture of flat-sheet and hollow-fiber membranes is closely related; the main difference is that there is no support prior to solidification of the hollow fiber.

Hollow-Fiber Spinning

There are three conventional hollow-fiber methods, all of them employing the phase inversion technique, dry spinning, wet-dry spinning, and melt spinning.

Dry spinning utilizes a low boiling solvent which evaporates rapidly over the drop height of the fiber [55]. The solvent must be evaporated inside and outside the fiber in order to maintain hollow-fiber geometry during the winding step. Fibers obtained by this method can be symmetric or asymmetric and with or without skin.

Most of today's HF hollow fibers are extruded by employing the *wet-dry spinning* method as shown in Fig. 1. The polymer solution consisting of the polymer in a water miscible solvent is filtered, degassed, and pumped into a spinning jet through the outer orifice with concomitant injection of the core medium (gas, liquid). In the case of hemofiltration membranes, a nonsolvent is used as a core medium and the interaction between this liquid and the polymer solution determines the membrane structure and the surface on the inner side of the hollow fiber. This step, which lasts only from less than a second to a couple of seconds, is the one mainly responsible for the membrane permeability.

The other important parameter in membrane formation is the medium on the outside of the fiber when the fiber leaves the yet. The fiber can either fall through gas (in most cases air) or can be spun directly into a liquid. These conditions will determine the outer surface and the outer membrane structure.

At this point the fiber has enough mechanical stability to be transported under moderate tension into subsequent tanks. These baths have the function of further stabilizing the hollow fiber structure as well as rinsing the fiber. For medical applications it is of utmost importance to wash the membrane free of all solvents and ad-

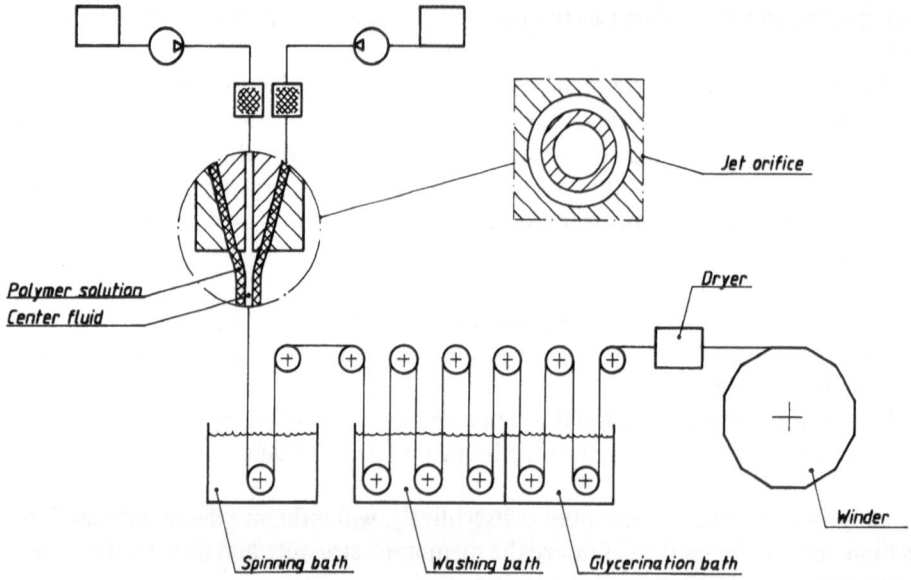

Fig. 1. Principle of fiber spinning

ditives. Therefore, the length of membrane in these baths might be as much as 100 m or more, and elevated bath temperatures are sometimes used.

In order to obtain a dry membrane, the water contained in it is replaced by agents such as glycerin. This stabilizes the membrane properties and prevents changes in permeabilities during air drying, which is normally done prior to winding the membrane. The glycerin prevents the shrinkage of the membrane pores which otherwise would occur when the water is removed by drying.

As a last step, the membrane is wound onto a bobbin, spool, or reel. Spinning velocity in wet-dry spinning can vary from 10 to approximately 80 m/min.

Heating a polymer to its melting point is often accompanied by thermal degradation, cross-linking, etc. *Melt spinning,* therefore, employs volatile or extractable plasticizers to decrease the melting point of the polymer. For example, cellulose acetate, which has a melting point at around 300 °C can be spun at temperatures of approximately 100 °C less when mixed with additives, such as dimethyl sulfoxide or glycerin.

A modification of melt spinning is to use polymer-additive combinations which are compatible at higher temperatures but not at lower temperatures. Phase separation occurs when, after extrusion, the fiber is allowed to solidify by cooling. The precipitated fiber consists then of two phases, the porous polymer matrix and the additive which has to be leached out.

Melt spinning tends to result in isotropic membrane structures.

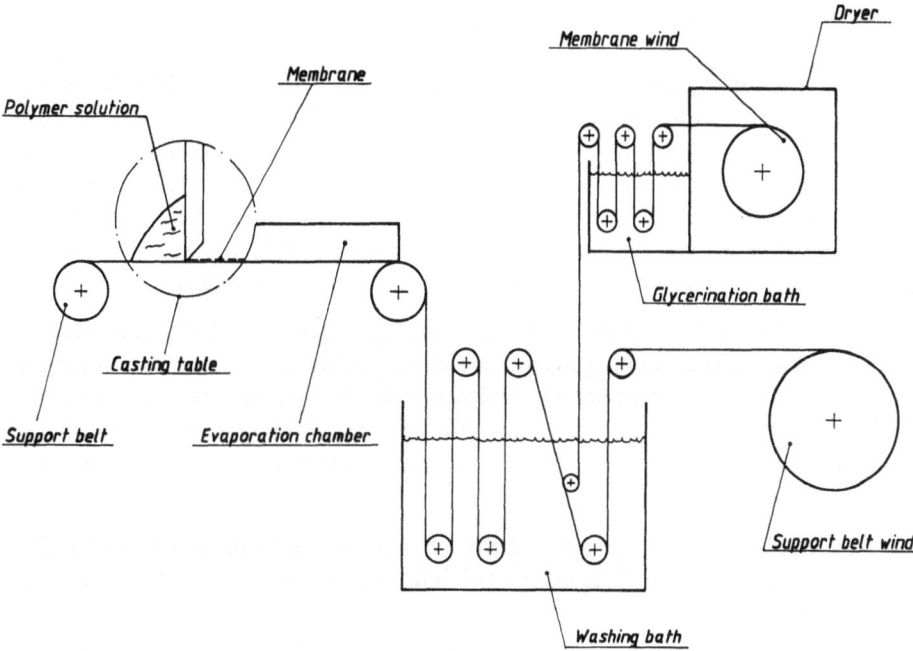

Fig. 2. Principle of flat-sheet membrane casting

Flat-Sheet Manufacturing

Flat-sheet membranes are produced in the same manner as hollow-fiber membranes in a dry, wet-dry, or melt process. However, two slightly different processes can be used (a) extrusion or (b) casting.

Extrusion of a flat sheet is the equivalent of spinning a hollow fiber except that instead of a spinnerette a slit-jet extruder is used. Extrusion can be done without support as in hollow-fiber spinning or onto a moving support belt as in flat-sheet casting. In membrane casting (Fig. 2) the polymer solution, after filtration and degassing, is pumped onto a moving support belt where the membrane casting thickness is determined by the distance of the so-called "doctor blade," which is adjustable in height, to the moving support belt. The support belt, which, for instance, can be a coated paper, a plastic film, or a stainless steel belt, is kept under tension to maintain a constant casting thickness. Again, as in wet-dry spinning, most HF membranes are obtained using a wet-dry casting process where a polymer film is allowed to partially dry by evaporating some of the solvent. Then the film is led through gelation and washing baths. After the membrane has been completely solidified, it is removed from the support belt, the water replaced by glycerin, and dried in a drying chamber. PA, PS, and CA membranes having asymmetric skinned sponge (or finger) structures can be produced this way.

Flat-sheet casting also offers the possibility of casting on a permeable support layer which becomes part of the final membrane. This method is used, for instance, in the manufacturing of CA membranes in order to improve the relatively low strength of the membrane film.

Examples of Manufacturing Processes

Polymethyl methacrylate. A mixture of syndiotactic and isotactic PMMA is dissolved in dimethyl sulfoxide of 120 °C. The solution is cooled to form a gel, then following solvent casting is further cooled to room temperature. Subsequently, the thin film of gel is immersed in an ice-water bath, whereby the dimethyl sulfoxide in the gel film is replaced by water to form the hydrogel structure of PMMA [98]. The membrane obtained by this process can be classified as a heteroporous gel membrane which is mostly suited for HDF and to a lesser extent for pure HF.

Cellulose Acetate. A casting solution is prepared by dissolving cellulose acetate in a solvent mixture and a swelling agent. The casting solution is cast onto a substrate and solvent is partially evaporated. Following this, the membrane is immersed in water to undergo gelation and to remove the solvent remaining in the membrane. If necessary, the membrane so formed is then heated to obtain the final desired properties.

Polyacrylonitrile. A solution of acrylonitrile in nitric acid is extruded into a coagulation bath containing up to 30% nitric acid. Subsequently, the membrane is washed free of nitric acid [36].

Polyethylene-polyvinyl alcohol. A solution of the copolymer is dissolved in dimethyl sulfoxide and extruded into an aqueous bath containing 20% dimethyl sulfoxide [103].

Formation of Hollow Fiber Membranes

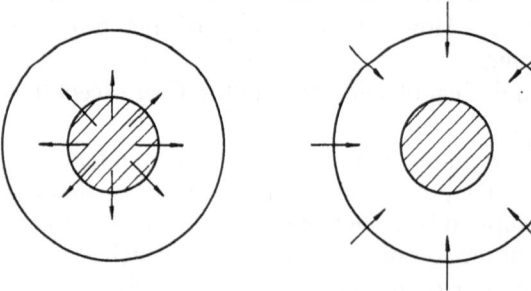

Inside Precipitation   Outside Precipitation

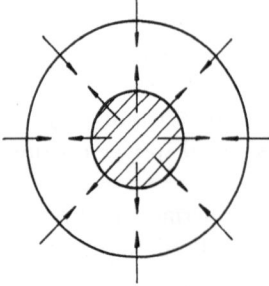

Outside and Inside Precipitation   **Fig. 3.** Schematic of hollow-fiber formation

Polyether-polycarbonate. A solution of the copolymer, together with polyethylene glycol as a swelling agent, is dissolved in a water miscible solvent. Following extrusion of the solution and partial evaporation of the solvent, the membrane is precipitated in water. The membrane is then washed, stabilized with glycerin, and dried with air [58].

Membrane Structure

Membranes for HF must fulfill the criteria of high plasma water flux and of a molecular weight cut-off of approximately 30000. Only membranes having certain structures can fulfill these criteria (see Figs. 4-9). As described in the previous sec-

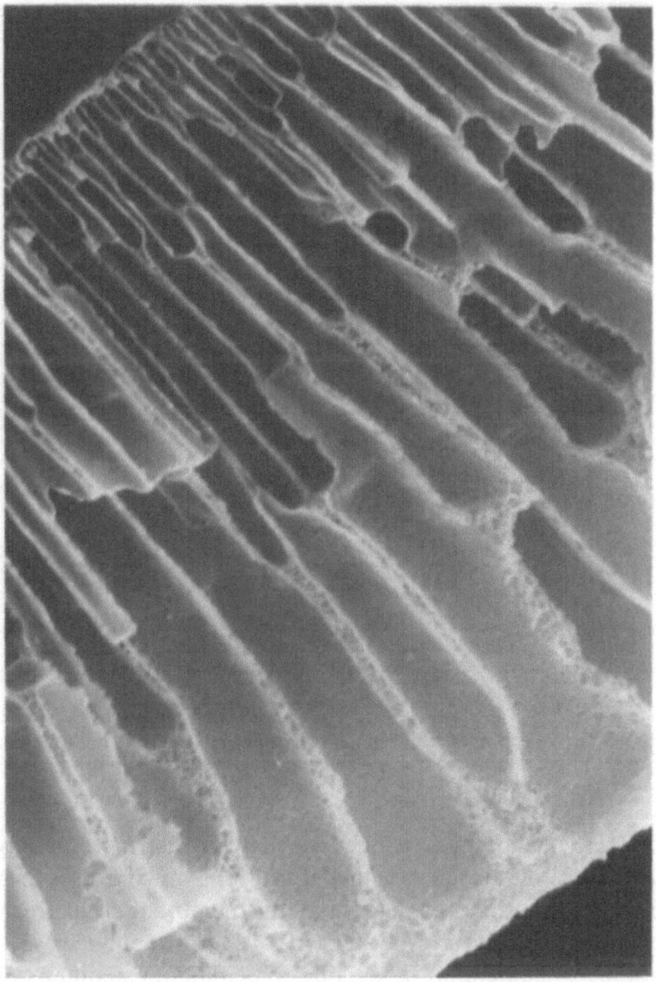

Skinned surface
in contact with blood

Finger-like support
structure
wall thickness 50 μm

Fig. 4. Cross section of a polyamide hollow fiber

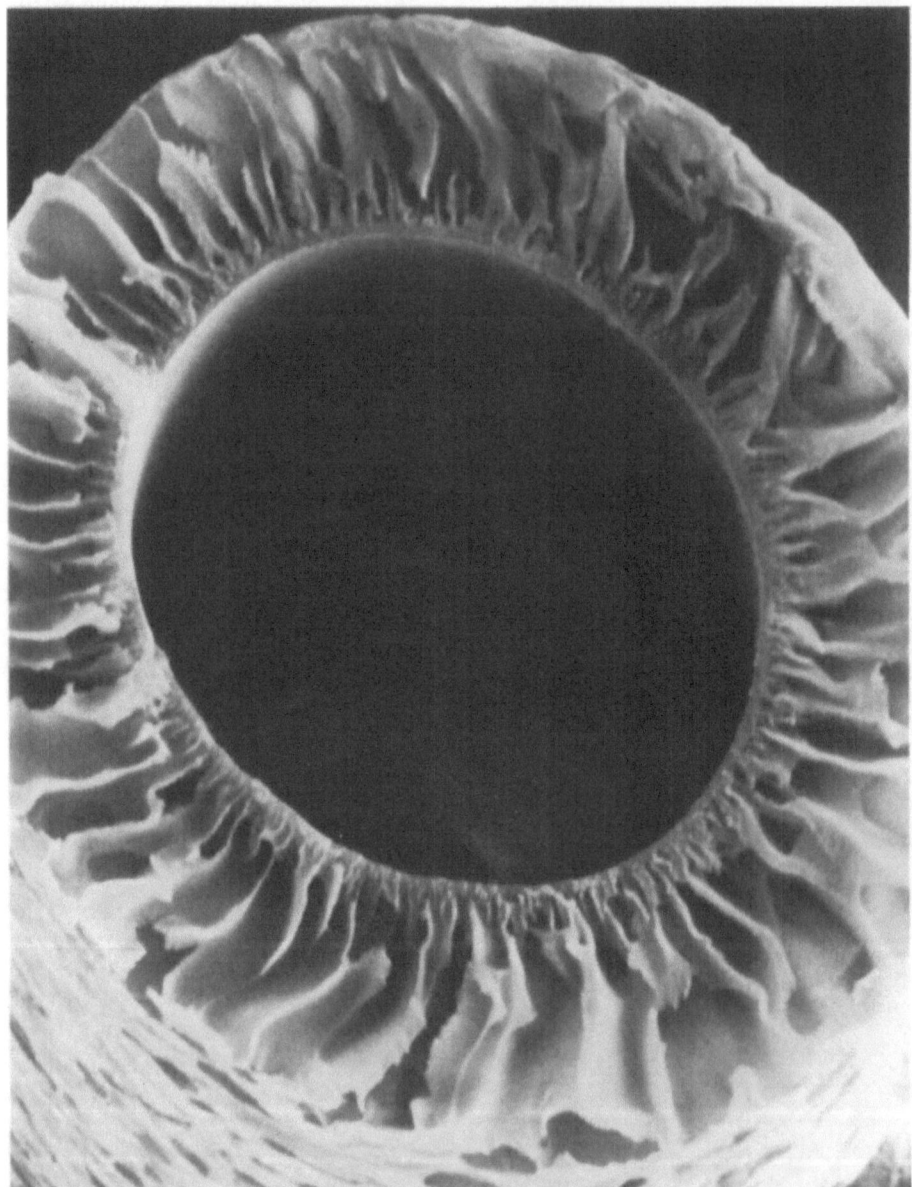

Fig.5. Cross section of an asymmetric skinned polysulfone hollow fiber

tion, HF membranes are made by phase inversion, i. e., a polymer dissolved in a solvent comes into contact with a nonsolvent which causes the polymer to precipitate. This precipitation step determines the membrane structure. Many parameters influence this step, such as type and concentration of polymer, solvents, solution viscosity, additives, temperature, and type of precipitation medium. For each membrane, optimum manufacturing parameters have to be developed to be used in HDF or HF.

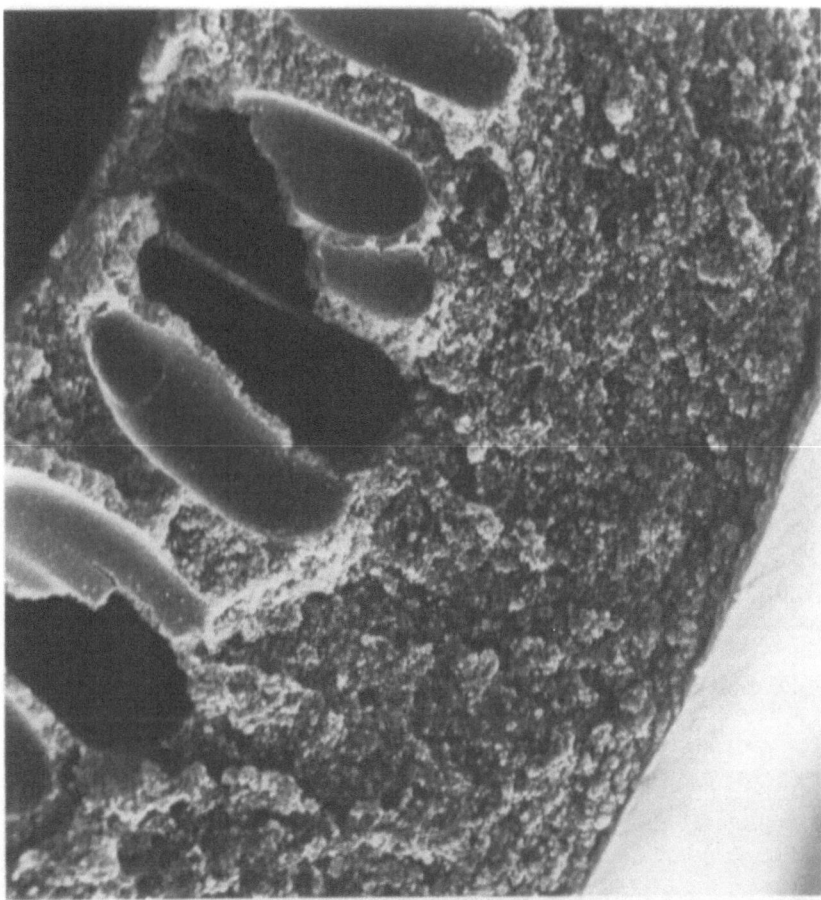

Fig. 6. Cross section through the wall of a polyacrylonitrile hollow fiber (PAN 200), wall thickness 50 μm

In the following, the precipitation of an asymmetric hollow-fiber membrane will be used to demonstrate the principles of membrane formation (Fig. 3). Hollow fibers can be precipitated from the inside, outside, or both sides, concomitantly. This results in asymmetric fibers with the skin either on the inside or outside, or, in the case of simultaneous precipitation from the inside and outside, in a symmetric membrane with skin structures both inside and outside. The mechanism of precipitating asymmetric membranes is described in detail by STRATHMANN [94, 95] and CABASSO et al. [16]. Most of the commercial HF membranes are asymmetric and most of them have a skin on the inside which is the part of the membrane exposed to the blood. Two examples of highly asymmetric structures with skins between 0.1 and 1 μm are shown in Figs. 4 and 5. This skin is the part of the membrane responsible for the permeability of the membrane, whereas the finger-like support structure is responsible for the mechanical stability of the membrane. The PAN membrane in Fig. 6 is mainly precipitated from the inside and only partly from the outside. This leads to a skin inside, sponge-like structures on the inside and outside, and finger-

Fig. 7. Cross section of a polyacrylonitrile flat sheet (AN 69) with symmetric structure

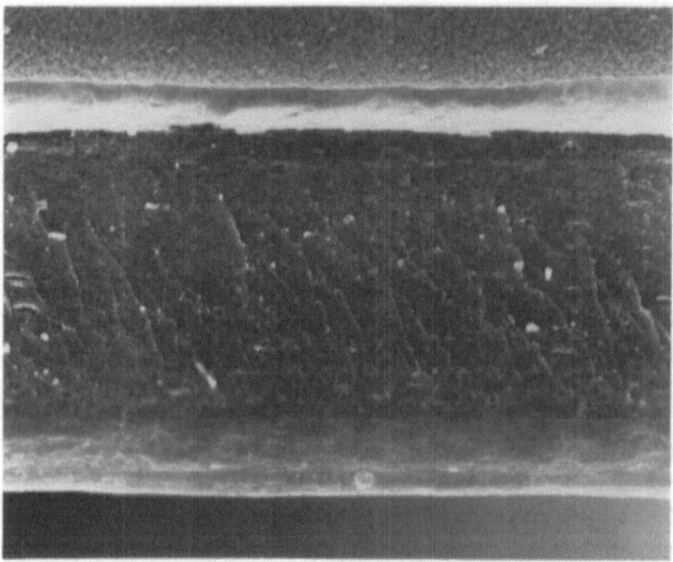

Fig. 8. Cross section through a homogeneous gel membrane (Cuprophan high flux)

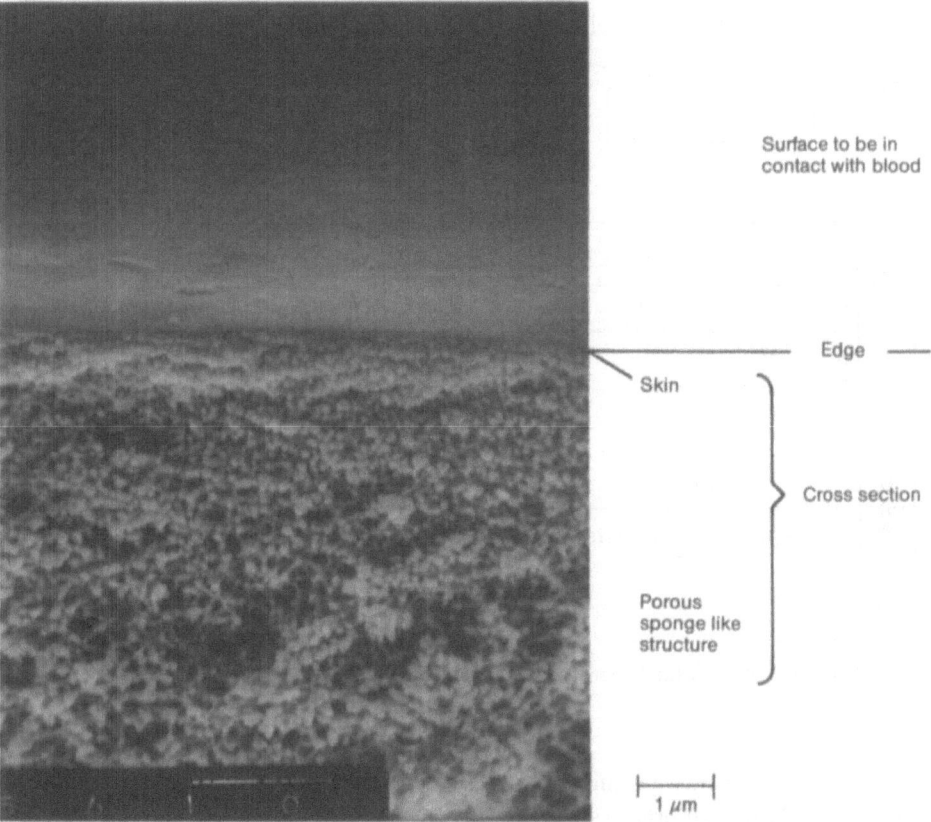

Surface to be in
contact with blood

Edge

Skin

Cross section

Porous
sponge like
structure

1 µm

Fig. 9. Cross section of a cellulose triacetate membrane

like voids in the middle. This formation of membrane structure has to take place in less than 1 s because immediately after leaving the jet the hollow fiber must be self-supporting.

In flat-sheet membrane manufacturing, it is not critical to have such a fast membrane formation because the membrane can be supported by a belt. But like in hollow-fiber manufacturing, the structure is determined by the mode of precipitation. Highly asymmetric structures can be obtained when the polymer film is quickly immersed into the precipitation bath. Symmetric structures can be obtained by slow precipitation. The membrane then needs the support of a support belt for up to a few minutes. Such a symmetric membrane, made from PAN, is shown in Fig. 7. Symmetric flat-sheet structures are also obtained when vertically extruding the polymer film into the precipitation bath (Cuprophan HDF [42], Fig. 8). An asymmetric flat-sheet membrane made from cellulose acetate is shown in Fig. 9. This membrane exhibits a skin with a sponge-like substructure.

Membranes can be divided into three groups: fluid membranes, finely porous membranes, and coarsely porous (microporous) membranes [80]. For HF, only finely porous membranes are used. As shown in Fig. 10, the finely porous membranes can be subdivided into gel membranes and heteroporous membranes [101]. Exam-

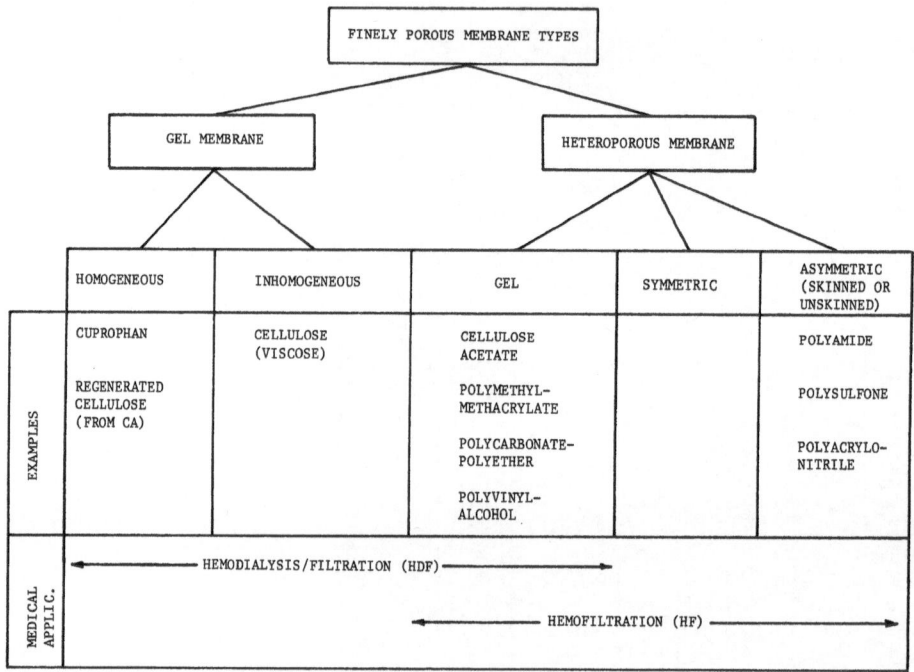

Fig. 10. Classification of finely porous membrane types with examples

ples of homogeneous gel membranes are Cuprophan and regenerated cellulose membranes. Gel membranes swell in water by incorporating water into the polymer matrix. The high flux types of these gel membranes (e. g., Cuprophan HDF) have a more open cellulose matrix (i.e., less cellulose per membrane thickness and area) which leads to higher permeability rates than the conventional cellulosic HD membranes (Cuprophan, regenerated cellulose from cellulose acetate, cellophane, viscose).

The heteroporous membranes possess still higher convective permeability. Again, different structures of heteroporous membranes exist. The heteroporous gel membranes are from hydrophilic polymers such as PVA, PE-PC, and cellulose acetate. Scanning electron micrographs of the heteroporous asymmetric membrane group were shown in Fig. 4–6 and Fig. 9. Examples for these are PA and PS.

Membrane Permeability

Whereas the previous section classified membranes according to their structures, this section describes the basic mechanism which governs the transport of solvent and solute through these membranes (Table 2) [79]. In a coarsely porous membrane, there is no interaction between fluid and membrane matrix. Consequently, the filtration is solely a function of the applied pressure. Solute transport is determined by a convective part and a diffusive part with convection as the main driving force. On the other hand, in a finely porous membrane there is an interaction between the

Table 2. Basic transport mechanism for the three typical membrane groups[a]

	Coarsely porous membranes	Finely porous membranes	Solution-diffu-sion (fluid) membranes
Solute flux	$\varnothing = I \cdot k \cdot c + \dfrac{P \cdot \Delta c}{d}$	$\varnothing = \dfrac{(1-\sigma) \cdot c \cdot -}{I + P \dfrac{\Delta c}{d}}$	$\varnothing = P \cdot \dfrac{\Delta c}{d}$
Solvent flux	$I = Lp \cdot \Delta P$	$I = Lp \, (\Delta P - \sigma \cdot \Delta \pi)$	$I = Lp(\Delta P - \Delta \pi)$

[a] See list of Nomenclature for explanation of symbols

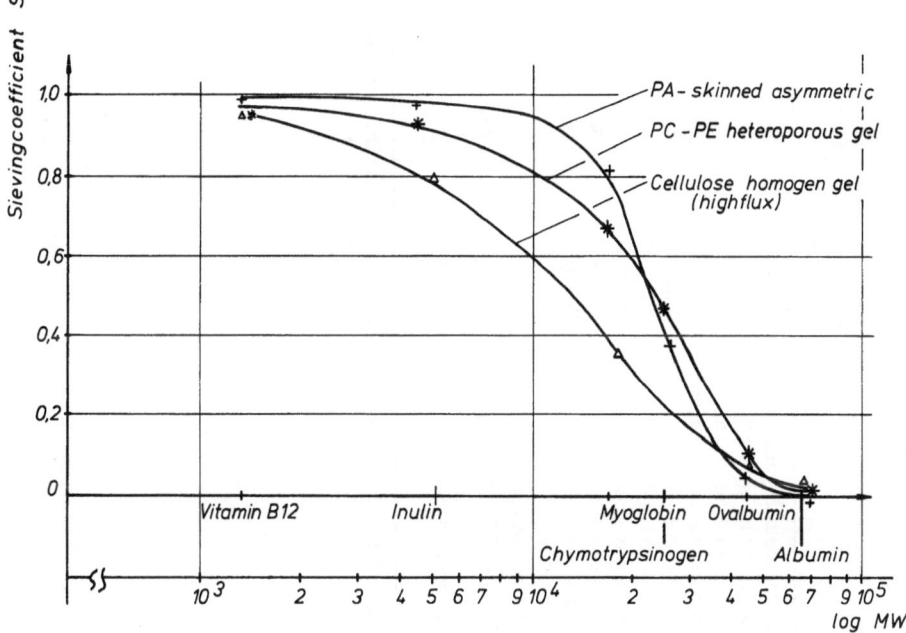

Fig. 11. Sieving coefficients vs log molecular weight for three flat-sheet membranes. Test conditions: concentration, 0.01%; filtration flux, 12 for PA, 4.0 for PC-PE, and 0.5 cm/s × 10⁻⁴ for cellulose homogeneous gel

membrane and the filtrate. This interaction is determined by the difference in osmotic pressure $\sigma \cdot \Delta \pi$ with σ as the STAVERMAN reflection coefficient which is a measure of the sieving properties of a membrane (see list of nomenclature).

To describe the important parameters of transport through a HF membrane, knowledge of the hydraulic permeability L_p of a membrane is required (Table 3).

$$L_p = I_v/(\Delta P - \sigma \cdot \Delta \pi) \tag{1}$$

One also needs the sieving coefficient S of a membrane (Table 4 and Fig. 11).

$$S = 1/R \tag{2}$$

Table 3. Description, application, and manufacturers of various polymer materials used in hemofiltration and hemodiafiltration

Polymer material	Membrane configuration	Membrane structure	Wet/dry membrane thickness (μm)	$L_P \times 10^5$ (ml/s at cm^2)	Main application	Manufacturer
Polyamide	F	Heteroporous, asymmetric	50/50	250	HF	Gambro
Polysulfone	F	Heteroporous, asymmetric	65/65	220	HF	Amicon
Polyacrylonitrile	F	Heteroporous, asymmetric	50/50	150	HF	Asahi
Polysulfone	F	Heteroporous, asymmetric	40/40	120	HDF	Fresenius
Polymethyl methacrylate	F	Heteroporous gel	40/40	21	HDF	Toray
Polyacrylonitrile	S	Heteroporous gel	30/30	55	HDF	Rhone Poulenc
Cellulose acetate	S	Heteroporous gel	125/120	150	HF	Sartorius
Cellulose triacetate	S	Heteroporous gel	85/85	150	HF	Daicel
Polysulfone	F	Heteroporous, asymmetric (hydrophilic)	70/70	300	HF	Kalle
Cuprophan high flux	F, S	Homogeneous gel	40/20	26	HDF	Enka
Regenerated cellulose	F	Homogenenous gel	45/40	18	HDF	Dow
Polycarbonate-polyether	F	Heteroporous gel	20/20	21	HDF	Gambro

F, hollow fiber; S, flat sheet; L_P, hydraulic permeability; HF, hemofiltration; HDF, hemodialysis/filtration; at, atmospheric pressure

Table 4. Sieving coefficients and corresponding flux

	Vitamin B12	Inulin	Myoglobin	Chymotryp-sinogen	Ovalbumin-Albumin	$J \times 10^4$ (cm/s)	$Lp \times 10^5$ (ml/s at.cm^2)
Polyacrylonitrile AN 69[a] Flat sheet 30 μm	0.75	0.65	0.30	-	-	7.0	55
Polycarbonate-polyether Flat sheet 20 μm	0.90	0.80	0.60	0.45	0.10	4.0	21
Cuprophan high flux[b] Hollow fiber ID = 215 μm	0.95	0.80	0.30			0.7	26
Cuprophan high flux Flat sheet 40 μm	0.95	0.78	0.35	0.20	0.08	0.5	15
Polyamide (skinned asymmetric) Hollow fiber ID = 215 μm	0.98	0.95	0.75	0.40	0.02	20.0	210
Polyamide (skinned asymmetric) Flat sheet 75 μm	0.95	0.95	0.80	0.25	0.03	12.0	100

[a] Data from [45]
[b] Data from [56]
J, flux tested in saline (0.01% concentration); Lp, hydraulic permeability; ID, inner diameter; at, atmospheric pressure

Table 5. Dimensions of commercially available hollow-fiber hemofilters

Type of filter	Manufacturer	Membrane area (m²)	Inner diameter (μm)	Blood volume (ml)	Fiber length (mm)	UF at QB (ml/min)			Membrane material	Steriliza-tion	Refer-ence
						100 TMP= 60 mmHg	200 TMP= 500 mmHg	400			
D 20[a]	Amicon	0.25	200	20	130	5–15	–	–	Polysulfone	ETO	4
D 30[a]		0.60	200	40	215	10–25	–	–		ETO	5
D 40		1.10	200	75	215	–	70–90	90–120			
PAN 150	Asahi	1.10	210	75	215	–	80–90	–	Polyacrylonitrile	ETO	6
PAN 200		1.40	210	100	240	–	80–100	–			
PAN 250		2.00	210	140	240	–	–	–			
FH 55[a]	Gambro	0.60	215	43	170	10–20	–	–	Polyamide	ETO	30
FH 77		1.35	215	90	280	–	80–90	100–140			
FH 88		1.95	215	137	280	–	80–100	120–120			
High flux dialysers which are used also as hemofilters											
B1-L	Toray	2.10	240	155	235	–	70–80	80–100	Polymethyl methacrylate	Gamma	44
Duoflux	Cordis Dow	1.80	200	135	250	–	60–80	80–100	Cellulose acetate	ETO	22
F 60	Fresenius	1.25	200	75	255	–	90–100	–	Polysulfone	ETO	28
D6	Fresenius	2.00	180 (dry)	100	255	–	70–90	90–120	Cuprophan HDF	ETO	

[a] Used for AV hemofiltration

TMP, transmembrane pressure; UF, ultrafiltrate; QB, mean blood flow

where R is the true solute rejection of a membrane.

The literature [45] gives an expression that relates the rejection to the volumetric flux.

$$1/S = R = \sigma(e^\beta - 1)/(e^\beta - \sigma) \tag{3}$$
$$\beta = J_v(1 - \sigma/P_m) \tag{4}$$

Since in HF the diffusive permeability P_m is of little importance, these values are not given in Table 4 which presents the sieving coefficients and corresponding volume fluxes of HF and HDF membranes in saline.

Hemofilters

The first device specially developed for HF was a hollow-fiber hemofilter by Amicon. Development took place in the late 1960s and first clinical use was reported by Hamilton et al. in 1971 [39].

QUELLHORST in 1972 published a study on the use of existing high flux dialysers (RP6, Rhône Poulenc) for HF [81]. His study, for the first time, involved a larger number of patients and initiated the spread of HF in Europe.

Table 6. Commercially available flat-sheet hemofilters

Filter	Manufacturer	Membrane area (m²)	UF at Q_B (ml/min)			Membrane material	Sterilization	Reference
			100 TMP= 60 mmHg	200 TMP= 500 mmHg	400			
SM 400 04	Sartorius	0.3	–	70- 95	80–110	Cellulose triacetate	ETO	85
SM 400 06		0.6	–	85–115	110–150			
SM 400 42		0.6		85–115	110–150			
Hemofresh[a]	Daicel	0.7		90–110	–	Cellulose triacetate	ETO	54
234	Secon	0.9	–	80–100	100–160	Polysulfone	Gamma	86
High flux dialysers which are used also as hemofilters								
1200 S[b]	Rhone Poulenc	0.5	10–25	–	–	Polyacrylonitrile (AN 69-S)	ETO+ Gamma	
2400 S		1.0				Polyacrylonitrile	ETO+ Gamma	
3000 S		1.2	–	70- 90	80–110			
GLM High Flux	Gambro	1.36	–	60- 90	80–110	Cuprophan HDF	ETO	30
H12–10	Rhone Poulenc	1.2	–	70- 90	81–110	Polyacrylonitrile (AN 69-N)	Gamma	46

[a] Not commercially available
[b] Used for AV hemofiltration
TMP, transmembrane pressure;   UF, ultrafiltrate; Q_B, mean blood flow

During the latter part of the 1970s, additional devices for HDF and HF were developed by various manufacturers (Tables 5, 6). At the same time, COLTON did theoretical work on the kinetics of HF [21]. Using the concentration polarization model [12], equations were derived describing the relationship between geometric dimensions of hollow-fiber and flat-sheet hemofilters and the filtration flux. The following equations, describing local filtration rate, mean wall-shear rate, and pressure drop, give approximate values for the basic parameters used in the design of a hemofilter device (see list of Nomenclature):

Hollow-fiber devices [12]:

$$Q_F = k_h \cdot \left(\frac{D^2 \cdot \gamma_w}{l} \right)^{1/3} \cdot \ln \frac{c_g}{c_b} \tag{5}$$

$$\gamma_w = \frac{32 \cdot Q_B}{n_h \, \pi \, d^3} \tag{6}$$

$$\Delta P = \frac{128 \cdot \pi \cdot l \cdot Q_B}{\pi \cdot n_h \cdot d^4} \tag{7}$$

Flat-sheet devices [50]:

$$Q_F = k_{fs} \cdot \left(\frac{b \cdot l}{h} \right)^{2/3} \cdot Q_B^{-1/3} \tag{8}$$

$$\gamma_w = \frac{6 \cdot Q_B}{b \cdot h^2 \cdot n_{fs}} \tag{9}$$

$$\Delta P = \frac{12 \cdot \eta \cdot l \cdot Q_B}{b \cdot h^3 \cdot n_{fs}} \tag{10}$$

The characteristic of protein concentration polarization is that with increasing transmembrane pressure (TMP) there is a linear increase in filtration flux. However, in a certain TMP range the filtration curve starts to flatten and at a certain pressure the maximum filtration flux is obtained. This plateau is reached at different TMPs depending on membrane, device dimensions, blood flow, and blood composition.

The complete theory of the concentration polarization phenomenon is described in more detail in the chapter by OFSTHUN, COLTON and LYSAGHT (see this volume).

Hollow-Fiber Devices

Hollow-fiber devices which are used in HF are summarized in Table 5. They can be divided into the following three groups:

1) Standard hemofilters (Fig. 12a), with hollow fibers of diameters between 200 and 215 μm, effective membrane areas of 1.0–2.0 m², and total fiber length of 210–280 mm

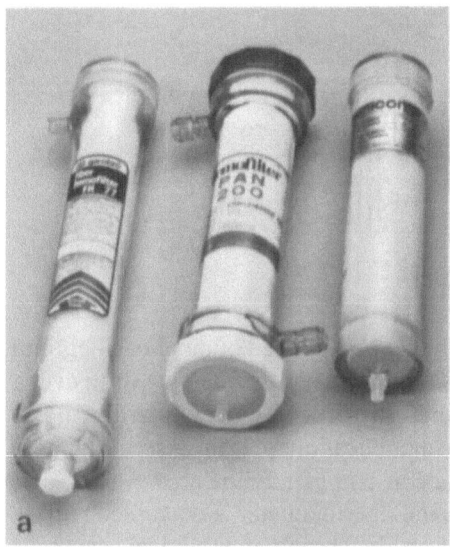
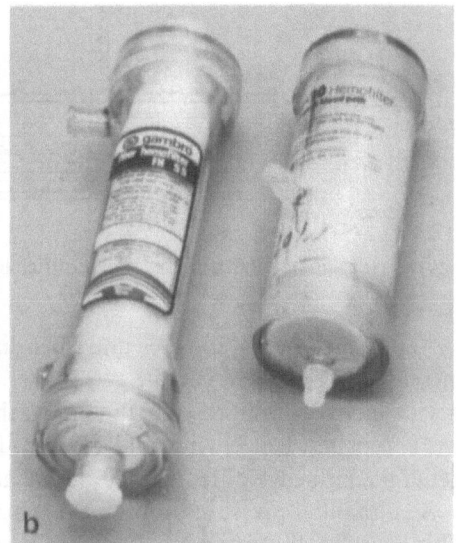
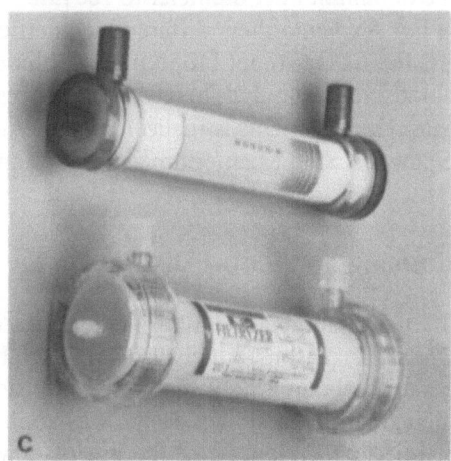

Fig. 12. Hollow-fiber hemofilter devices.
a Standard hemofilters. **b** AV hemofilters.
c HDF dialysers

2) AV hemofilters (Fig. 12b; used for arteriovenous or spontaneous HF applied without a blood pump [24, 60], with smaller surface areas (0.25–0.6 m^2) and shorter fiber lengths (100–150 mm)

3) High flux dialysers or hemodiafilters (Fig. 12c; also used in HF, characterized by membranes combining high filtration rate and high diffusive permeability, with surface areas of 1.2–2.1 m^2

Design Characteristics

One of the variables of a hollow-fiber device is the membrane surface area which can be changed by changing the total number of fibers, the length of fibers, or the fiber diameter. The influence of membrane surface area upon the performance data of a device is studied in several publications and is described in more detail below.

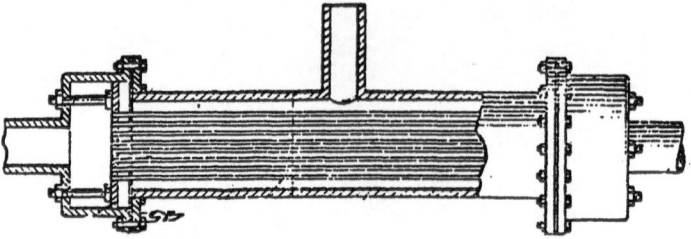

Fig. 13. Housing of the first hollow-fiber artificial kidney [70]

At constant membrane area and fiber diameter but reduced number of fibers and increased length, the shear rate gets higher. Simultaneously, the pressure drop over a device increases with the length (Eq. 3); therefore, the length of standard hemofilters is kept between 210 mm and 280 mm. Two publications [47, 88] describe in more detail the influence of length of a device at a constant membrane area.

A substantial pressure drop occurs when the fiber diameter is decreased (Eq. 3). This, and the ability to rinse the fiber free of residual blood after clinical use, limits the minimum fiber diameter to 180 μm.

For AV hemofilters different geometric dimensions are required. Since these filters are used without blood pumps, blood flow is maintained by using the arterial blood pressure only. Therefore, it is necessary for AV filters to possess a low pressure resistance. This is realized by either reduced filter length or by increased fiber diameters. Studies on optimization of dimensions are published [68].

Housing and Blood Distribution

In all available hollow-fiber hemofilters, the fibers are potted in tubular housings. One of the reasons, which also applies to hemodialyzers, is that in a round tube, it is easier to obtain a tight seal between header and housing. The first patent [70] for such an artificial kidney design was applied for in 1960 (Fig. 13). The development of injection molding and the use of newly developed plastics allowed design of smaller parts which were optimized for better blood flow distribution.

For even blood flow distribution, the blood inlet and outlet have to be designed in such a way that the same blood flow velocity and the same pressure are obtained in all fibers. Two examples for flow distributors where blood enters from the center are shown in Fig. 14. Another design is the "tangential flow distribution" where the blood enters tangentially (Fig. 15).

A design for a square hollow-fiber or flat-sheet device is described in a US patent [25]; but it is not currently used commercially. Having calculated the flow volume over the header's length (Fig. 16), the header gap is declined exponentially with the distance to the inlet in order to effect the same flow rate in each fiber.

As mentioned before, an increase in wall shear rate decreases the concentration polarization and thereby increases the filtration rate. One patent [20] suggests increasing the shear rate by dividing the blood compartment into two chambers connected in series (Fig. 17). This increases the shear rate; however, the pressure drop between inlet and outlet becomes very high.

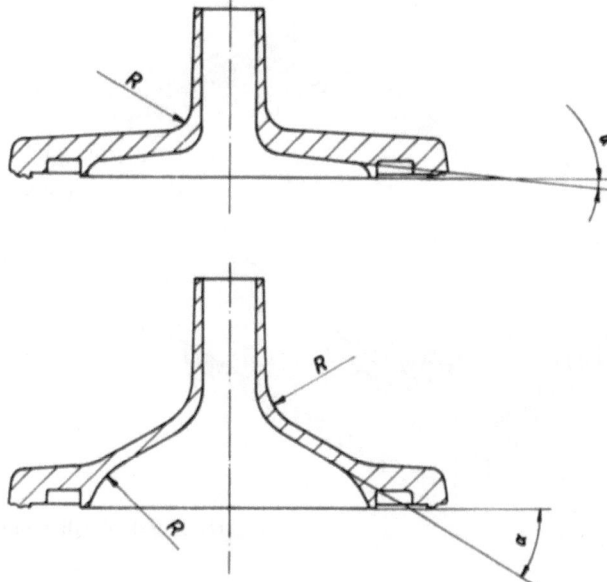

Fig. 14. Examples of blood
flow distributors with central flow

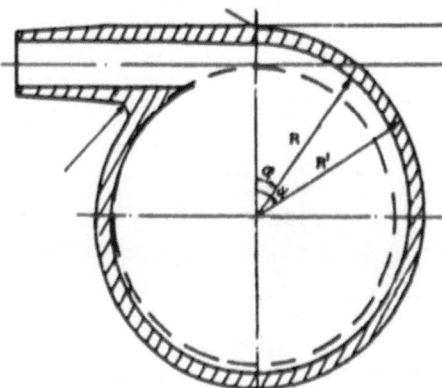

Fig. 15. Tangential blood flow distribution

Filter Manufacturing and Assembly

Several steps are involved in the assembly of hollow-fiber hemofilters. The last step
of hollow-fiber manufacturing, (Fig. 1) the winding of the membrane onto a reel, also represents the first step of hollow-fiber device assembly. After cutting the fiber to
length, bundles of several thousand fibers are obtained. These bundles are put into
the housing, then at both ends the potting material (polyurethane, epoxy) is inject-
ed. While the resin hardens, which normally takes a couple of minutes, centrifuga-
tion is used to equally distribute resin between the fibers at each end of the housing
and to prevent the flow of resin into the bore of the fiber. After the material has
hardened completely, both ends are cut to the length of the housing. In the last step,

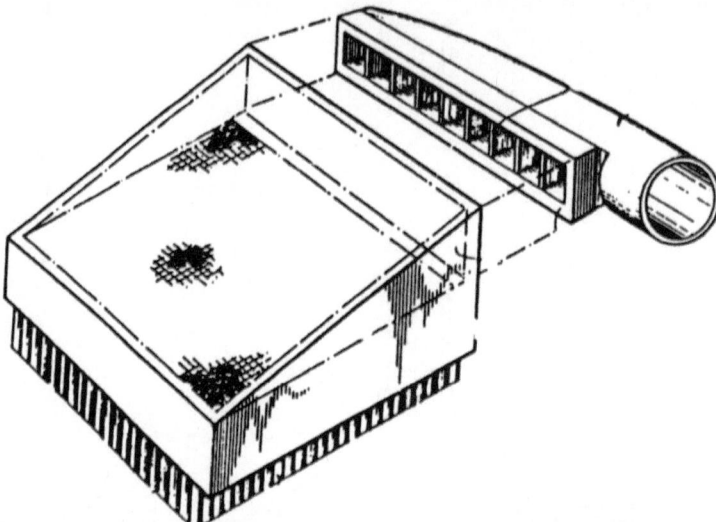

Fig. 16. Blood flow distribution with convergent profile [25]

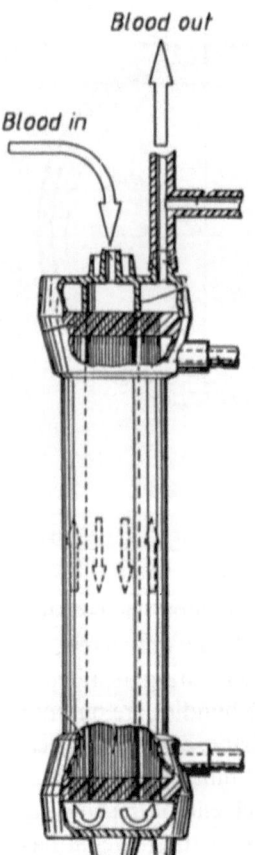

Fig. 17. Diagram showing a method of increasing the shear rate in a hollow-fiber hemofilter. The device is divided at the blood side into two chambers in series [20]

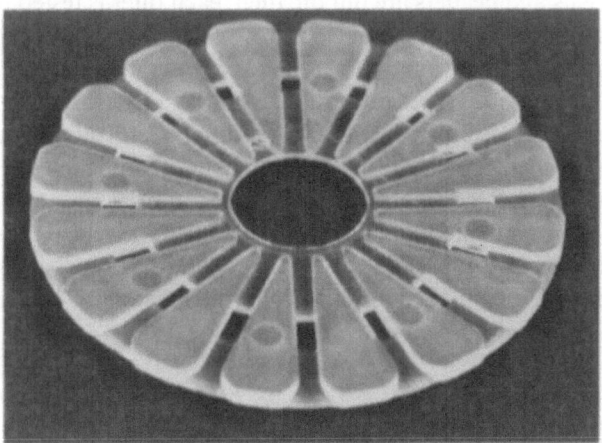

Fig. 18. Blood distribution ring for flat-sheet hemofilters

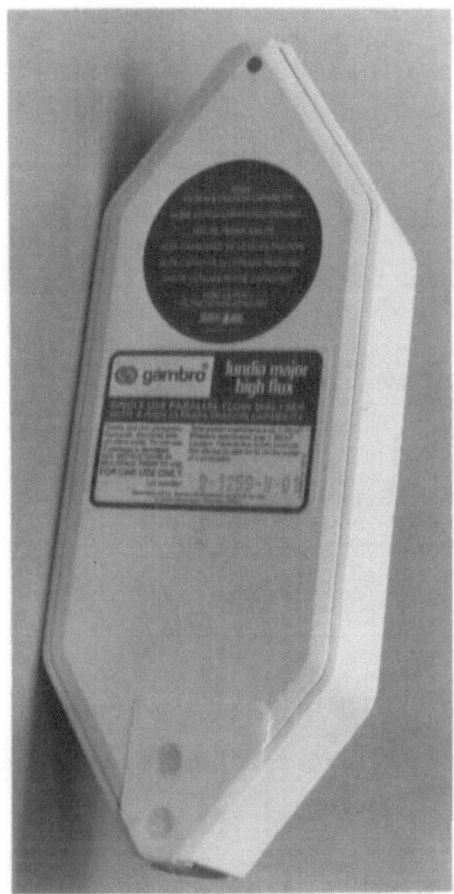

Fig. 19. Parallel flow, flat-sheet, high flux dialyser

seals and headers are put on, then, each filter is tested by a special leak test to guarantee integrity of the device.

The different, mainly synthetic polymer materials used for hemofilter membranes allow various types of sterilization methods. Most of the available devices are ethylene-oxide sterilized. But also radiation sterilization is used (PMMA) and some of the others are heat resistant enough to theoretically allow the use of steam sterilization (PS, PA, PC, glass).

All single steps of assembly are done under clean room conditions. Prior to distribution of a finished device, quality controls according to good manufacturing practices are employed – statistically taking samples and testing each lot for sterility, apyrogenicity, and performance.

Flat-Sheet Membrane Hemofilters

Commercially available hemofilters with flat-sheet membrane are listed in Table 6. Some of them are also used for high flux dialysis or for HDF (see Figs. 18–22).

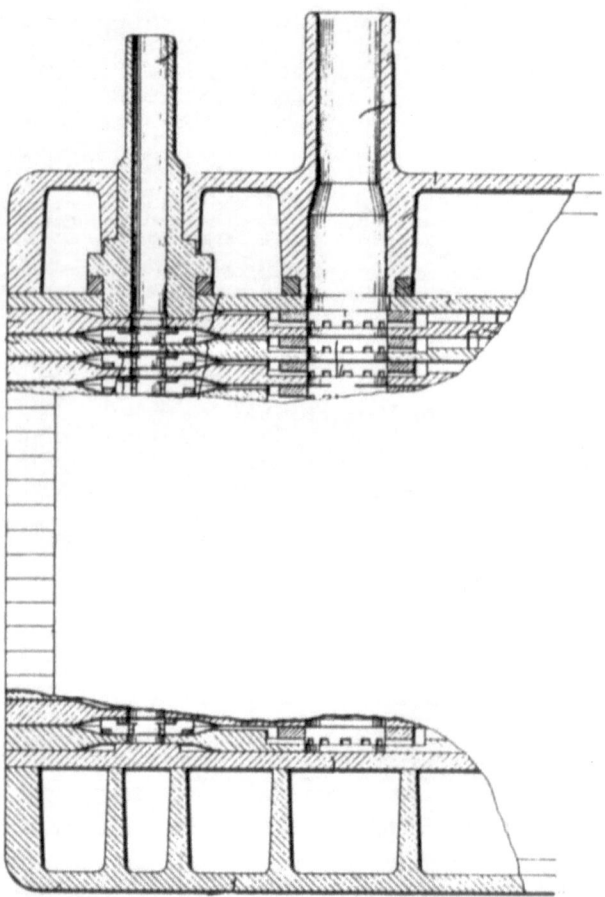

Fig. 20. Cross-section through a flat plate HDF dialyser with the blood distribution and the filtrate outlet [83]

Blood Flow Distribution

Whereas all hollow-fiber filters are made in very similar configurations, flat-sheet devices allow more variations in the design of blood flow distributors and in the design of membrane supports. An example of a device where the blood is distributed through rings is shown in Fig. 21 top. Figures 18 and 19 show the design of such a ring-type distributor and the corresponding device. Inside the device, the blood flows through a blood channel and from there, via a number of these rings (dependent on the number of layers), the blood enters the single layers radially (Fig. 20).

Another device, shown in the middle of Fig. 21, and schematically in Fig. 22, distributes the blood with a header similar to those in hollow-fiber devices. The blood enters each membrane layer which is kept open by a corrugated film [54].

Membrane Support

The first flat-sheet hemofilters used the techniques of flat-sheet hemodialyzers [34]. Examples for these are Rhone Poulenc's RP6 containing AN 69 membrane and Gambro's GLM containing Cuprophan HDF. The membrane layers, between two endplates are stacked in a sandwich-like manner and held together by special side plates or screws. This type of design allows adjusting the blood film thickness and by using, for instance, multipoint or sine-wave shaped support plates it is possible to influence the blood flow [83]. The so-called vortex system is such a design which has been investigated extensively. The membrane support is designed in a way to

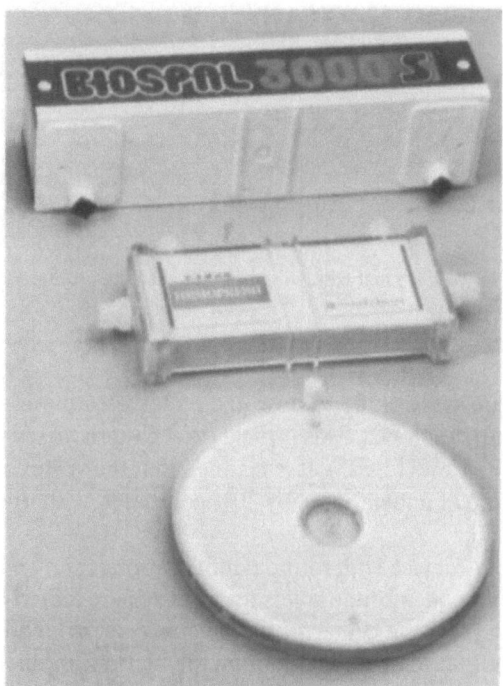

Fig. 21. Flat-sheet hemofilters

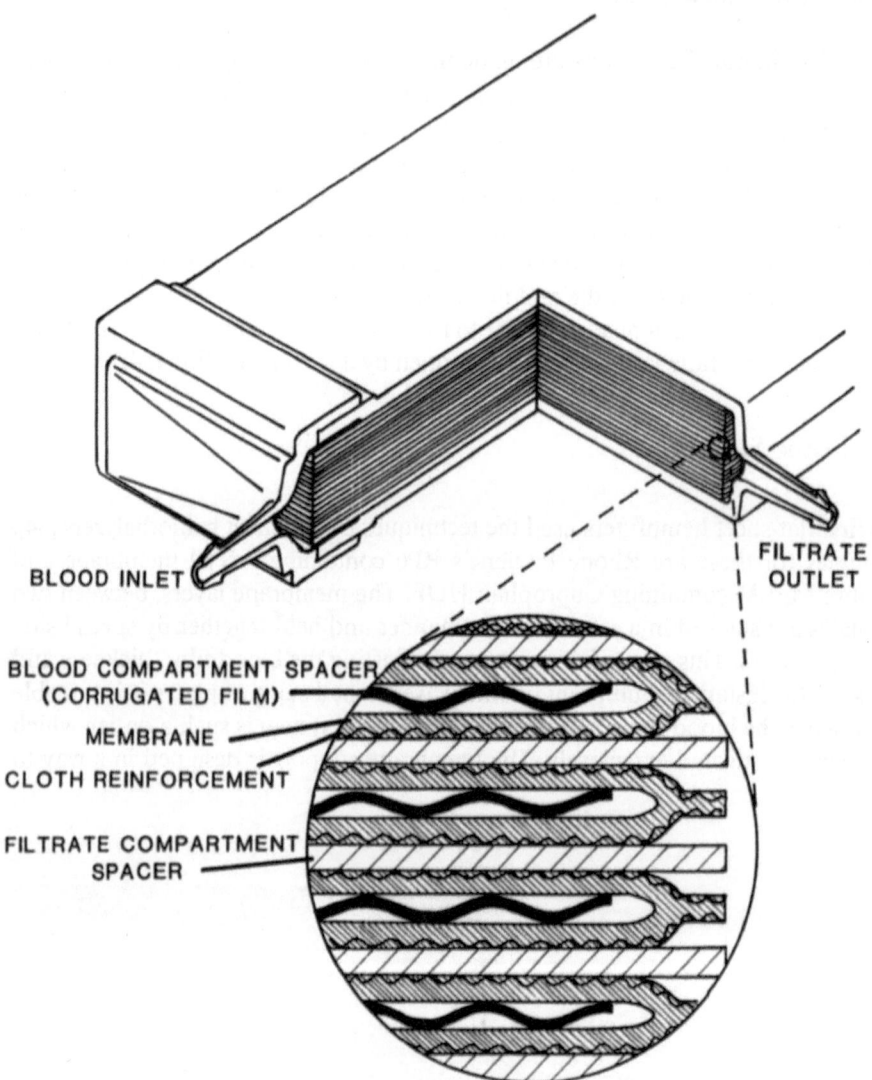

BLOOD INLET

FILTRATE
OUTLET

BLOOD COMPARTMENT SPACER
(CORRUGATED FILM)

MEMBRANE

CLOTH REINFORCEMENT

FILTRATE COMPARTMENT
SPACER

Fig. 22. Schematic drawing of a flat-sheet hemofilter with folded membrame

cause the blood to flow in circular streamlines which reduces the concentration polarization [52]. This typical flow pattern arises when blood is pumped with a pulsatile flow (Fig. 23). It is claimed that the vortex mixing system increases the filtration rate of a membrane by 30% compared with the same membrane in a normal device [57].

A device with round configuration is shown in Fig. 21, bottom. In this disk hemofilter, membrane layers and spacers are sealed outside. The blood is directed radially from the center to the outside (Fig. 24). During use, the disc has to be kept in a holder in order to maintain the blood film thickness.

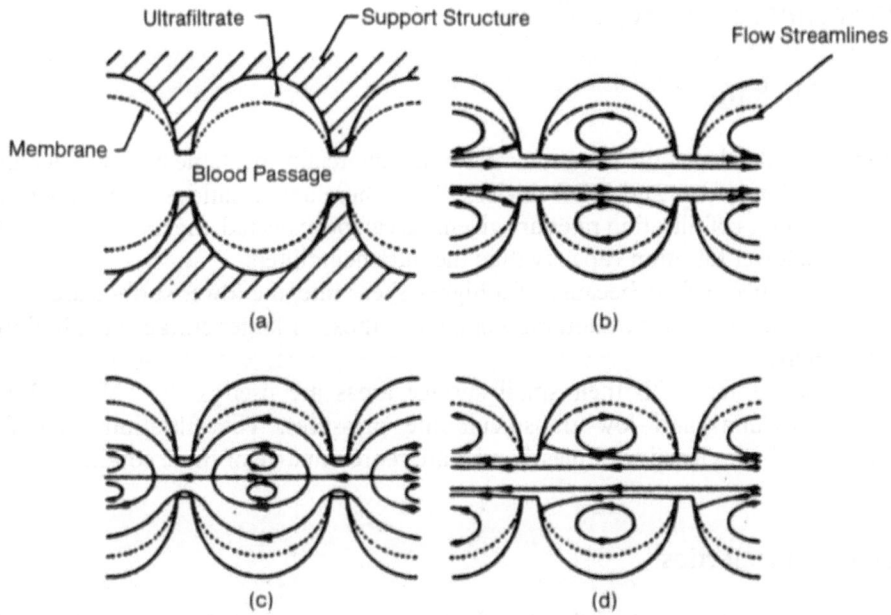

Fig. 23 a–d. Principle of the vortex mixing flat-sheet hemofilter

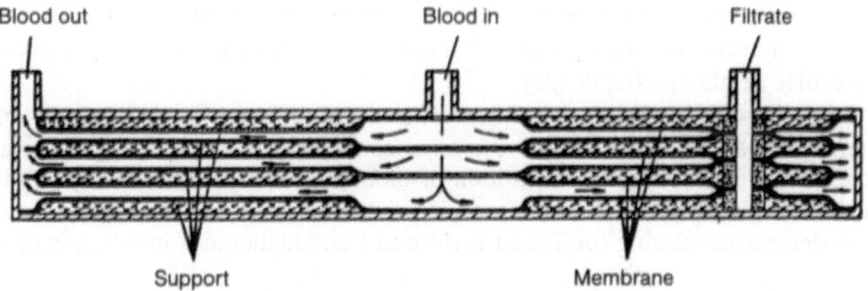

Fig. 24. Schematic drawing of a thin blood flow disc hemofilter [74]

Most of the flat-sheet devices have lower surface areas than the hollow-fiber de-vices. This is because the membrane layer design allows a smaller blood film thick-ness which leads to higher shear rates. However, as a consequence, the higher shear rate results in a higher pressure drop. Since in practical application, parameters, such as blood flow, hematocrit, and protein concentration, which also influence the pressure drop, vary considerably, a compromise between shear rate and pressure drop on the optimum design has to be made in all filters [51].

Looking into the future, a hemofilter could be imagined in which the optimum shear rate is automatically obtained by constantly checking clinical parameters such as blood flow, pressure, and even blood composition. For example, at a low blood flow, the blood film thickness is automatically reduced, thereby increasing the shear rate. At a high blood flow, the reverse takes place. A similarly operating device is al-ready available as a filter in plasma separation.

Performance of Hemofilters

Filtration Rate

Tables 5 and 6 depict the filtration rates of commercially available hollow-fiber and flat-sheet hemofilter and HDF devices. Since there are variations from patient to patient, ranges of filtration rates are given. As can be expected, the high flux devices exhibit a lower filtration capacity than the pure hemofilters.

As described before, because of a higher shear rate, the lower surface area flat-sheet devices possess filtration rates similar to those of larger surface area hollow-fiber filters.

AV hemofilters with their small surface areas are used at low blood flows (30–100 ml/min) and low transmembrane pressures. The filtration rates for $Q_B = 100$ ml/min listed in Tables 5 and 6 are representative of these conditions.

Sieving Properties

The sieving coefficient S, defined as the concentration of a solute in the filtrate divided by the concentration in blood, is used to evaluate the performance of a hemofilter. In addition to membrane properties, sieving coefficients depend very much on the test solution. Sieving coefficients measured in water are about 1.0 for solutes up to a molecular weight range of 10000 to 15000. Figure 11 shows typical sieving coefficient curves for substances with molecular weights from 1300 to 66000, the molecular weight of albumin [32].

It is important to note that sieving coefficients of different filters should be only compared when measured under the same conditions (filtration flux per surface area, shear rate, type and composition of blood, pressure). Table 7 compares the sieving coefficient of insulin measured in saline and in blood. As can be seen for most devices, the sieving coefficient is close to 1 and higher in water than in blood

Table 7. Typical sieving properties, measured in saline and in whole blood or plasma

Type of filter	Manufacturer	Sieving coefficient measured in saline Inulin (MW 5200)	Sieving coefficient[a] measured in whole blood Inulin (MW 5200)	Sieving coefficient in vivo β_2-microglobulin (MW 11800)	Reference
D 30	Amicon	0.99	0.52		84
PAN-15	Asahi	0.87	0.33	<0.1	82, 84
Hemofresh	Daicel	0.99	0.78	0.35	54
FH 202	Gambro	0.99	0.18–0.60	0.41	82, 84
40042	Sartorius		0.60	–	85
GLM highflux	Gambro	0.8	0.75	0.60	84
F 60	Fresenius	1.0	0.99	0.53	28
610/AN 69	Hospal	0.77–0.80	0.79	0.47	82

[a] Sieving coefficient in blood depends also on filtration rate; corresponding filtration rate could not be taken from the reference

[82, 84, 92]. One of the factors causing different values between saline and blood is the adsorption of proteins onto the surface of the membrane.

There are presently no data available on how filtration flux through the membrane or blood flow influences sieving coefficients of proteins under clinical conditions. However, it can be concluded from in vitro experiments [41, 61] that as the filtration rate increases the sieving coefficient decreases.

When sieving coefficients are known, it is possible to predict solute clearances. The plasma clearance K_P can be calculated using the following equation:

$$K_P = \frac{Q_F \cdot C_F}{C_{Pi}} \tag{11}$$

For urea, where the sieving coefficient is 1, the clearance is equal to the filtration rate of the device and with high filtration rate hemofilters it is, therefore, possible to achieve clearances almost as high as with conventional dialyzers [13, 90].

The whole blood clearance of a solute is defined as:

$$K_B = \frac{C_{Bi} - C_{Bo}}{C_{Bi}} \times \left(Q_B + \frac{Q_F \cdot C_{Bo}}{C_{Bi}} \right) \tag{12}$$

In those cases where solute concentrations in plasma and whole blood are equivalent, the equations for K_P and K_B become identical. For solutes, which have a lower concentration in erythrocytes than in plasma (C_{Pi} exceeding C_{Bi}), whole blood clearances will be numerically greater (10%–40%) than plasma clearances.

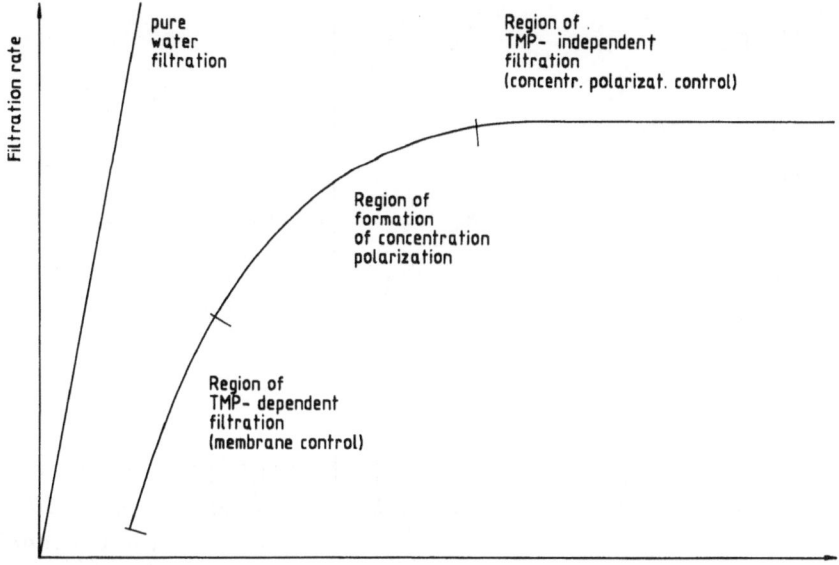

Fig. 25. Filtration rate vs transmembrane pressure (TMP) for blood is influenced by concentration polarization (pure water filtration shown for reference)

Parameters Influencing Hemofilter Performance

Transmembrane Pressure (TMP). Adjustment of the TMP controls the filtration rate. Figure 25 depicts a typical curve of filtration rate vs TMP. At a low TMP, the filtration rate increases almost linearly with TMP. Then the slope decreases and finally a plateau is reached where an increase in TMP does not result in a higher filtration rate. At what TMP this plateau is reached depends on various factors, such as membrane characteristics, composition of blood (hematocrit, protein concentration), and on flow conditions (blood flow, shear rate, membrane area) [26, 40, 66, 78].

Influence of Composition of Blood. Several publications [21, 27, 31, 75] demonstrate the correlation of the specific filtration rate of blood (UF/cm^2) and total protein concentration (Fig. 26). These findings are in agreement with the previously described concentration polarization model which describes a correlation between

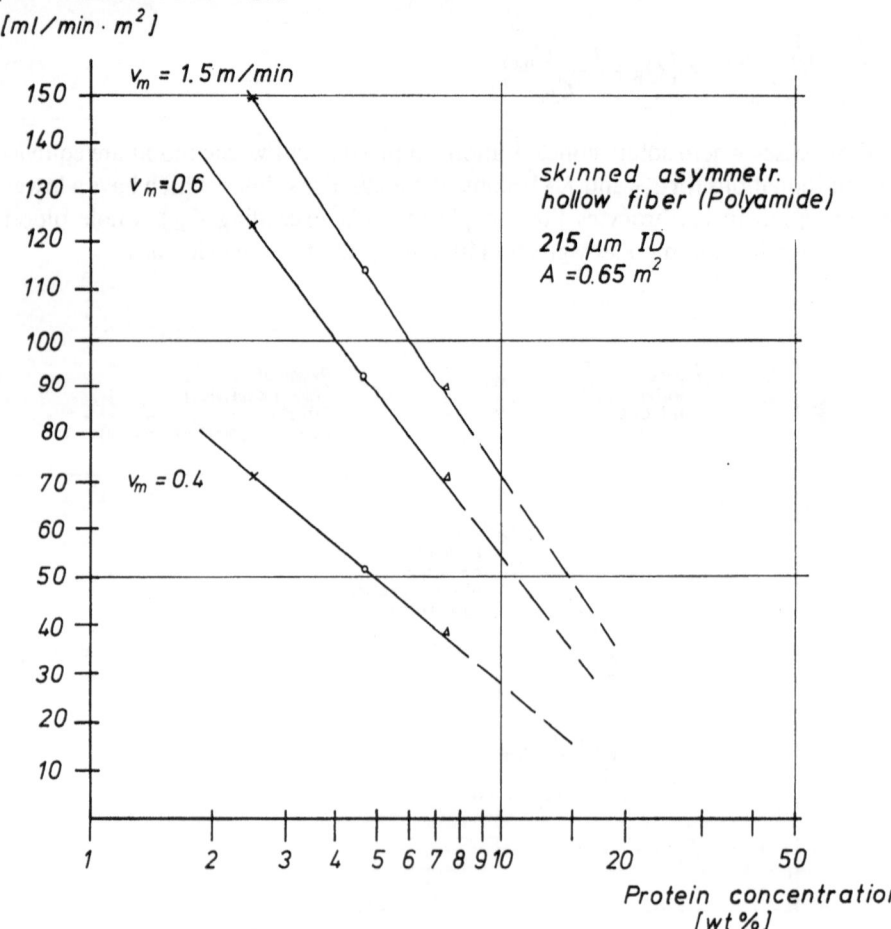

Fig. 26. Specific ultrafiltration rate vs protein concentration at different blood flow velocities v_m. Bovine blood, 25% Hct, 2.5–7.0 wt% protein, temp. 37 °C, TMP 500 mmHg

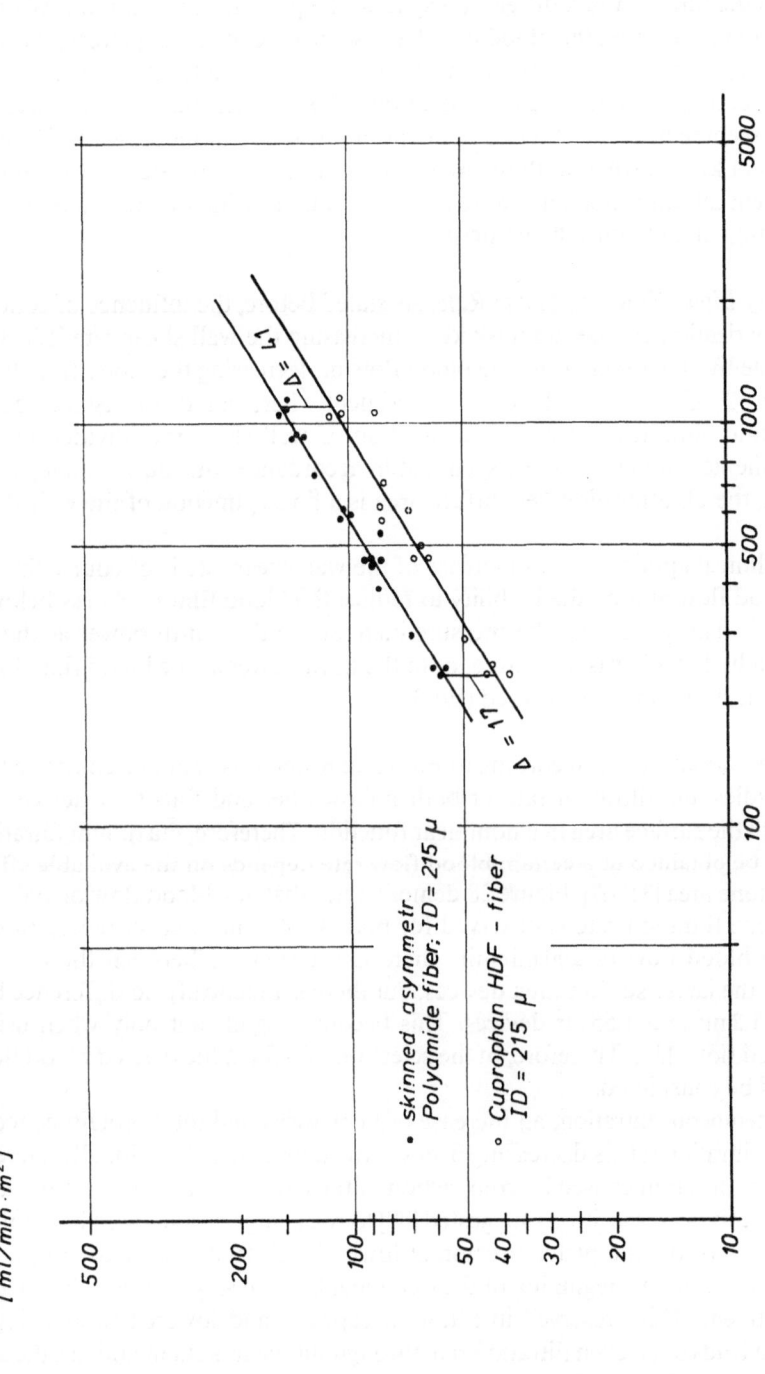

Fig. 27. Specific ultrafiltration rate vs $\dfrac{\text{wall shear rate}}{\text{effective fiber length}}$

Bovine blood, 25% Hct, 70 g/l protein, TMP 600 mmHg

UF and natural logarithm of protein concentration (Eq. 1). The hematocrit of blood influences the filtration in a different way than the protein concentration. With increasing blood flow rate, the blood cells have some type of stirring effect [75]. That means the higher the hematocrit, the greater the increase in ultrafiltration as a function of increasing blood flow rate. In addition to hematocrit and protein concentration there seem to be some other components in the blood influencing the filtration rate. It is not known whether these are proteins or microaggregates, but in clinical use, different ultrafiltration rates were found on patients with identical total protein concentration and identical hematocrit.

Influence of Blood Flow and Shear Rate. As stated before, the influence of concentration polarization can be diminished by increasing the wall shear rate [12]. This can be done by either increasing the blood flow or decreasing the blood film thickness. Figure 27 gives the results of an experiment where blood was used to determine specific ultrafiltration rate as a function of wall shear rate divided by the length of the hemofilter. It can be seen that in accordance with Eq. 2, in a logarithmic graph, the ultrafiltration per surface area is a linear function of the wall shear rate.

In the clinical application, an increase of the wall shear rate is of course limited by the blood flow and by the inability to reduce the blood film thickness below a certain limit. This is because the pressure increases to the fourth power as the diameter of a hollow fiber is decreased, or to the third power as the blood film thickness in a flat sheet device is lowered (Eq. 3, 6).

Influence of Surface Area. According to Eq. 5 and 8, and this could be confirmed by clinical studies, the filtration rate of both hollow-fiber and flat-sheet devices increases with the surface area in a nonlinear function. Therefore, maximum filtration which can be obtained at a certain blood flow rate depends on the available effective membrane area [31, 67]. Figure 28 demonstrates that at a blood flow of 100 ml/min the same filtration rate is observed for both small and large surface area devices. At a blood flow of 200 ml/min, there is a difference between the 0.65 m² device and the larger surface area devices, but there is practically no difference between the 1.2 m² and 1.55 m² devices. This becomes significant only when using higher blood flows [32]. Therefore, in the selection of a filter, the desired blood flow rate should be considered.

Due to hemoconcentration, an increase of hematocrit and total protein concentration, the filtration rate is decreasing over the treatment time. Additionally, there is a decrease of filtration caused by compaction of the concentration polarization layer. To avoid this decrease, it was suggested [89] to use a large surface area hemofilter and operate is below the plateau region at lower TMP. That means, the filtration rate will be lower in the beginning of the treatment but will stay constant during the whole treatment. This "reserve" in filtration capacity and lowered protein layer compaction leads to an even filtration rate throughout the treatment and has the advantage that a good estimation of how much plasma water will be removed during the treatment time can be made in advance.

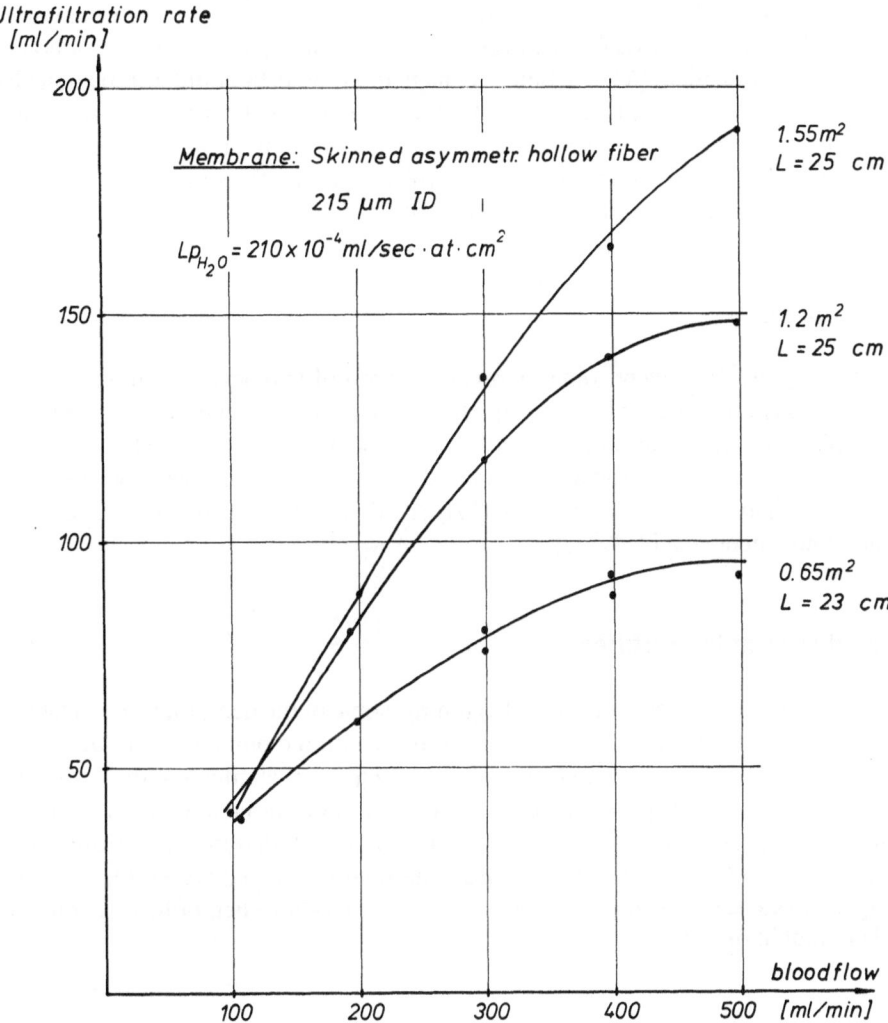

Ultrafiltration rate
[ml/min]

Fig. 28. Ultrafiltration rate vs blood flow for different surface areas. Bovine blood, 25% Hct, 70 g/l protein, 37 °C, TMP 600 mmHg

Blood/Device Interactions

Thrombogenicity

There are no reports of clotting occurring in the devices but thrombus formation can occur in spite of adequate heparinization. The mechanism of thrombus formation in extracorporeal circulation is complex and has been poorly investigated. From investigations done in hemodialyzers it was found that two factors play important roles, the flow in a device [10, 11] and the membrane [65, 96]. The individual patient's blood as well as the administered dose of heparin and its half-life in that patient influences these two factors. In general, hemofilters need the same amounts of heparin as hemodialyzers; however, the demand of heparin varies considerably from patient to patient [62, 64]. Some damage to blood cells could also be done by blood pumps. One study [10] investigates the influence of shear rates on red blood cells and concludes that under laminar flow the damage to erythrocytes is not significant. Also, the higher pressure of 300–700 mmHg in HF compared with HD is not reported to have an influence on red blood cell damage [102].

Leucopenia

In recent years there were some reports on a drop of leukocytes during the initial phase (0–30 min) of hemodialysis [23]. The authors agree that the type of membrane used plays a major role on the extent of leucopenia in dialysis. Cellulosic membranes, which are the ones mainly used in dialysis, induce leucopenia, whereas the mostly synthetic materials used in HF (PA, PMMA, PAN, PS) are reported to cause little or no leucopenia [2, 49, 87].

Blood Loss in Hemofilters

As in dialyzer manufacturing, in the beginning, some of the hemofilters had leakage problems. These problems could be traced to membrane pinholes and potting defects. Nowadays, these problems are almost completely eliminated, thus, the leak rate of hemofilters is approximately the same as found in hemodialyzers. Since a higher TMP is used and since no dilution of filtrate with dialysis fluid is done, it is generally easier to detect a microleak in a hemofilter than in a dialyzer. Also, when a proper rinse-back procedure is used, the residual blood in hemofilters is comparable to that in dialyzers.

Acknowledgment

The authors are grateful to Roswitha Kunas and Janice Elkin for assistance in the preparation of this manuscript.

References

1. Abel JJ, Rountree LG, Turner BB (1913) On the removal of diffusive substances from the circulating blood of living animals by means of dialysis. Trans Am Physicians 28: 51
2. Aljama P, Bird PAE, Ward MK, Feest TG, Walker W, Tanboga H, Sussman M, Kerr DNS (1978) Haemodialysis-induced leucopenia and activation of complement: Effects of different membranes; Proc Eur Dial Transplant Assoc 15: 144
3. Alwall N, Herner B (1948) On the artificial kidney, VI. Acta Med Scand 132: 572

4. Amicon Corporation Innovative kidney replacement therapy, continuous arteriovenous hemofiltration and other effective ultrafiltration techniques, manufacturer's technical information, Amicon Corp, Scientific Systems Division, Danvers, MA 01923/USA
5. Amicon Corporation (1979) Diafilter for hemofiltration. Technical information, April 1979. Amicon Corporation, Lexington, Massachusetts/USA
6. Asahi Medical Hemofilter PAN 150, PAN 200, Manufacturer's technical information. Asahi Medical Co. Ltd., Hibiya-Mitsui-Building 1-2, Yurakucho 1-Chome, Chiyda-ku, Tokyo, Japan
7. v. Baeyer H, Schnabel R, Vaulont W, Kaczmarczyk G (1980) Properties of porous glass membranes with respect to application in blood purification. Trans Am Soc Artif Intern Organs XXVI: 309
8. Bianchi R, Bionda A, Carmassi F, Palla R, Donadio C, Galli M, Chiellini E, Molea N, Mariani G (1979) Evaluation of new membranes for hemodialysis: preliminary studies with a polycarbonate membrane. J Dial 3: 383
9. Bixler HJ, Nelsen LM, Bluemle LW jr (1968) The development of a diafiltration system for blood purification. Trans Am Soc Artif Intern Organs 14: 99
10. Blackshear PL jr, Forstrom RJ (1975) Fluid dynamics of blood cells and applications to hemodialysis. In: Mackey BB (ed) Proceedings 8th annual contractor's conference, Artificial kidney program of NIAMDD. DHEW Publication No. (NIH) 75-248: 59. DHEW, Washington
11. Blackshear PL jr, Patankar SV (1978) Fluid dynamics of blood cells and applications to hemodialysis. In: Mackey BB (ed) Proceedings 11th annual contractor's conference, Artificial kidney program of NIAMDD. DHEW Publication No. (NIH) 79-1442: 97
12. Blatt WF, Dravid A, Michaels AS, Nelsen L (1970) Solute polarization and cake formation in membrane ultrafiltration: causes, consequences and control techniques. Flinn JE (ed) Membrane science and technology. Plenum, New York
13. Bosch JP, Geronemus R, Glabman S, Lysaght M, Kalm T, v Albertini B (1978) High flux hemofiltration. Artif Organs 2: 339
14. Brull L (1928) L'ultrafiltration in vivo. CR Séance Soc Biol 99: 1607
15. Cabasso I, Tamvakis AP (1979) Composite hollow fiber membranes J Appl Polym Sci 23: 1509
16. Cabasso I, Klein E, Smith JK (1976) Polysulfone hollow fibers. J Appl Polym Sci 20: 2377
17. Chang R, Liu C, Daly W (1979) Anionic hemofiltration membranes. Artif Organs 3 [Suppl]: 463
18. Christen G et al. (Rhone Poulenc) (1975) Membrane of copolymer acrylonitrile/olefinically unsaturated comonomer. US patent 3,930,105, Dec 30, 1975
19. Christen G, et al. (Rhone Poulenc) (1977) Membrane of copolymer acrylonitrile/olefinically unsaturated comonomer. US patent 4,056,467, Nov 1, 1977
20. Christopherson K, Falkvall T, Mattison U, Shaldon S (1982) Filtering device. Eur Patent 0076422, Sept 24, 1982
21. Colton CK, Henderson LW, Ford CA, Lysaght MJ (1975) Kinetics of hemodiafiltration. I. In vitro transport characteristics of a hollow fiber blood ultrafilter. J Lab Clin Med 8: 353-371
22. Cordis Dow GmbH: Duo-flux künstliche Niere. Manufacturer's technical information. Fürstenriedstraße 69, D-8000 München 21
23. Craddock PR, Fehr J, Dalmasso AP, Birgham KL, Jacob HS (1977) Hemodialysis leukopenia. Pulmonary vascular leucostasis resulting from complement activation by dialyzer cellophane membranes. J Clin Invest 59: 879
24. Darup J, Bleese N, Kalmar P, Lutz G, Pokar H, Polonius MJ (1979) Hemofiltration during extracorporeal circulation (ECC). Thorac Cardiovasc Surg 27/4: 227-230
25. Davis HR, Brockely CHA, Parkinson GV, Price JDE (1977) Manifold for ultrafiltration machine. US patent 4038191
26. Dorson WJ jr et al (1978) Quantitation of membrane-protein-solute interactions during ultrafiltration. Trans Am Soc Artif Intern Organs XXIV: 155
27. Fernando T (1981) Concentration of animal blood by ultrafiltration. Biotechnol Bioeng 23/1: 19
28. Fresenius AG Hemflow F. Manufacturer's technical information. Fresenius AG, D-6370 Oberursel
29. Funck-Brentano JL (1972) Experience with a new 'open membrane'. Proceedings workshop on dialysis and transplantation. Am Soc Artif Intern Organs 18: 80

30. Gambro Lundia AB Fiber Hemofilter FH77. Manufacturer's technical information. Gambro Lundia AB, S-22010 Lund/Sweden
31. Goehl H, Schaefer K, Gullberg CA (1979) Hemofiltration with different types of membranes. Proc Eur Soc Artif Organs 6: 180
32. Goehl H, Konstantin P, Gullberg CA (1982) Hemofiltration membranes. Contrib Nephrol 32:20
33. Göhl H, Mayer G, Geiling G, Gullberg CA (1982) Filtration membrane and process of producing the membrane Europ Pat Appl 0098392, 1982
34. Gullberg CA, et al (1979) A new hemofiltration system. Proc Eur Soc Artif Organs 4: 56
35. Haas G (1928) Über Blutwaschung. Klin Wochenschr 7: 1356
36. Hashino Y et al (1975) Acrylonitrile-polymer Hollow Fibers. US patent 3,871,950, March 18, 1975
37. Hashino Y, Yoshino M, Sawabu H, Konno T (1980) Method for producing hollow fibers of acrylonitrile polymers for ultrafilter. US patent 4,181,694, 1980
38. Hashino Y et al (1980) Polyacryl-ether-sulfones. US patent 4,208,508, June 17, 1980
39. Hamilton R, Ford C, Colton C, Cross R, Steinmuller S, Henderson L (1971) Blood cleaning by diafiltration in uremic dog and man. Trans Am Soc Artif Intern Organs 17: 259
40. Henderson LW, Colton CK, Ford CA (1975) Kinetics of hemodiafiltration, II. Clinical characterization of a new blood cleansing modality. J Lab Clin Med 85 (3): 372
41. Henderson LW, Leypoldt JK, Frigon RP, Uyeji SN, Alford M (1984) Slow flow hemofiltration improves solute transport. 2nd Annual Workshop on ISH, Milano, July 1984
42. Henne W, Duenweg G, Bandel W (1979) A new cellulose membrane generation for hemodialysis and hemofiltration. Artif Organs [Suppl] 3: 466
43. Higley WS, Cantor PA, Fisher BS (1976) Thin polycarbonate membrane for use in hemodialysis. US patent 4,069,151, 1976
44. Hoechst AG Manufacturer's technical information. Toray Industries Inc, Verkauf Pharma, D-6230 Frankfurt 80
45. Holland FF jr, Klein E, Wendt RP, Eberle K (1978) Rejection of solutes by hemodialysis/hemofiltration membranes. Trans Am Soc Artif Intern Organs 24: 662
46. Hospal Medical Corporation. H12-10 Plate hemodialyzer-AN69. Manufacturer's technical information. Hospal Medical Corporation, East Brunswick, NJ 08816/USA
47. Hüfler M, Schaefer K, v Herrath D (1982) Modifications of hemofiltration. Contrib Nephrol 32: 154
48. Ishii K, Honda Z, Tsugaya H (1981) Process of preparing semipermeable membrane having selective permeability. US patent 4,279,846, 1981
49. Jacob AI, Gavellas G, Zarco R, Perez G, Bourgoignie JJ (1980) Leukopenia, hypoxia, and complement function with different hemodialysis membranes. Kidney Intern 18: 505
50. Jaffrin MY et al (1978) Factors governing hemofiltration in a parallel-plate exchanger with highly permeable membranes. Trans Am Soc Artif Intern Organs 24: 448
51. Jaffrin MY (1981) Design analysis of parallel plate and hollow fibers haemofilters. Med Biol Eng Comp 19: 321
52. Jefree MA et al (1981) Increased maximum haemofiltration rates in a vortex mixing hemofilter; Proceedings ESAO VIII: 150
53. Jitsuhara J, Kumura S (1983) Structure and properties of charged ultrafiltration membranes made of sulfonated polysulfone; J Chem Eng Jpn 16/5: 389
54. Kai M, et al, Maekawa M, et al (1981) Development of a cellulose acetate membrane and a module for hemofiltration. In: Turbak AF (ed) Synthetic membranes, vol II. ACS Symposium Series No 154
55. Kesting RE (1977) Dry spun asymmetric hollow fiber. US patent 4,035,459, July 12, 1977
56. Klein E, Holland FF, Eberle K (1978) Rejection of solutes by hemofiltration membranes. ASAIO-J 1/1: 15–23
57. Klein E, Holland FF (1978) Evaluation of membranes for use in hemofiltration. Gulf South Research Institute, New Orleans, XI. Ann Contractors Conference, Contract No NO1-AM-7-2209, Proceedings 1978, p 175
58. Konstantin P, Goehl H, Gullberg CA (1981) A new copolymer material for diffusion and filtration. Proc ISAO Artif Organs [Suppl] 5: 691
59. Konstantin P, Goehl H, Ohmayer MT, Buck RJ, Gullberg CA (1982) Membrane and process for producing the membrane. Eur Pat Appl 0111663, 1982

60. Kramer P, Wigger W, Rieger J, Matthaei D, Schelo F (1977) A new and simple method for treatment of overhydrated patients resistant to diuretics. Klin Wochenschr 55: 1121
61. Leypoldt JK, Frigon RP, Henderson LW (1983) Dextran sieving coefficients of hemofiltration membranes. Trans Am Soc Artif Intern Organs 29: 678
62. Lindsay RM (1980) Variable heparin requirements during hemodialysis. Why? ASAIO J 3: 81
63. Loeb S, Sourirajan S (1962) Adv Chem Ser 38: 117
64. Luttinger M, Cooper CW, Leininger RI (1968) Preparation of novel hemodialysis membranes. Trans Am Soc Artif Intern Organs 14: 5
65. Lyman DJ, Knutson K, McNeill B, Shibatani K (1975) The effects of chemical structure and surface properties of synthetic polymers on the coagulation of blood. IV. The relation between polymer morphology and protein adsorption. Trans Am Soc Artif Intern Organs 21: 49
66. Lysaght MJ, Colton CK, Ford CA, Stone RA, Henderson LW (1977) Mass transfer in clinical blood ultrafiltration devices in technical aspects of renal dialysis. Pittman Medical, London
67. Lysaght MJ, Albertini BV, Bosch JP, Ford CA, Geronemus R (1978) Relationship between surface area and ultrafiltration rate in capillary hemofilters. Proceedings ESAO 5: 178
68. Lysaght MJ (1981) Selection of optimal capillary internal diameter in blood ultrafilters. Proc ESAO 8: 130
69. Man NK et al (1975) Die Polyacrylonitril-Membran: Eine neue Hämodialyse-Membran mit hoher Permeabilität. Klin Nephrol 1, 2: 48
70. Mahon HJ (1960) Permeability separatory apparatus, US-Patent 3,228,876, Sept 1960
71. Marze X, Quentin JP (1974) Acrylonitrile copolymers. US-Patent 3,795,635 1974
72. Michaels AS (1971) High flow membrane, US-Patent 3,615,024, Oct 26, 1971
73. v Mylius U, Streicher E, Schneider HW (1976) Kapillarmembranen zur Blutdiafiltration. Biomed Tech 21: 306
74. Nussbaumer DG, Perl H (1978) Einflußgrößen bei der Hemofiltration. Wissenschaftliche Information Fresenius, Nephrologie Heft 2/78 page 145–155
75. Okazaki M, Yoshida F (1976) Ultrafiltration of blood: Effect of hematocrit on ultrafiltration rate. Ann Biomed Eng 4: 138
76. Ota K et al (1975) Polymethylmethacrylate capillary kidney highly permeable to middle molecules. Proc Eur Dial Transplant Assoc 12: 559
77. Ota K et al (1978) Short-time hemodiafiltration using polymethylmethacrylate hemodiafilter. Trans Am Soc Artif Intern Organs 24: 454
78. Pasternack A (1973) Zur Blutdetoxikation nach dem Prinzip der Ultrafiltration. Thesis, Technische Hochschule Aachen
79. Pusch W (1980) Synthetic membranes, state of the art. Desalination 35: 5
80. Pusch W, Walch A (1982) Synthetische Membranen – Herstellung, Struktur und Anwendung. Angew Chem 9: 670
81. Quellhorst E, Fernandez E, Scheler F (1972) Treatment of uremia using an ultrafiltration system. Proc Eur Dial Transplant Assoc 9: 584
82. Ramenofsky J, Lai F, Schroeder P, Hosokawa S, Kato Y, Henderson L (1981) Comparison of hemofiltration membrane performance: Sieving coefficients (Abstr) Am Soc Artif Intern Organs 10: 55
83. Riede G, Hagström O (1973) Dialysevorrichtung. Patent DE 23 19 949
84. Röckel A, Gilge U, Ohl B, Liewald A, Heidland A (1982) Elimination of low molecular weight proteins during hemofiltration. Contrib Nephrol 32: 40
85. Sartorius GmbH Hemofilter. Manufacturer's technical information. Sartorius GmbH, D-3400 Göttingen
86. Secon GmbH. Hämo-Dia-Filter für die Hämofiltration und die Hämodiafiltration. Manufacturer's technical information. Secon GmbH, D-3400 Göttingen
87. Schaefer K, v Herrath D, Hüfler M (1982) Stable PO_2 during hemofiltration in spite of a drop in leucocytes. Nephron 32: 377
88. Schneider H, Streicher E, v Mylius U (1979) A theoretical and experimental approach towards optimal dimensions for capillary hemofilters. J Artif Organs [Suppl] 3: 114
89. Shaldon S, Deschodt G, Granollerus C, Oules R, Gullberg CA, Mayr (to be published) Experience with on-line hemofiltration. Artif Organs
90. Shaldon S, Beau MC, Deschodt G, Mion C (1981) Mixed hemofiltration (MHF): 18 months experience with ultrashort treatment time. Trans Am Soc Artif Intern Organs 27: 610

91. Sonoda T et al (1980) Polymethylmethacrylatmembran, De OS 3125980 A1, July 1980
92. Smeby LC, Jørstad S, Widerøe TE (1980) Design analyses of a new selective filtration system for removal of uremic toxins. Clin Nephrol 13 (3): 125
93. Stone W (1977) Polycarbonate membrane for hemodialysis and hemofiltration. Dial Transplant 6 (4): 10
94. Strathmann H (1975) Struktur und Funktion von Kunststoffmembranen. Mitt Klin Nephrol 4: 14
95. Strathmann H (1980) Development of new membranes. Desalination 35: 39
96. Sreeharan N et al (1982) Membrane effect on platelet function during hemodialysis: A comparison of Cuprophan and polycarbonate. Artif Organs 6/3: 324
97. Streicher E, Schneider H (1977) Asymmetric polyamide hollow fiber filters in the hemofiltration system. J Dial 1 (7): 727
98. Tanzawa H et al (1975) Semi-permeable membranes, their preparation and their use. US patent 3,896,061, July 22, 1975
99. Walch A (1978) Hämofiltrationsmembran auf Basis von Polyamid, Verfahren zu ihrer Herstellung und ihre Verwendung. Eur Pat App 0002053 A3, Nov 1978
100. Walch A (1981) Makroporöse asymmetrische hydrophile Membran aus synthetischem Polymerisat. European Patent 3149976
101. Walch A, Wildhardt J, Beissel D (1982) Membranes in hemodialysis – Development and structure. Annual Sifra Meeting on New Dialysis Trends, Cortina d'Ampezzo, July 1982
102. Walpoth B et al (1980) Surface changes in experimental hemofiltration. Proceedings ESAO 7: 156
103. Yamashita A, Kawai S, Tanii K, Takakura K (1981) Ethylene-vinyl alcohol copolymer membrane and a method for producing the same. US patent 4,269,713, 1981

Equipment for Hemofiltration

B. VON ALBERTINI

Table of Contents

Introduction

For hemofiltration to be a practical alternative to routine hemodialysis, it must be delivered by fail-safe automated equipment, which provides the essential functions of the treatment and, at any time, maintains the patient's safety without the necessity of human intervention. A variety of hemofiltration machines are available which perform this task reliably and accurately.

Hemofiltration lowers the concentration of uremic solutes in the patients with end-stage renal disease by the periodic removal of a large fraction of total body water and its solutes by ultrafiltration and the simultaneous replacement with a physiologic solution. For this purpose, the patient's blood circulates during the treatment through an extracorporeal circuit where an ultrafiltrate of plasma is removed in a hemofilter and the blood volume is simultaneously reconstituted with replacement fluid. The total volume of exchange ranges from 20-40 liters per treatment, which is typically carried out in 4-5 h three times weekly.

Operational Features

The equipment for hemofiltration has to meet three basic operational requirements:

a) it must safely accomodate the extracorporeal blood circuit,
b) it must provide the pressure for ultrafiltration in the hemofilter, and
c) blood volume must be accurately reconstituted by delivering substitution fluid.

While different technical approaches have been made to meet these requirements, all hemofiltration machines in use have these features in common:

Extracorporeal Blood Circuit

Analogous to hemodialysis, blood gained from the patient's vascular access is pumped to the hemofilter and returned to the patient through a disposable plastic tubing set. Ultrafiltration is achieved in the hemofilter by exerting a hydrostatic pressure gradient across the membrane, resulting in the transfer of plasma water and solutes. Substitution fluid is delivered either proximally to the hemofilter (predilution) or into the venous drip chamber (postdilution).

The features of the equipment needed to operate the extracorporeal circuit are essentially identical to those of hemodialysis machines. During the treatment, 50–100 liters of heparinized blood are carried through the circuit by a peristaltic roller pump in the arterial line which, in conjunction with the resistance to flow, provides the driving force for the positive component of the transmembrane pressure gradient in the hemofilter. Safety features in the circuit include pressure monitors in the arterial and venous blood lines and an air detector linked to an automatic clamping device in the venous line. The machines are wired internally to shut off extracorporeal circulation whenever preset pressure values are exceeded or a line disruption occurs.

Hydraulic Circuit

In contrast to the complex hydraulic components of hemodialysis machines necessary for the preparation of dialysate, this aspect of hemofiltration machines consists of two separate, comparatively simple circuits for ultrafiltrate and substitution fluid. A roller pump creates the negative component of the transmembrane pressure and carries the ultrafiltrate through a disposable tubing set from the hemofilter to a collection cannister. A negative pressure monitor in this circuit prevents preset transmembrane pressure limits from being exceeded, and a blood leak detector activates an alarm condition, which shuts off extracorporeal circulation, should a major membrane rupture occur.

In a separate circuit, substitution fluid is delivered from its containers into the blood line by another roller pump, which operates under the control of the balancing system. Other features of the circuit include a flow-through heater with thermostatic control and a thermometer for overheat alarm. The disposable sterile tubing set used in this circuit contains a segment for the heater and usually has multiple attachments for the collapsible plastic bags in which the fluid is purchased, thus permitting a completely sealed sterile circuit and preventing the accidental pumping of air into the blood circulation. Batch-prepared substitution fluid from a single open cannister has also been successfully used in recent years.

Balancing System

The functionally most genuine part of the hemofiltration apparatus is the balance control, providing the matching of the volumes of substitution fluid and ultrafiltrate. Large volumes are exchanged in a short time during the treatment, and accurate control of fluid balance is of critical importance. Imbalance of ultrafiltration and substitution could rapidly lead to life-threatening volume depletion or overhydration of the patient. The pace of exchange is determined by the ultrafiltration rate obtained in the hemofilter. Since ultrafiltration rate changes during the treatment, it must be continuously monitored and the rate of fluid replacement adjusted accordingly. Moreover, the machine has to be programmable to remove the patient's weight gain between treatments by replacing the ultrafiltrate with a proportionally smaller volume of substitution fluid throughout the treatment.

Solutions to Technical Problems

Early clinical investigators of hemofiltration had to rely on manual control of fluid balance while using components of hemodialysis machines for the extracorporeal blood circuit. Fluid balance was achieved with the help of bed scales and manual adjustment of the substitution pump, requiring constant supervision of the treatment. Most of the automated equipment available today originates from early prototypes developed in close association with key investigators. These developments occurred independently, and the various technical approaches in use reflect the different preferences and philosophies of these early investigators. A description of the various conceptual approaches can be found in some of the earliest publications on hemofiltration [1, 2].

Three different conceptual methods to achieve fluid balance in hemofiltration have been explored:

a) by volumetric control,
b) by gravimetric control, and
c) with control of flows.

Volumetric Control

In this approach, fluid balance is achieved by measurement of volumes. Since both ultrafiltrate and substitution fluid are liquids, the displacement by volume of the ultrafiltrate is used to deliver an identical volume of substitution fluid to the patient. This concept is illustrated by the example of a single pump with two identical, separate tubing segments for ultrafiltrate and for substitution fluid, which ideally deliver identical volumes with each stroke. Similarly, volume control can be achieved by the alternate filling of a double cylinder with a single piston or a sealed chamber separated into two compartments by a flexible membrane. Such a system operates by means of the ultrafiltrate filling a previously empty compartment and displacing the separating piston or membrane, thereby forcing an identical volume of substitution fluid out of its previously full compartment.

While conceptually simple, accurate fluid balance by volumetric control in hemofiltration is difficult to achieve technically. Many of the technical problems result from the disparity of pressures in the two hydraulic circuits. Substitution fluid is delivered under positive pressure into the blood circuit, while ultrafiltrate is generated under negative pressure. The high ultrafiltration rates necessary to accomplish an adequate exchange within a reasonable time in hemofiltration cannot be obtained without exerting substantial negative pressures downstream of the membrane. As a result, dissolved air, which crosses the membrane with plasma water, forms gas bubbles which interfere with volumetric control of the ultrafiltrate. In order for such systems to operate accurately, the ultrafiltrate must be degassed in a separate step and the pressures within the control circuits carefully matched. Additionally, a set of valves is required to switch between alternate cycles for filling and emptying of the volume controller. Due to their technical complexity, volumetric hemofiltration systems have not found widespread acceptance. It is noteworthy, however, that the technical explorations of this approach in the past have substantially influenced the development of modern hemodialysis equipment. The newest generation of hemodialysis machines with volumetric ultrafiltration control is at least in part the result of efforts to develop such a system for hemofiltration.

Gravimetric Control

Monitoring of fluid balance by weight instead of volume is the basis of this technique, which is used in the majority of available hemofiltration machines. Both ultrafiltrate and substitution fluid have similar specific weights, permitting effective control of the exchange with scales. Since the total volume of the ultrafiltrate and substitution fluid can be conveniently placed on the scale, accuracy of control is maintained throughout the treatment and is not influenced by differences in pressure and air bubbles. Technically, gravimetric control is achieved by either one single scale or two individual scales for ultrafiltrate and substitution fluid in combination with a microprocessor.

Single-scale systems operate by maintaining the weight of combined ultrafiltrate and substitution fluid constant throughout the treatment. At the onset, the container for ultrafiltrate is empty and the one for substitution fluid full. Both are on the same scale and the combined weight is entered into an electronic or mechanical control as zero value. During the treatment, ultrafiltrate gradually fills is container. This is sensed by the scale as an increase in weight, which in turn activates a pump to remove substitution fluid from its container, deliver it to the patient, and thereby maintain the total weight on the scale constant. Desired weight loss during the treatment can be programmed either by diverting that volume of ultrafiltrate with a small preset pump from the circuit before reaching the scale or by mechanically diminishing the weight of the ultrafiltrate sensed by the scale. Both electronic and mechanical scales are used in gravimetric systems of this type and provide good accuracy of fluid balance.

A microprocessor operates hemofiltration machines with two independent electronic scales for ultrafiltrate and substitution fluid. The advantage of such equipment is that it is fully programmable and that the rates of ultrafiltration and substitution can be individually monitored throughout the treatment. The disadvantages relate to the complex electronics required and the need for costly electronic scales operating with sufficient accuracy within a wide weight range.

Control by Flow

Fluid balance with this approach is achieved by monitoring the respective fluid flows in the ultrafiltrate and substitution circuits. Both flotation-type mechanical and electromagnetic flowmeters have been used experimentally for this purpose. For the same reasons as with volumetric systems, accurate, continuous control is difficult to achieve technically.

Available Equipment

Volumetric Systems

The first balance equipment for hemofiltration was developed for L. W. HENDERSON in 1973 at the University of Pennsylvania by G. KLIGER and E. HORN in association with D. CLEVELAND of Amicon [3]. Designed for the predilution mode, this system operated reliably with a reciprocating, paired piston pump matching the volumes of ultrafiltrate and substitution fluid. A float control in a separate reservoir under negative pressure prevented air from entering the volume controller with ultrafiltrate (Fig. 1).

An operational prototype for volumetric control of postdilution hemofiltration was developed around 1976 by E. STREICHER and H. SCHNEIDER in Stuttgart, West Germany [4]. Its key component is a small chamber divided by a flexible membrane into one compartment for ultrafiltrate and another one for substitution fluid. A set

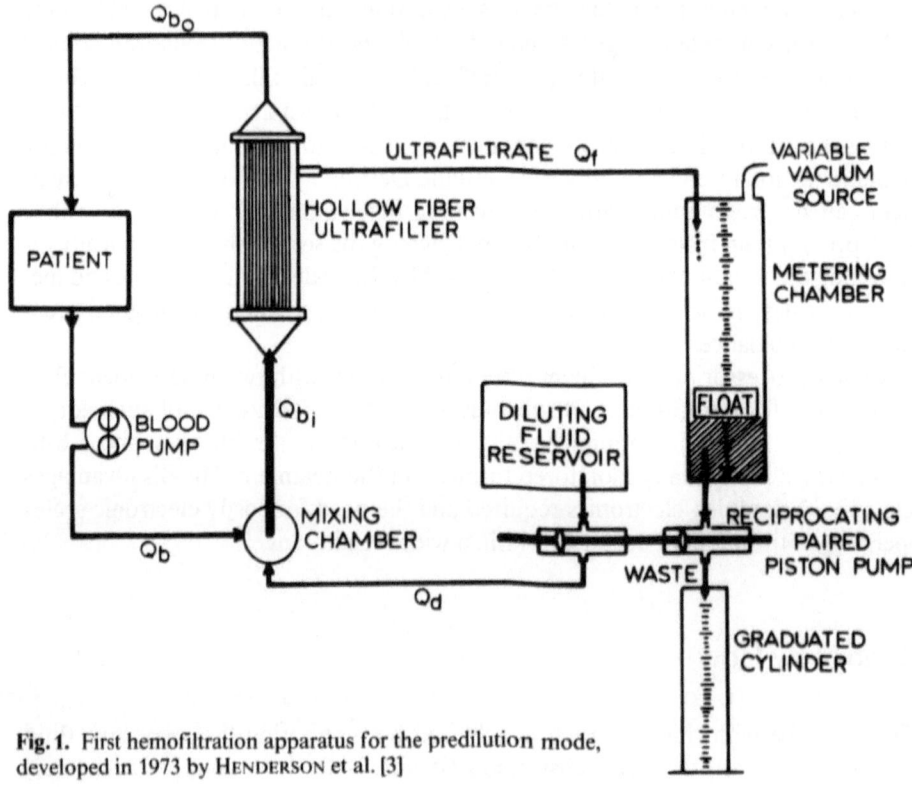

Fig. 1. First hemofiltration apparatus for the predilution mode, developed in 1973 by HENDERSON et al. [3]

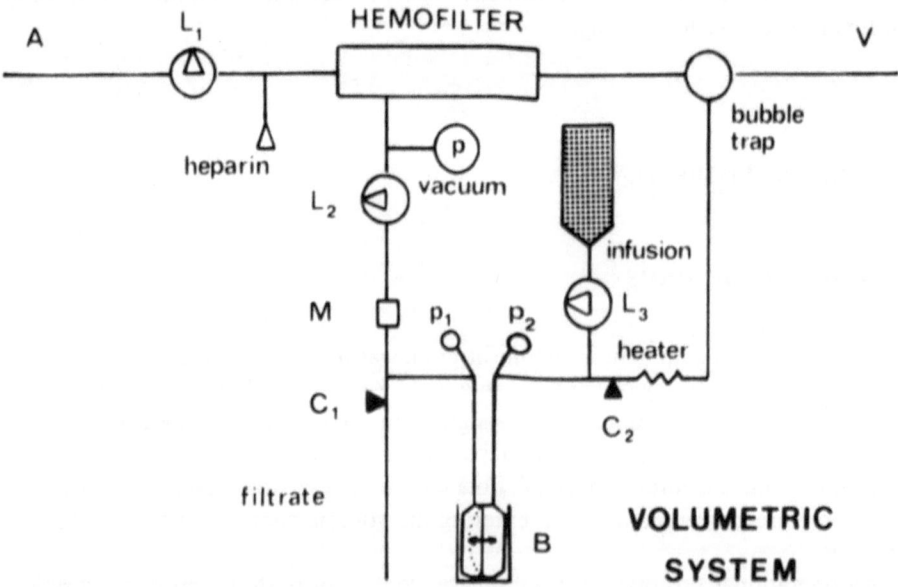

Fig. 2. Prototype for volumetric control of hemofiltration developed by STREICHER et al. [4]. A balancing chamber ((B) is alternatively filled and emptied by the ultrafiltrate and substitution fluid. (L_1, L_2, L_3, pumps; p, p_1, p_2, pressure monitors; C_1, C_2, valve clamps; M, deaerator)

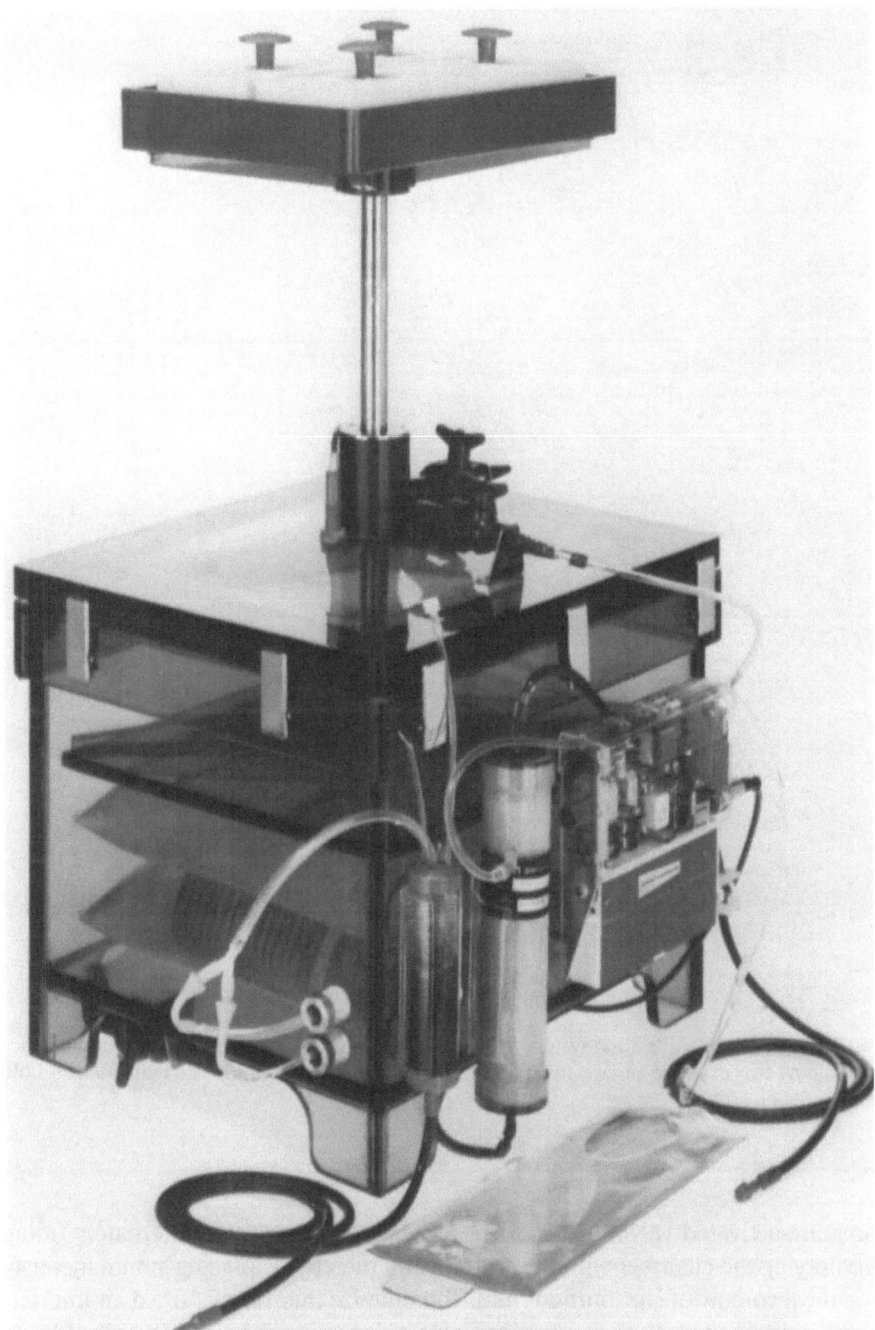

Fig. 3. Weight-driven volumetric balancing system for slow arteriovenous hemofiltration, developed by P. KRAMER and manufactured by Schi-Wa Arzneimittelwerk, Bad Laehr, West Germany

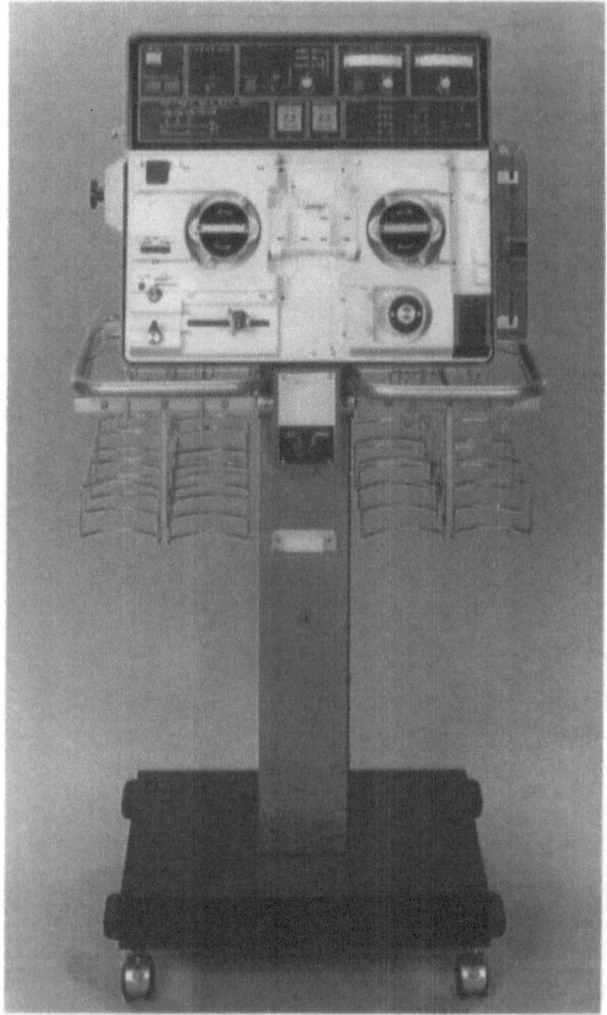

Fig. 4. Nipro NY-3 hemofiltration system (Nipro Medical Industries, Tokyo, Japan). Fluid balance is achieved by two matched pumps for ultrafiltrate and substitution fluid. The machine can hold 20 l-liter infusion bottles

of pressure-activated valves switches the system into two cycles, alternately filling and emptying the chamber with ultrafiltrate and thereby displacing simultaneously an identical volume of substitution fluid. To minimize the effect of freed air interfering with volume control, the system contains a degassing device in the ultrafiltrate circuit and operates under matched positive pressures (Fig. 2). Because of minor technical problems and lack of support, this project was later abandoned. This innovative approach, nevertheless, must be regarded as the forerunner of the newest generation of hemodialysis machines. Available only recently, these machines control ultrafiltration during dialysis by an essentially identical volumetric system.

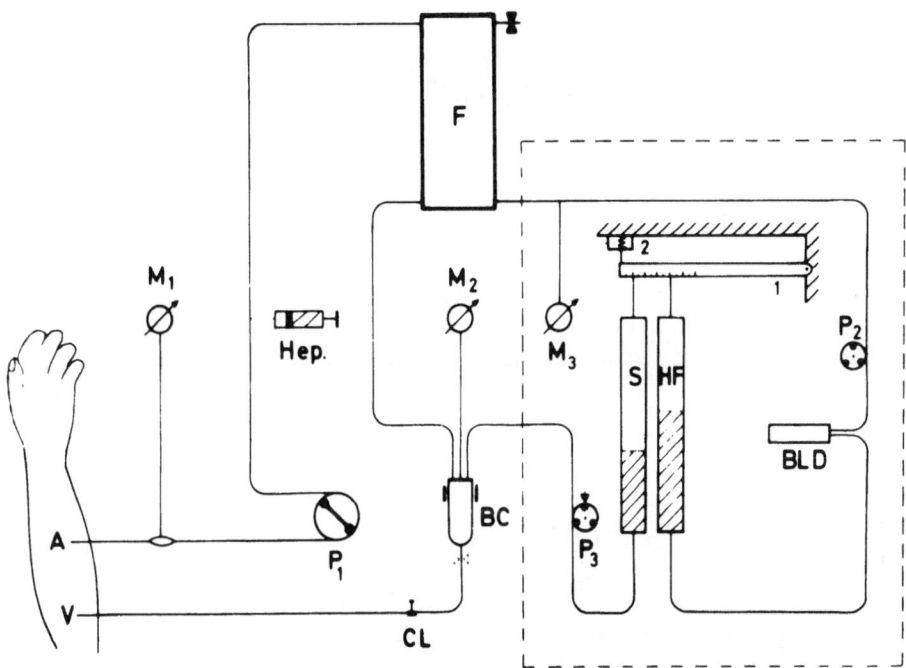

Fig. 5. Schematic diagram of first gravimetric hemofiltration system developed by DOHT, KLEIN, and QUELLHORST. Sustitution Fluid *(S)* and ultrafiltrate *(HF)* hang on a single scale with an electronic weight cell *(2)*. Proportional weight loss is programmed by the relative position of the ultrafiltration cannister *(HF)* on the lever *(1)*. (*F*, hemofilter; P_1, P_2, $P3$, pumps; M_1, M_2, pressure monitors; *BLD*, blood leak detector)

An attractively simple volumetric balancing system for slow arteriovenous hemofiltration was developed around 1978 by P. KRAMER at the University of Göttingen and manufactured by Schi-Wa Arzneimittelwerk, 4518 Bad Laer, West Germany [5] (Fig. 3). This weight-driven system operates entirely without pumps. It consists of a flexible bag for substitution fluid in a hermetically sealed box open only to the ultrafiltrate line. A weight pushes on this bag and forces substitution fluid out, thereby creating the negative pressure for ultrafiltration. As the substitution fluid bag empties, the box is gradually filled with ultrafiltrate. The apparatus contains also an electronically controlled valve, which bypasses the ultrafiltrate at timed intervals for programmable weight loss. Despite its simplicity, only a few units of this type have been built.

A unique volumetric hemofiltration machine was developed and manufactured by Nipro Medical Industries, Tokyo, Japan (Fig. 4). Volumetric control of balance in the Nipro NY-3 hemofiltration system is achieved by a roller pump with identical pump segments for ultrafiltrate and substitution fluid. A sophisticated circuit matches the positive pressures in the pump segments and prevents the interference of air with the volumetric control. Another unique feature of this machine is that it is designed to draw the substitution fluid from a large number of 1-liter glass bottles. This equipment has found only little use outside Japan.

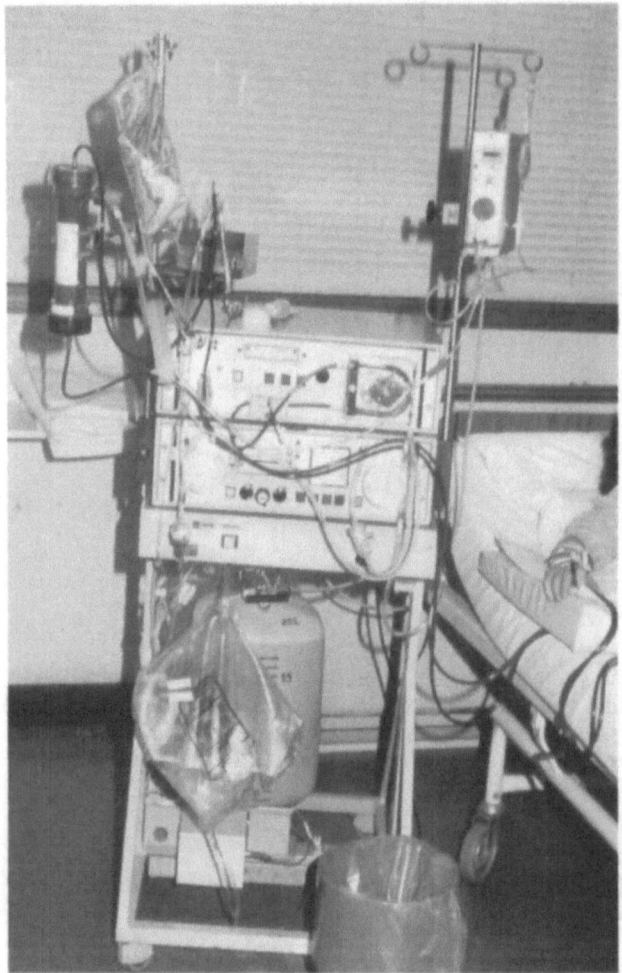

Fig. 6. Hemofiltration system BF 911 (Bellco-Deutschland GmbH, Freiburg, West Germany) in use at the Nephrologisches Zentrum Niedersachsen

Gravimetric Systems

The first workable gravimetric system for hemofiltration was developed in 1976 by B. DOHT and E. KLEIN with E. QUELLHORST in Hann. Münden, West Germany [6], (Figs. 5, 6). It was later manufactured as BF 910 and BF 911 by August Fischer KG in Göttingen, West Germany (now defunct), and distributed by Bellco-Deutschland GmbH, 7800 Freiburg, West Germany. The balancing system consists of a single scale with a transducer-type weight cell and operates by maintaining constant weight throughout the treatment. At the onset, the scale is electronically zeroed at the weight of the empty container for ultrafiltrate and the full one for substitution fluid. As ultrafiltrate is generated during the treatment, the weight on the scale increases. This in turn activates the substitution pump to draw substitution fluid from

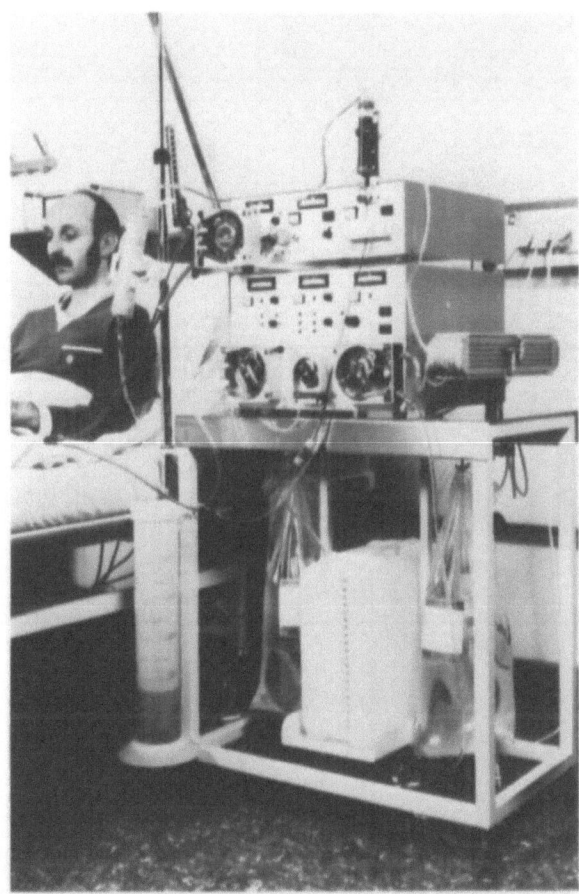

Fig. 7. Hemofiltration system
AFG 02 (Dialyse Technik
GmbH, Karlsruhe-Forchheim,
West Germany)

the scale and deliver it to the patient. Programmable weight loss is achieved mechanically in a simple, imaginative fashion: The scale hangs on the weight cell by a lever, which articulates in a joint fixed to the frame of the machine. While the substitution fluid hangs directly under the weight cell, the cannister for the ultrafiltrate can be moved on this lever, thereby reducing the weight momentum sensed by the scale. Proportional gradual weight loss is achieved by this approach throughout the treatment. The maximal capacity for exchange, primarily dictated by the dimension of the ultrafiltrate container, was 20 liters for the model BF 910 and was later increased to 30 liters for the BF 911. These sturdy machines operate with good reliability and accuracy and have been in use in Hann. Münden, Hannover, Milan, and New York. A total of about 25 such machines have been built.

A similar gravimetric machine was developed around the same time at the Technische Hochschule Aachen, West Germany, and later manufactured as Hemofiltration System DT and AFG 02 by Dialyse Technik GmbH, 7512 Karlsruhe-Forchheim, West Germany. It uses the same single-scale approach for balancing control. It differs, however, in the way the programmed weight loss is achieved: A separate small pump removes ultrafiltrate at a preset rate from its circuit before it

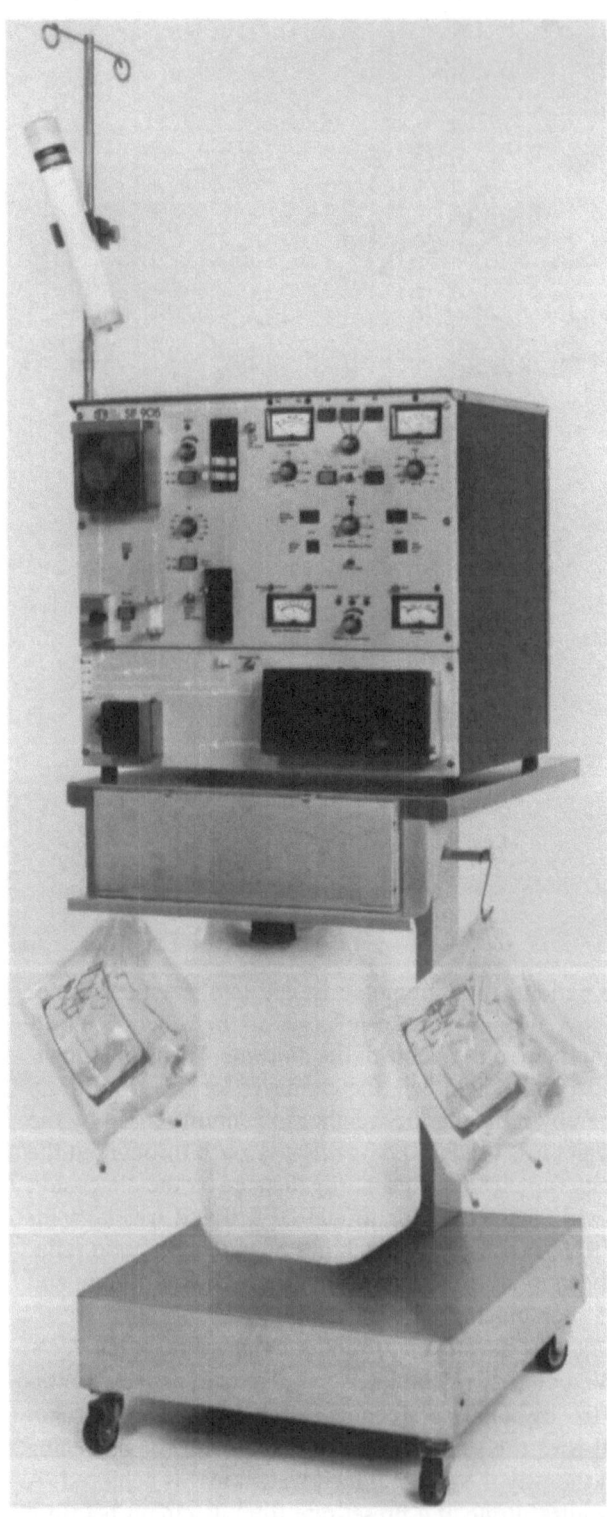

Fig. 8. Hemofiltration system SIF 905 (SIFRA, Società Italiana Farmaceutici Ravizza, Isola della Scala, Italy)

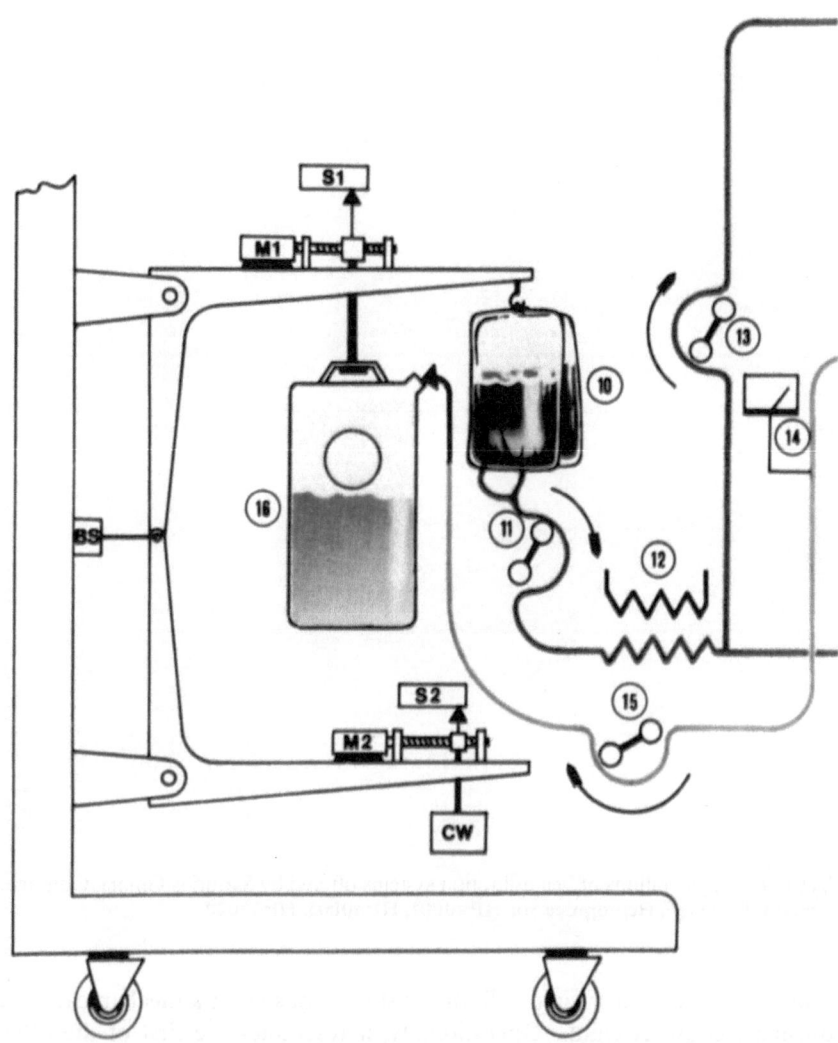

Fig. 9. Schematic diagram of the gravimetric control in the SIF 905 hemofiltration machine. Fluid balance is achieved by automated positioning of the ultrafiltrate cannister and a counterweight *(CW)* on a mechanical scale. (M = electric motors, s = sensors, BS = potentiometer controlling substitution pump, 10 = substitution fluid, 11 = substitution pump, 12 = heater, 13 = predilution pump, 14 = pressure monitor, 15 = ultrafiltrate pump, 16 = ultrafiltrate container)

reaches the container on the scale. While total volume of weight loss is conveniently collected in this approach, imbalance between ultrafiltration and substitution may be disproportionate towards the end of the treatment, when ultrafiltration rates are lower. The maximal capacity of exchange is 20 liters. The system is still manufactured and is used mainly in West Germany (Fig. 7). A newer model AFG 04 operates with two microprocessor-controlled scales and alleviates the above drawback.

A functionally entirely mechanical single-scale gravimetric hemofiltration machine was developed in 1979 by G. FRIGATO and B. VON ALBERTINI and manufactured as SIF 905 and SIF 907 by SIFRA, Isola della Scala (VR), Italy (Figs. 8, 9). In-

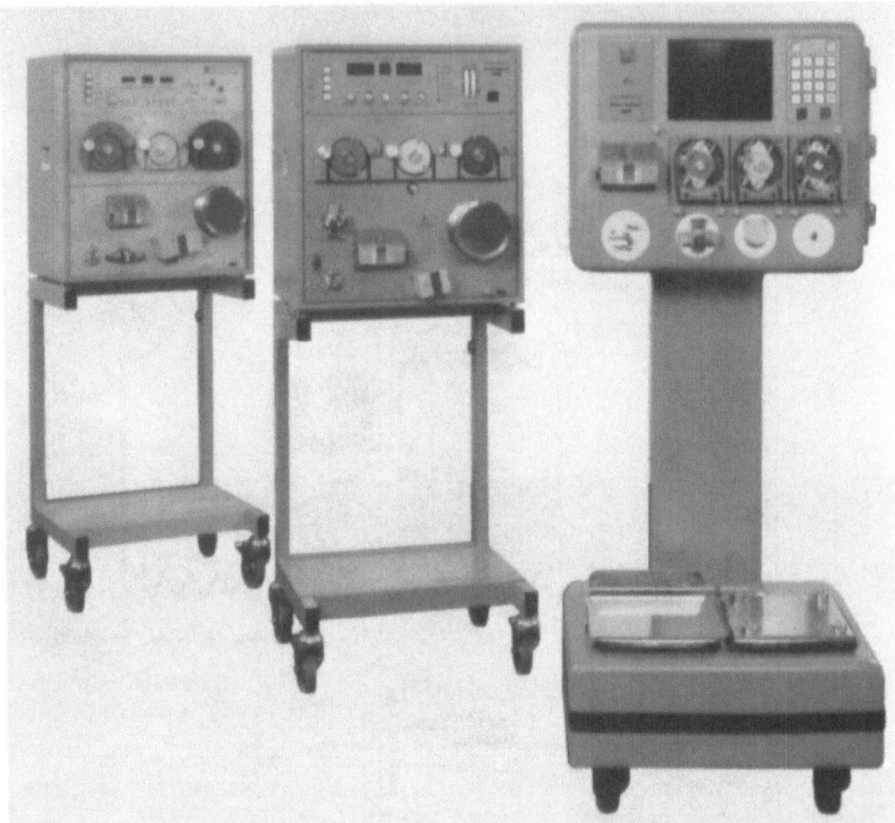

Fig. 10. Three generations of hemofiltration systems offered by Sartorius GmbH, Göttingen, West Germany. From *left,* Hemoprocessor HP 40001, HP 40005, HP 40020

stead of an electronic weight cell, this system is based on a mechanical scale with adjustable counterweights. Operationally, it resembles the first of the aforementioned gravimetric systems. The position of the counterweight for zeroing the scale at the onset and the relative position of the ultrafiltrate container on the lever arm of the scale are achieved by electric motors, which at the same time provide the information for the electronic display of total exchange, weight loss, and substitution rates. In its operation, the rate of the substitution pump is determined by a simple potentiometer, which is activated by the tilting of the scale under the weight of the incoming ultrafiltrate. The mechanical functioning of this system prevents malfunctions and alleviates the complex circuits needed for the amplification and processing of electronic weight cells. Unique features of this system are the total exchange capacity of 36 liters and a predilution pump specifically designed for high-performance, combined pre- and postdilution. Close to 100 machines of this type have been built and are in use throughout Italy.

The first microprocessor-controlled hemofiltration system with two separate scales for ultrafiltrate and substitution fluid was developed in 1976 by a leading manufacturer of precision scales, Sartorius GmbH, 3400 Göttingen, West Germany,

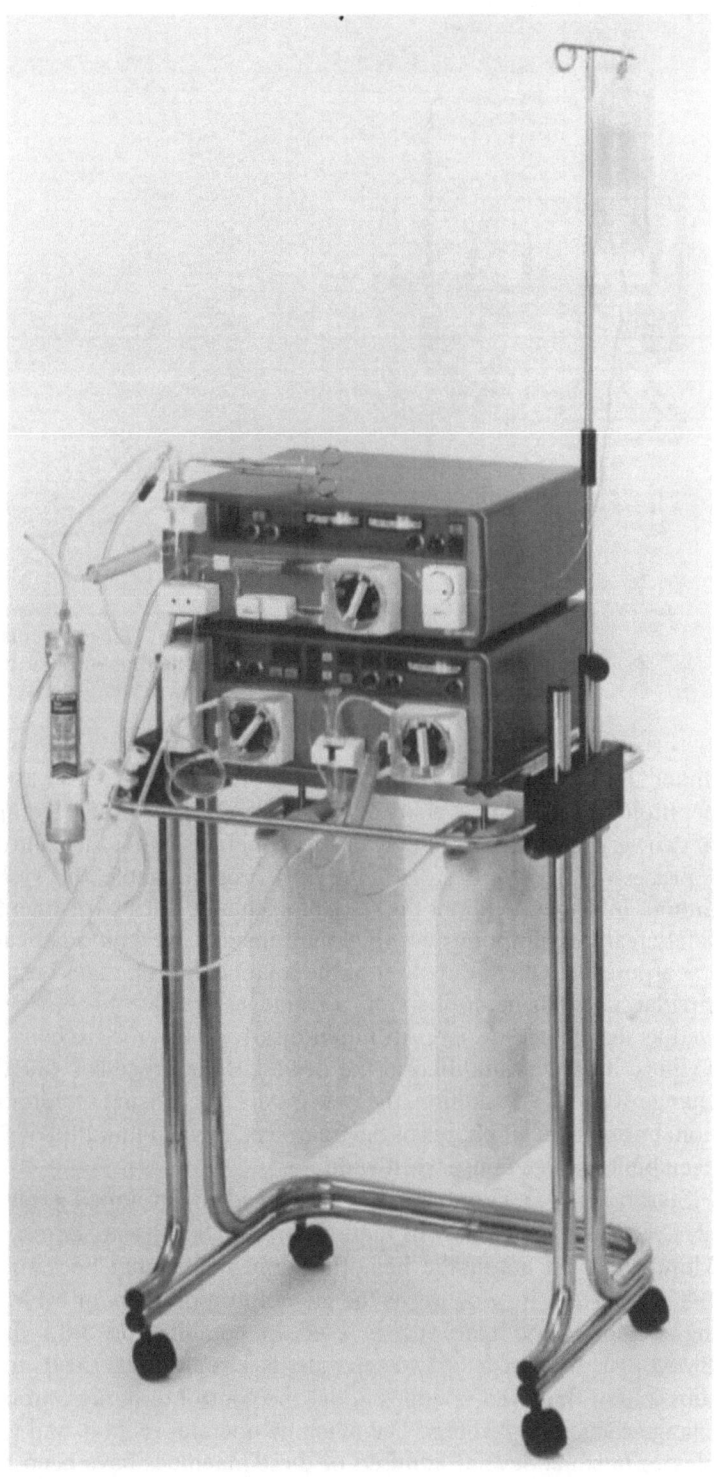

Fig. 11. Gambro (Lund, Sweden) system for hemofiltration, showing the blood monitor BMM 10-1, the hemofiltration monitor HFM 10-1, and the hemofilter FH 77

During hemofiltration

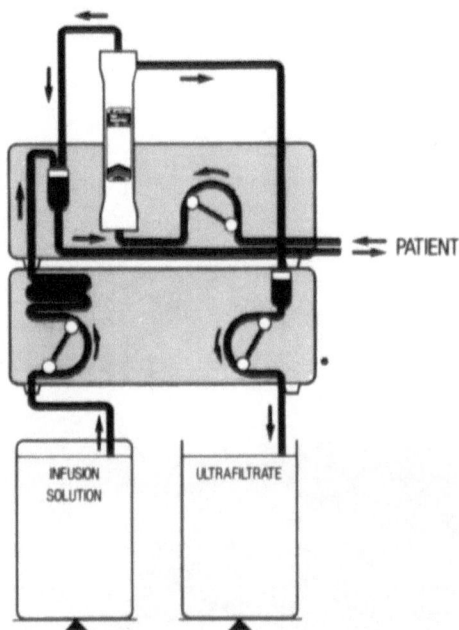

≒ PATIENT

INFUSION
SOLUTION

ULTRAFILTRATE

Fig. 12. Operating diagram of the Gambro hemofiltration system

under the leadership of E. KNOTHE and V. REICHE in close association with the nephrologists at the University of Göttingen. The Sartorius Hemoprocessor consists of two very precise electronic scales and operates under the control of a digital microprocessor (Fig. 10). Besides being fully programmable, this system provides continuous information about the rates of exchange during treatment, monitors all the safety features, pinpoints eventual malfunctions, and automatically primes the extracorporeal circuit at the onset of the treatment. It operates best with the flat-plate circular Sartorius hemofilters. Its advantages are its convenience and precision, as well as the elegant design. An initial disadvantage, the exchange capacity of only 15 liters, has been modified in the newest Hemoprocessor 400 020, which can exchange 30 liters. In addition, the new model has a visual monitor displaying operational priming in all phases of the treatment. Several hundred of these systems have been built and are in use worldwide.

Starting in 1977, Gambro AB, Lund, Sweden, developed under the moving force of C. GULBERG and in consultation with K. SCHAEFER, Berlin, and S. SHALDON, Montpellier, an automatic hemofiltration system that became available around 1980 and is now in wide use as the Hemofiltration monitor HFM 10-1. The balancing system is modular and is used in combination with the blood monitor BMM 10-1. It consists of two separate, electronic weight cells for ultrafiltrate and substitution fluid and operates under the control of a microprocessor. Its total exchange capacity is 35 liters. The machine operates reliably and is not unduly complex to operate. Several hundred of these machines have been built and are used worldwide (Figs. 11, 12).

Flow Control Systems

Experimental flotation-type and electromagnetic flow meters for monitoring fluid balance have been used clinically with predilution-hemofiltration, where ultrafiltration rates are relatively high and constant throughout the treatment [7]. A system operating with electromagnetic differential flow meters is under development by Gambro for a machine with in-line fluid production for hemofiltration.

References

1. Quellhorst E, Scheler F (eds) (1976) Aktuelle Nephrologie. Wissenschaftliche Informationen, Fresenius Stiftung 4: 85–103
2. Mackey B (ed) (1977) Proceedings of the 10th Annual Contractors' Conference, Bethesda, Maryland. Department of Health Education, and Welfare (NIH) 77-1442
3. Henderson LW, Colton CK, Ford CA (1975) Kinetics of hemodiafiltration. II. Clinical characterization of a new blood cleansing modality. J Lab Clin Med 85: 372
4. Streicher E, Schneider H (1978) Theoretische und technische Grundlagen der Hämofiltration. Nieren Hochdruckkrankh. 1: 9
5. Trautmann M, Groene HJ, Heuer E, Kramer P (1982) Intestinale Substitution bei arteriovenöser Hämofiltration. In: Kramer P (ed) (1982) Arteriovenöse Hämofiltration. Vandenhoek and Ruprecht, Göttingen, p 259
6. Quellhorst E (1983) Ultrafiltration and haemofiltration, practical applications. In: Drukker W, Parsons FM, Maher JF (eds) (1983) Replacement of renal function by dialysis. Martinus Nijhoff, Boston, p 265
7. Cheung AC, Kato Y, Leypolt JK, Henderson LW (1982) Hemodiafiltration using a hybrid membrane system for self-generation of diluting fluid. Trans Am Soc Artif Intern Organs 28: 61

Substitution Fluid for Hemofiltration

G. M. EISENBACH and S. SHALDON

Table of Contents

Introduction

New therapies in medicine offer benefits but often have inherent dangers which are only evident after the passage of time has tempered initial enthusiasm. Since the introduction of long-term end-stage renal therapy in 1960, the patient has been exposed to increasingly larger volumes of parenteral fluids. Thus, the patient on hemodialysis and hemodiafiltration is exposed to 25 000 l of dialysate fluid per year, while the patient on hemofiltration or peritoneal dialysis receives only about 5000 l per annum. As there are now patients alive who have undergone 20 years of hemodialysis and 10 years of hemofiltration or peritoneal dialysis, the cumulative magnitude of trace contamination with toxic elements of these fluids and its subsequent effect on the patient are slowly becoming better understood.

In this chapter, we will briefly discuss the evolution of quality control in parenteral fluids as a consequence of epidemics of shock, septicemia, and death associated with contaminated fluid. We will then address in more detail the specific problems associated with the production of hemofiltration replacement fluids, where historically the same mistakes have been made as previously for IV fluids. Hopefully, as we learn from our mistakes, we will make progress.

Intravenous Parenterals

The first reported use of IV fluid therapy was in the treatment of cholera in 1831 [1]. Since that time, problems associated with the quality of fluids for parenteral administration, particularly as they relate to sterility, nonpyrogenicity, and trace element contamination, have been subject to government regulation via pharmacopoeias worldwide. As early as 1942, USP XII [2] required parenteral solutions to be tested for pyrogens. As medicine and surgery evolved, increasing use of IV fluid therapy resulted in numerous reports of sporadic or epidemic outbreaks of fever, shock, or septicemia owing to contamination of parenteral fluids [3-10]. Classic examples were the "Abbot epidemic" [7, 8], and the "Davenport incident" [6], both of which occurred in the early seventies. Apart from the financial implications for the IV fluid industry, the improvement in quality control resulted in many recalls of fluids produced for parenteral use [11].

From these reports, it became evident that most of the germs involved were gram-negative bacteria not normally found in everyday clinical experience. The microorganisms identified during these episodes were *Enterobacter agglomerans, Enterobacter cloacae, Pseudomonas cepacia* and coryneform organisms. Because of some special characteristics, these bacteria are dangerous and difficult to detect. FELTS [4] demonstrated that these bacteria stored at 4 °C are able to grow in isotonic saline and in 5% dextrose when inoculated, whereas a microorganism like *E. coli* shows no relevant growth. As growth was limited to 10^6 germs/ml in most of the reported instances, the solutions remained crystal clear, and contamination could not be monitored by observation of cloudiness of the fluid. MEERS [6] showed that the aforementioned bacteria – when inoculated in 5% dextrose – are able to survive for 11 months [12].

Sources of contamination have been discovered in some of the epidemics [6-8], being mostly in-process failures in manufacturing parenterals. Possible faults arising in the container-manufacturing process, such as pinhole leaks or hairline cracks [8, 9], have also been reported.

Thus, the consequence of these unfortunate failings has been to emphasize the difference between intrinsic and extrinsic contamination [8]. The recognition of the type of bacteria involved – mostly slow-growing, gram-negative germs with a great capacity for endotoxin production – elicited a growing interest in how to cope with endotoxin- or pyrogen-related problems: New concepts of understanding the mechanisms of the pyrogenic response were developed [13-17]. The conventional in vivo rabbit pyrogen test was compared with in vitro tests like the limulus amebocyte lysate (LAL) test [18, 19], which was further refined to increase sensitivity and reliability [20-22] and is now commercially available in several modalities. The threshold pyrogenic dose for rabbit and man was compared and established to be approximately 1.0 ng/kg BW for *E. coli* and 50-70 ng/kg BW for *Pseudomonas* in man [23, 24]. Purified endotoxin standards as reference for evaluation of the LAL assay were set [25, 26], since the potency of endotoxin varies from species to species owing to differences in the lipopolysaccharide (LPS) molecule [27].

In addition, the pharmaceutical industry took up the challenge of pyrogen-related matters. With respect to sterilizing procedures, it is very difficult to remove pyrogens from parenterals, since they are very stable thermally and very insensitive to pH changes [28]. Since the commonest pyrogen is a LPS, a negatively charged substance, removal with cationically charged adsorbents was first tried [29, 30], but was rather erratic and highly dependent on both the concentration of pyrogens in solution and the ionic charge of the solution [31]. Therefore, filtration using different size-discriminating filter media was an obvious second approach [36, 37]. The technical literature on pyrogens indicates that LPS molecules are present in a wide range of aggregated states, depending on the composition of the solvent, the basic subunit being in the order of 10000–20000 daltons. In water and crystalloid solvents, particularly in the presence of divalent cations, LPS molecules aggregate into rather large vesicles [32]. Breakdown of the aggregates can be achieved by removing divalent ions or by adding detergents or bile salts [33–35]. There are also water-soluble pyrogens as small as approximately 2000 daltons (lipid A) [16], which are able to induce production of interleukin 1 [17].

NELSEN [38] conducted experiments in which different filter media (0.2-µm filters to filters for a nominal molecular weight limit of 10000) were challenged with pyrogens in different solvents (water and saline with and without bile salts added). It was found that a log reduction value (LRV) of 4 occurred using a filter of 0.025 µm, but on adding bile salts (i.e., the most disaggregate state of pyrogens) a filter with a nominal molecular weight limit of 10000 was necessary to achieve a similar LRV. This finding was consistent and independent of feed volume. According to these results, it seems possible to remove pyrogens from parenterals by means of ultrafiltration. However, using bacterial filtrate rather than pure endotoxin, DINARELLO and SHALDON [39] have suggested more recently that anisotropic ultrafilters remove pyrogens by a combined process of adsorption (related to the hydrophobic qualities of the membrane) and surface rejection.

Preparation of Substitution Fluid for Hemofiltration

With the introduction of the concept hemofiltration by HENDERSON in 1967 [40] and its first long-term clinical application by QUELLHORST in 1976 [41], the preparation of substitution fluid became a major issue, particularly when it was realized that the amount of fluid to be substituted in order to achieve adequate small molecular weight clearance was in the range of 75–100 l weekly, or some 5000 l annually.

Some of the requirements for the preparation of substitution fluid include (a) variable but reproducible constituents, (b) absence of bacterial or fungal contaminants, (c) nonpyrogenic properties, (d) absence of organic or inorganic particulate matter, (e) acceptable levels of trace metals, and (f) low cost.

In the early days of hemofiltration [41–44] substitution fluid was given by means of 1-l bottles, a very labor-intensive process with a high risk of contamination when the bottles were connected.

With advances in membrane technology and the use of blood flows exceeding 350 ml/min, ultrafiltration rates increased, necessitating infusion rates of up to 200 ml/min in the postdilution mode. In this context, not only the total amount of fluid exchanged per treatment session, but also the amount of fluid given per unit time has to be considered. This had – and continues to have – a number of serious drawbacks. Even small concentrations of pyrogens, bacteria, or unwanted organic or inorganic material might be detrimental to the patient because of the large volumes applied parenterally per unit of time.

The large volume turnover necessitated the development of automatic balancing control systems. After a short period of trials with volumetric systems, gravimetric systems were developed [45]. With the availability of gravimetric balancing systems, plastic bags containing 4.5–10 l came into use; they are collapsible, represent reasonably large aliquots, and have a low intrinsic weight.

Commercially Prepared Substitution Fluid

The common basis of all techniques for producing substitution fluid is the production of water of the highest quality [46]. That means a very low content of particulate matter and solutes as well as minimal bacterial and pyrogenic concentration. This water can be further processed by autoclaving, filtration sterilization, or other means. The efficacy of all sterilizing systems depends on the bioburden, because a sterilizing system can only reduce bacterial counts by a certain order of magnitude for a given setting. Therefore, the quality of the water entering the sterilizing process is of the greatest importance.

Table 1. Bacteriology of severe pyrogenic reactions resulting from hemofiltration performed with commercial substitution fluid [12]

Case	Blood culture	Infusate culture	Outcome
1		E. agglomerans + P. cepacia	dead
2		E. agglomerans	survived
3	sterile	E. agglomerans	survived
4	sterile	E. agglomerans[a]	survived
5		Providentia	dead
6		A. muconis	dead
7		Xanthomonas	dead
8	sterile	Pasteurella species	survived
9	P. aeruginosa	P. aeruginosa + Coryne-bacterium + staphylococci	survived
10	β-hemolyzing streptococci	sterile	dead
11		Pseudomonas group	dead
12		B. megaterium[a]	survived
13		sterile	survived
14	not investigated	E. coli	survived
15	not investigated	saphrophytic spore-forming germ[a]	dead
16	S. lutea + S. albus +2 gram-negative bacteria	not investigated	survived
17	sterile	not investigated[a]	survived
18	sterile	not investigated	survived
19	sterile	not investigated	survived

[a] Vacuum-packed infusate bags

Some plants manufacturing substitution fluid use municipal water, which is regularly checked for drinking water quality. This water is fed through a deionizer, a particle filter system, and is finally distilled. Filter system and distillery are steamed daily and checked for microbiological and pyrogenic (limulus) contamination. In a blending unit, preweighed solutes and distilled water are mixed together. The resulting solution is then pumped through a sterilizing filter into the final tank, where it is diluted with distilled water to the desired concentration. The sterilizing filter is subjected regularly to an integrity test. Finally, 4.5-l bags are filled with substitution fluid. After being vacuum-wrapped in a second bag, the filled bags are autoclaved. After that, random samples are taken for the rabbit pyrogen test and for sterility tests using the disc filtration mode to detect bacteria. Each autoclaved lot is stored at least 4 weeks, and every bag controlled visually before distribution. All blending and filling equipment is steamed daily and tested for microbiological and pyrogenic contamination. In this way, using a distillery as the main sterilizing means, chemical disinfection of the equipment is avoided.

Despite these precautions in the production of commercial substitution fluid, febrile complications have occurred [12, 47–49], as summarized in Table 1. The reported fever and shock episodes could have been due either to contamination during assembly of lines, bags, and hemofilters on the hemofiltration monitor or to bacteria contained in the bags before use that grow slowly and produce pyrogens during storage. The introduction of vacuum wrapping did not totally prevent the occurrence of these episodes. In view of the fact that industry guarantee of sterility ceases once the fluid bag is opened and subsequent safety is the responsibility of the user, the potential hazards of using fluid bags for conventional hemofiltration become very difficult to assess at the time of use and may be a good reason for abandoning this method [12].

Pyrogen Content

As mentioned earlier, the threshold pyrogenic dose for man is in the order of 1 ng/ kg BW for *E. coli* [23]. Therefore, it was concluded that it was reasonable to set 0.1 ng/ml pyrogen as a release criterion for medical devices [24, 25]. However, it should be noted that LAL-positive results may be obtained from substances of cuprophan dialyzers [51, 52] or polyamide dialyzers. These substances do not cause a rabbit fever response, but are still from two to ten times higher than the rabbit threshold pyrogenic dose [51, 53]. Also, these substances do not stimulate the human monocyte to produce interleukin 1 and cannot be considered true pyrogens [51]. However, the presence of positive LAL tests at low concentrations in IV fluids cannot be attributed solely to so-called environmental endotoxins [50], since when concentrated they stimulate monocytes to produce interleukin 1.

In a revised draft guideline, the FDA clearly established endotoxin limits based on endotoxin dose and endotoxin units (EU) referenced to the U.S. standard endotoxin EC-5 [54]. The endotoxin tolerance limit – taken as the maximum human dose of noncontaminated hemofiltration solution (35 l/4 h) in a worst case condition – is about 8 pg/ml endotoxin. PEARSON [53], however, feels that an acceptable release criterion for hemofiltration substitution fluid is about 16 pg/ml, since he believes that he is measuring mainly environmental toxins, substances with a high reactivity to the LAL test, but with low pyrogenicity. The subject is still open to debate, and we believe that the presence of 16 pg/ml of LAL-reacting material may not be without danger to the patient in the long run, in view of the recently proposed interleukin 1 hypothesis on the potential long-term effects of repeated activation of the acute phase response [55].

Until rather recently, however, a LAL test setting with a sensitivity as low as 8 pg/ml was not commonly available either to the manufacturer during production or to the user at the time of use. In addition, the methodology of reliable disc filters permitting total volume examination of parenteral fluids for bacterial contamination had not been developed [56].

Conventional hemofiltration, which uses substitution fluid stored in containers, is still performed despite serious warnings against it [12]. However, as suggested by some investigators [12, 48, 49] most users have put into the substitution fluid line a bacterial filter, an ultrafilter, or both in order to remove possible bacterial or pyrogenic contamination in the stored fluid.

On-Site Devices for the Preparation of Substitution Fluid

To overcome the necessity of purchasing costly commercial infusate potentially burdened by contamination, HENDERSON [57–59] developed in 1978 an on-line infusate-producing system using a polysulfone ultrafilter as a bacterial filter which was also capable of removing pyrogens. However, the manufacturer of the ultrafilter was not able to guarantee the physical integrity of the device, and there was no nondestructive testing method available. As a solution, SHALDON [45] introduced in 1981 an in-line dextran blue loop within the main ultrafiltering unit and a blue detector downstream in order to detect possible pinhole leaks. In addition, he installed a second ultrafilter downstream from the detector. By combining this sterilizing system with already available gravimetric balancing systems. SHALDON developed the first on-line batch-blending system for clinical use [45, 60–62].

Subsequently, the dextran blue loop was removed, as it was found to store pyrogens. However, two ultrafilters in series were retained, and, in addition, a bacterial filter – checked by an appropriate physical integrity test – was employed to lessen the probability of a bacterial or pyrogenic breakthrough.

With the same intent of reducing the need to purchase substitution fluid, QUELLHORST and his group [63] have used a different approach based on the same principle. Reverse osmosis water sterilized by a double-layered sterilizing filter is pumped into the mixing chamber, where the final solution is prepared. This fluid flows through a pyrogen filter before being filled into 10-l bags. This device is based on a commercially available filtering system, specifically designed as a sterilizing filter for the production of sterile and nonpyrogenic solutions, which can be tested by a built-in integrity testing system. With this system, the socalled cow, QUELLHORST produces both substitution fluid for hemofiltration and peritoneal dialysate. In principle, his apparatus is another batch-blending device that retains the disadvan-

Table 2. Findings of on-site preparation of substitution fluid using ultrafiltration and the batch-blending method

Author	Water treatment	Findings		
		Bacterial	Pyrogens	Clinical
HENDERSON and BEANS [57]	RO	negative	negative	no adverse reactions
SHALDON et al. [60–62]	RO	positive	negative	no adverse reactions
PIERIDES et al. [66]	RO	positive	negative	no adverse reactions
KESHAVIAH et al. [68, 69]	RO	n.g.	negative	febrile reactions (7/3841)[a]
HILDEBRAND et al. [63]	RO	negative	negative	no adverse reactions
EISENBACH [67]	RO	positive	negative	no adverse reactions
HAAS et al. [64]	RO	negative	negative	pyrogenic reactions (4/1300)[a]

Samples for microbiological and pyrogenic examination are taken after the main water-processing unit and after the main pyrogen filter. RO, reverse osmosis; n.g., not given
[a] number of episodes/number of treatment sessions

tages of possible contamination through handling of the bags and the potential bacterial growth in the bags. An additional ultrafilter is installed in the substitution fluid line before the substitution fluid enters the blood stream. Similar systems have been described by others [71, 73].

Table 2 compiles some of the results of on-site batch preparation of substitution fluid based on ultrafiltration sterilization. The common principle is ultrafiltration, mostly using hemofilters made of polysulfone, polyamide, polyacrylonitrile, or triacetate, which are able to remove bacteria and pyrogens. To increase safety, most users install a final ultrafiltering device in the substitution fluid line before the fluid enters the blood stream. All these on-site devices, including those used for water preparation, are sterilized chemically between runs. The clinical results look very promising. No adverse reactions [57, 60–63, 66, 67] except for seven mild febrile reactions in 3800 treatment sessions at one center [68–70] and four pyrogenic reactions in 1300 sessions at another center [64] have been reported thus far. On-site batch-preparation thus seems to be a reliable, safe, and relatively inexpensive method for the noncommercial preparation of substitution fluid.

Nevertheless, a number of issues relating to his method of preparation remain to be settled. Most of the on-site preparation systems for producing substitution fluid described above depend on ultrafilters as a sterilizing unit. A unit of this type cannot be subjected to a pressure integrity test. There are, however, commercially available filtering systems specifically designed to remove bacteria and pyrogens which can be tested and even autoclaved. Whereas the ability of these systems to remove bacteria is satisfactory, there is a lack of sufficient data proving their reliability as a pyrogen filter. So far, the device QUELLHORST uses has produced satisfactory results [63].

As mentioned above, other disadvantages of batch-blending are contamination during assembly and intermediary storage of the containers with its opportunity for bacterial growth. The findings listed in Table 2 refer to measurements made after the fluid has passed through the main ultrafiltration-sterilization unit. The danger of contamination by connection or handling is demonstrated by the results of some studies in which mostly gram-positive bacteria were detected, such as can be expected when contamination during handling has occurred. Not surprisingly, since gram-positive germs prevail, pyrogen measurements by the limulus assay were reported to be negative in all studies.

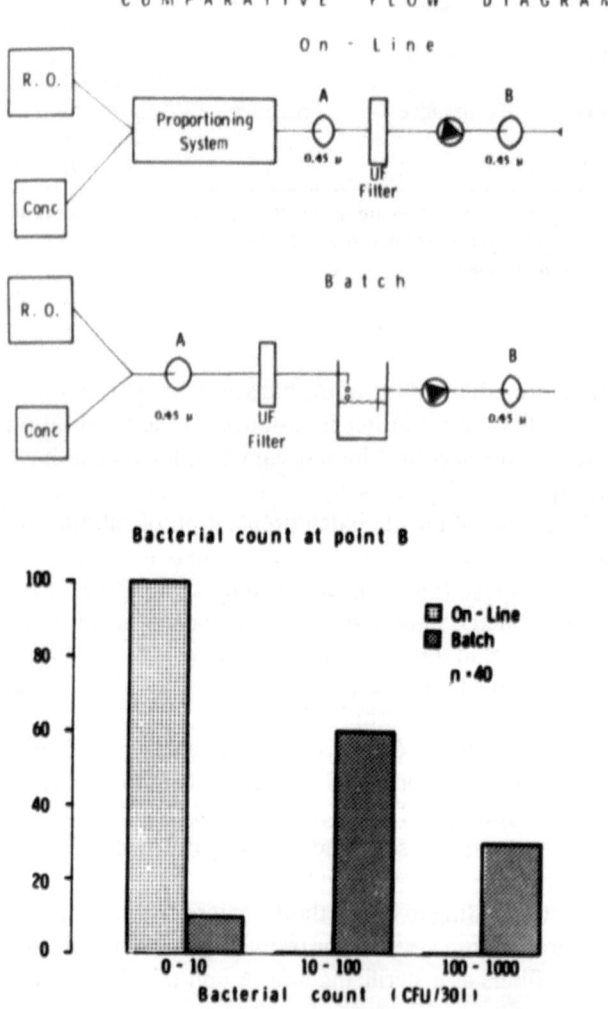

Fig. 1. Frequency distribution of bacterial counts in colony-forming units *(CFU)* per 30 l *(bottom)* of full-stream samples taken at point *B* using continuous preparation *(On-line)* and batch-blending preparation *(Batch)* of substitution fluid

To improve the situation, in 1978 HENDERSON [58], and more recently, Shaldon [71-74] suggested and developed a continuous proportioning system which eliminates connections and intermediary storage. SHALDON [73, 74] (Fig. 1) compared this continuous proportioning system with his original batch-blending device. The number of colony-forming units grown on a filterdisc in a Swinnex filter holder downstream from the main ultrafiltering unit was measured at point B. Samples with high bacterial counts were found only in the batch blending device and not in the continuous proportioning system.

Most of the requirements for substitution fluid listed above are met by existing on-site devices, particularly continuous proportioning systems. The criterion of variable but reproducible constituents can be met by continuous proportioning systems even during runs. Using a reverse osmosis unit in the water preparation cycle and ultrafilters during final preparation as outlined above eliminates bacterial and fungal contaminants, pyrogenic agents, and organic or inorganic particulate matter. Indeed, using an ultrafilter, pyrogen levels below 3 pg/ml are routinely obtained. This indicates the clear superiority of on-site devices over commercial bag fluid. Production costs are reasonable, and the product is safe for the patient.

The remaining problem concerns the achievement of acceptable levels of trace metals. Special care has to be taken here with regard to aluminum. Not only the plastic disposables but also the salts or salt concentrates used should be aluminum free. This of course also applies to hemodialysis materials and equipment [48, 63, 75-81].

Conclusion

For the present time, the use of commercial substitution fluid in single bags is an appropriate method, if a final pyrogen filter is employed, preferably a built-in disposable one. While this is a rather expensive method, it does reduce residual pyrogenic content.

On-site preparation based on ultrafiltration-sterilization in conjunction with a batch-blending device is a safe method, if a final disposable pyrogen filter is used.

Both an integrity test for the main pyrogen filter and the results of pyrogenic challenge tests [82] should be routinely available for all filters used as pyrogen filters.

The on-site continuous proportioning system, which also implements ultrafiltration-sterilization together with an automatic volumetric control, appears superior to all other hemofiltration techniques. It eliminates connections and intermediary storage, thereby lessening the potential for bacterial contamination and pyrogen production, and may reduce the load of potentially toxic substances that leach out off plastic materials.

In treating patients with end-stage renal disease by means of hemodialysis, hemodiafiltration, or hemofiltration, exposure to large amounts of fluid is unavoidable. However, the system with the smallest volume exposure per patient and the least potential for contamination in all areas discussed should be considered the most appropriate treatment modality in the long run.

References

1. Lewins R (1831) Injection of saline solution in extraordinary quantities into the veins in cases of malignant cholera. Lancet ii: 243–244
2. Pharmacopeia of the United States of America, 12th Revision (USP XII). From Nov. 1, 1942, Easton, Pa.
3. Duma RJ, Warner JF, Dalton HP (1971) Septicemia from intravenous infusions. N Engl J Med 284: 257
4. Felts SK, Schaffner W, Melli MA, Koenig MG (1972) Sepsis caused by contaminated intravenous fluids. Ann Intern Med 77: 881
5. Maki DG, Goldman DA, Rhame FS (1973) Infection control in intravenous therapy. Ann Intern Med 9: 867
6. Meers PD, Calder MW, Mazhar MM, Lawry GM (1973) Intravenous infusion of contaminated dextrose solution. Lancet ii: 1189
7. Mackel DC, Maki G, Anderson RL, Rhame TS, Bennet JV (1975) Nationwide epidemic of septicemia caused by by contaminated intravenous products: Mechanisms of intrinsic contamination. J Clin Microbiol 2: 486
8. Maki DG, Rhame FS, Mackel DC, Bennet JV (1976) Nationwide epidemic of septicemia caused by contaminated intravenous products. Am J Med 60: 471
9. Editorial (1976) Thomas Latta, what have we done? – The hazards of intravenous therapy. N Engl J Med 294: 1178–1180
10. Maki DG (1981) Nosocomial bacteremia. An epidemiologic overview. Am J Med 70: 719–732
11. Report of the Comptroller General the US (1976) Recalls of large volume parenterals (Liquid drugs administered intravenously or by other non-oral means). March 12, 1976 (MSD-76-67)
12. Frei U, Koch KM (1983) Fever and shock during hemofiltration. Contrib Nephrol 36: 107–114
13. Snell ES (1975) Gram-negative bacterial endotoxin and the pathogenesis of fever. Prog Drug Res 19: 402–411
14. Dinarello CA, Wolff SM (1978) Pathogenesis of fever in man. N Engl Med 298: 607–612
15. Morrison DC, Ulevitch RJ (1978) The effects of bacterial endotoxins in host mediation systems. Am J Pathol 93: 527–617
16. Dinarello CA (1983) Pathogenesis of fever during hemodialysis. Contrib Nephrol 36: 90–99
17. Dinarello CA, Wolff SM (1982) Molecular basis of fever in humans. Am J Med 72: 799–819
18. Levin J, Bang FB (1964) The role of endotoxin in the extracellular coagulation of Limulus blood. Bull John Hopkins Hosp 115: 265–274
19. Levin J, Bang FB (1964) A description of cellular coagulation in the Limulus. Bull John Hopkins Hosp 115: 337
20. Nandan R, Brown DR (1977) An improved in vitro pyrogen test: To detect picograms of endotoxin contamination in intravenous fluids using Limulus amebocyte lysate. J Lab Clin Med 89: 910–918
21. Dubczak J, Cotter R, Dastoli F (1979) Quantitative detection of endotoxin by nephelometry. In: Cohen E (ed) Biomedical applications of the horseshoe crab (Limulidae). Liss, New York, pp 403
22. Gardi A, Arpagaus GR (1980) Improved microtechnique for endotoxin assay by the limulus amebocyte lysate test. Anal Biochem 109: 382–385
23. Greisman SE, Hornick B (1969) Comparative reactivity of rabbit and man to bacterial endotoxin. Proc Soc Biol Med 131: 1154
24. Dabbah R, Ferry E, Gunther DA (1980) Pyrogenicity of E. coli 055: B 5 endotoxin by the USP rabbit test - a HIMA colloborative study. J Parent Drug Assoc 34: 212
25. Parenteral Drug Association, Interindustry Communication (1980) A response to the Federal Register (Jan. 18, 1980) 45: 3668
26. U.S. Food and Drug Administration (1980) Human and veterinary drugs; availability of draft guidelines for use of Limulus amebocyte lysate. Fed Reg 45: 3668
27. Tominaga H, Tanaka S, Tominaga N (to be published) Endotoxin level of sterile injection solutions and substitution fluid for haemofiltration in Japan and Australia. Nephron
28. Elin RJ, Wolff SM (1973) Bacterial endotoxins. In: Laskin AP, Lechevalier P (eds) CRC Handbook on microbiology, vol II. CRC Press Cleveland, pp 215–239

29. Nolan JP, McDevitt JJ, Goldman GS (1975) Endotoxin binding by charged and uncharged resins. Proc Soc Exp Biol 149: 766-770
30. Kaden H (1975) The use of asbestos filter beds in the production of sterile and pyrogen-free solutions. Pharmazie 29: 752-753
31. Koppensteiner G, Kruger D, Osmers K, Woog H, Zimmermann G (1976) An experimental investigation of the elimination of pyrogens from parenteral medicines. Drugs Made Ger 19: 113-123
32. Hannecart-Pokorny E, Dekegel D, Dupuydt F (1973) Macromolecular structure of lipopolysaccharides from gram-negative bacteria. Eur J Biochem 38: 6-13
33. Ribi E, Anacker RL, Brown R, Haskins WT, Malmgren B, Milner KC, Rudback JS (1966) Reaction of endotoxin and surfactants in physical and biological properties of endotoxin treated with sodium deoxycholate. J Bacteriol 92: 1493-1509
34. Rogers SW, Gilleland HE jr, Eagon RG (1969) Characterization of a protein lipopolysaccharide complex released from cell walls of pseudomonas aeruginosa by ethylendiamintetraacetic acid. Can J Microbiol 15: 743-748
35. Rudback JA, Milner KC (1968) Reaction of endotoxin and surfactants III. Effect of sodium lauryl sulfate on the structure and pyrogenicity of endotoxin. Can J Microbiol 14: 1173-1178
36. Sweadner KJ, Forte M, Nelsen LL (1977) Filtration removal of endotoxin (pyrogens) in solution in different states of aggregation. Appl Exp Microbiol 34: 382-385
37. Zimmermann G, Kruger D, Woog H (1976) Pyrogen elimination from parenteral medicines by means of molecular filtration. Drugs Made Ger 19: 123-128
38. Nelsen LL (1978) Removal of pyrogens from parenteral solutions by ultrafiltration. Pharm Tech May: 47-50
39. Dinarello CA, Shaldon S (1985) Pyrogen removal my membrane filtration. Blood Purification (in press)
40. Henderson LW, Besarab A, Michaels A, Bluemle LW jr (1967) Blood purification by ultrafiltration and fluid replacement (diafiltration). Trans Am Soc Artif Intern Org 13: 216
41. Quellhorst E, Rieger J, Doht B, Beckmann H, Jakob J, Kraft B, Scheler F (1976) Treatment of chronic uremia by an ultrafiltration kidney. First clinical experience. Proc Eur Dial Transplant Assoc 13: 314-321
42. Hamilton R, Ford C, Colton C, Cross R, Steinmüller S, Henderson LW (1971) Blood cleaning by diafiltration in uremic dogs and man. Trans Am Soc Artif Intern Org 17: 259
43. Quellhorst E, Fernandez E, Scheler F (1972) Treatment of uremia using an ultrafiltration-filtration unit. Proc Eur Dial Transplant Assoc 9: 584
44. Henderson LW (1982) The beginning of hemofiltration. Contrib Nephrol 32: 1-19
45. Ramperez D, Beau MG, Deschodt G, Flavier JL, Nielsson L, Mion C, Shaldon S (1981) Economic preparation of sterile pyrogen-free infusate for hemofiltration. Proc Eur Dial Transplant Assoc 18: 293-296
46. Keshaviah P, Luehmann D (to be published) The importance of water treatment in haemodialysis and haemofiltration
47. Daul A, Graben N, Bock KD (1981) Septicaemie als Komplikation der Haemofiltration. Diagn Intensivther 6: 284-294
48. Herrath D v, Schaefer K, Huefler M, Pauls A, Koch KM (1982) Complications of Hemofiltration. Contrib Nephrol 32: 146-153
49. Herrath D v, Schaefer K, Huefler M, Pauls A, Koch KM, Goehl H, Ljuggren L, Gardiner P (1983) Complications of hemofiltration. Int J Artif Organs 6: 49-52
50. Pearson FC, Weary ME, Bohon J, Dabbah R (1982) Relative potency of "environmental" endotoxin as measured by the Limulus amebocyte lysate test and the USP rabbit pyrogen test. In: Watson SW, Levin J, Novitsky TJ (eds) Endotoxins and their detection with the Limulus amebocyte lysate test. Riss, New York, pp 65-77
51. Pearson FC, Bohon J, Lee W, Bruszer G, Sagona M, Dawe R, Jakubowski G, Morrison D, Dinarello C (1984) Comparison of chemical analyses of hollow-fiber dialyzer extracts. Art Org 8: 291-298
52. Henne W, Schulze H, Pelger W, Tretzel J, Sengbusch G v (1984) Hollow-fiber dialyzers and their pyrogenicity by Limulus amebocyte lysate. Artif Organs 8: 299-305
53. Pearson FC (1983) The preparation of hemofiltration solution and quality assurance issues. 1st annual meeting International Society of Hemofiltration, Frankfurt, 1983

54. FDA (1983) Draft guideline for validation of the limulus amebocyte lysate test as an endproduct endotoxin test for human and parenteral drugs, biological products and medical devices. Pharmacopeial Forum 9: 3012–3021
55. Henderson LW, Dinarello CA, Koch KM, Shaldon S (1983) Interleukin 1 hypothesis. Blood Purification 1: 1
56. Mayr HU, Stec F, Canaud B, Mion CM, Shaldon S (to be published) Microbiological aspects of the batch preparation of replacement fluid for hemofiltration. Blood Purification
57. Henderson LW, Beans F (1978) Successful production of sterile pyrogenfree electrolyte solution by ultrafiltration. Kidney Int 14: 522–525
58. Henderson LW, Sanfelippo ML, Beans E (1978) "On-line" preparation of sterile pyrogen-free electrolyte solution. Trans Am Soc Artif Intern Organs 24: 465–467
59. Henderson LW (1980) Hemofiltration for the treatment of hypertensions associ associated with end-stage renal failure. Artif Organs 4: 103–107
60. Shaldon S, Beau MC, Deschodt G, Flavier JL, Ramperez P, Nielsson L, Mion C (1982) Three years of experience with on-line preparation of sterile pyrogen-free infusate for hemofiltration. Contrib Nephrol 32: 161–164
61. Shaldon S, Beau MC, Branger B, Deschodt G, Delisle Nichols HF, Oules R, Ramperez P, Mion C (1983) Economic preparation of sterile non-pyrogenic infusate for hemofiltration. Dialysis Transplantation 12: 792–793
62. Shaldon S, Beau MC, Deschodt G, Flavier JL, Nielsson L, Ramperez P, Mion C (1983) Three years of experience with on-line preparation of sterile pyrogen-free infusate for hemofiltration. Intern J Artif Organs 6: 25–26
63. Hildebrand U, Quellhorst E (1983) Central proportioning system for the production of substitution fluid. Oral presentation at the International Workshop of Hemofiltration, Frankfurt, 1983
64. Haas T, Villeboeuf F, Fournier JF, Mayrand B, DeViel E, Dongradi G (1984) The extemporaneous preparation of sterile, pyrogen-free reinjection fluid for hemofiltration. Dial Transplant 13: 559–562
65. Yamagami S, Kishimoto T, Tanaka H, Mackawa M (1982) On-line preparation of substitution fluid for hemofiltration (Abstr). Eur Dialysis Transplant Assoc abstr 19: 154
66. Pierides AM, Schniepp B, Johnson WJ (1981) Two year experience with over 500 sessions of postdilution hemofiltration. Trans Am Soc Artif Intern Organs 17: 618–622
67. Eisenbach GM (1984) Hemofiltration substitution fluid preparation: Past, present and some future aspects. 2nd Annual workshop of the International Society of Hemofiltration, Milan
68. Keshaviah P, Ebben J, Hirsch D, Luehmann D, Collins A, Shapiro F (1983) On-site preparation of substitution fluid for large scale delivery of hemofiltration (HF) (Abstr). Am Soc Nephrol annual meeting, p 49 A
69. Keshaviah P, Luehmann D, Hirsch J, Ebben J, Collins A, Shapiro F (1984) Central on-site preparation of substitution fluid for hemofiltration (Abstr). Am Soc Artif Intern Organs, 30th annual meeting 13: 46
70. Luehmann D, Hirsch D, Ebben J, Collins A, Shapiro F, Keshaviah P (1984) Central on-site preparation of substitution fluid for hemofiltration. Trans Am Soc Artif Intern Organs 30: 195–198
71. Shaldon S, Deschodt G, Branger B, Oules R, Gullberg CA, Mion C (1983) Experience with on-line haemofiltration (Abstr). Artif Organs 7: 57
72. Shaldon S, Beau BC, Mayr H, Gullberg CA (1984) In-line hemofiltration. Am Soc Artif Intern Organs, 30th annual meeting, 13: 55
73. Shaldon S, Beau BC, Mayr H, Gullberg CA (1984) In-line hemofiltration. Int Soc Nephrol, 9th int congress, Los Angeles, p 189 A
74. Shaldon S, Deschodt G, Granolleras C, Oules R, Gullberg CA, Mayr H (to be published) Experience with on-line hemofiltration. Artif Organs
75. Fuchs C, Quellhorst E, Scheler F (1984) Prophylaxis and methods for early recognition of aluminium intoxication. Contrib Nephrol 38: 81–91
76. Salvadeo H, Minoia C, Segagni S, Villa G (1979) Trace metal changes in dialysis fluid and blood of patients on hemodialysis. Intern J Artif Organs 2: 17–21
77. Sancipriano GP, Fidelio T, Squiccimarro G, Ragni R (1983) Aluminium (Al) in bags for HF: critical limits. International workshop on hemofiltration, Frankfurt, 1983

78. Mason JC, Jones NF, Hilton PJ (1983) Aluminium in hemofiltration solutions. Lancet 1: 762–763
79. Cumming AD, Simpson G, Bell D, Cowie J, Winney RJ (1982) Acute aluminium intoxication in patients on continous ambulatory peritoneal dialysis. Lancet 1: 103–104
80. Herrath D v, Schaefer K, Hüfler M, Gawlik D, Gardiner PE (1983) Spurenelemente im off-line hergestellten Infusat für die Hämofiltration. Nieren- Hochdruckkr 12: 175–178
81. Fuchs C, Quellhorst E, Scheler F (1983) Einfluß verschiedener Behandlungsverfahren auf die Plasma-Aluminiumkonzentration bei chronisch niereninsuffizienten Patienten. Nieren- Hochdruckkr 12: 179–185
82. Klinkmann H, Falkenhagen D, Smollich BP (to be published) Investigation of the permeability of highly permeable polysulfone membranes for pyrogen. Contrib Nephrol

Selection of Patients for Hemofiltration

S. GLABMAN and A. LAUER

During the past 25 years a number of modalities have been developed for the treatment of end-stage renal disease (ESRD). In addition to conventional hemodialysis (HD) and transplantation, continuous ambulatory peritoneal dialysis (CAPD) and hemofiltration (HF) have become alternatives for the treatment of ESRD. HF has become particularly popular in Europe. The purpose of this chapter is to identify those types of patients who might be best suited for chronic HF.

Patients with cardiomyopathies, autonomic dysfunction, ischemic heart disease, and the elderly may not tolerate fluid removal during conventional HD [1]. The removal of the interdialytic weight gain in these patients may be accompanied by the development of hypotension, cramps, nausea, and vomiting [2]. Hemofiltration is associated with fewer of these symptoms than conventional HD [3, 4]. The reasons for this reduction in symptoms have been speculative. It has been suggested that variations in membrane biocompatibility, removal of vasoactive middle molecules, and differences in renin or appropriate noradrenalin release may be factors. Better refilling of the intravascular space might also account for the improved tolerance of HF over HD [3, 4]. Although there is published data to support many of these hypotheses, the last explanation is most intriguing. Conceivably, as large volumes of fluid are removed from the vascular space by HF, the plasma protein concentration increases. The retention of these negatively charged plasma proteins obligates the retention of cations, in particular sodium, to maintain electrical neutrality. The rise in plasma sodium concentration results in an increase in plasma tonicity and water shifts from the intracellular space to the extracellular space. This shift of fluid preserve the intravascular volume and limits the development of the symptoms frequently associated with hypotension [5].

It is controversial as to whether HF is more effective than other treatment modalities in the control of hypertension. Bosch et al., in a cross-over study did not observe significant changes in pretreatment with either HF or HD [6]. Alternatively, JAHN et al., studied 12 patients with ESRD complicated by drug-resistant, volume-independent, hypertension [7]. Patients received either hemodialysis or HF for 6 months. Systemic vascular resistance was lower in patients on HF than in patients on HD. The decreased systemic vascular resistance appeared to correlate with lower plasma renin and lower plasma dopamine hydroxylase concentrations [7]. It would be difficult to categorically claim that HF is more effective for blood pressure control than HD. However, there may be a subset of patients with refractory hypertension who could benefit from HF. The proof of this supposition requires additional investigation.

HF appears to have a role in the control of secondary hyperparathyroidism. The capacity of this type of treatment because of higher membrane sieving to remove fragments of parathyroid hormone (PTH), as well as the intact hormone, may account for its effectiveness in controlling renal osteodystrophy [8]. By contrast, patients on chronic hemodialysis do not undergo a reduction in PTH levels and frequently plasma levels of this hormone increase with time. In an ABA (A, hemodialysis; B, hemofiltration) study involving HF and HD, the authors observed a significant fall in plasma phosphorous levels in ten patients after 4 months of HF [6, 9]. This combined effect of removing middle molecules, such as parathyroid and its circulating fragments, as well as better control of plasma phosphorous levels, suggests a role for HF in selected individuals. Conceivably, patients with uncontrollable metabolic bone disease could benefit from chronic HF.

Glucose intolerance is frequently observed in patients with ESRD. The mechanism for the impaired glucose intolerance is probably multifactorial and has in part been attributed to:

a) a circulating insulin antagonist,
b) decreased insulin release following a glucose load,
c) abnormalities in glucose utilization, and
d) defects in glycogen storage [10].

The disappearance of glucose following an intravenous load is similar whether the patient is treated with HF or HD [11]. Of interest is the fact that lower levels of plasma insulin are required to reduce plasma glucose levels in patients undergoing chronic hemofiltration than in those on chronic HD [11]. This observation might be indicative of an increased peripheral insulin sensitivity in patients on HF. It is difficult to know whether the improved insulin sensitivity observed in patients on HF has a significant impact on patient morbidity and/or mortality.

Disorders in plasma lipid concentration are well-documented in patients with ESRD [12]. Recent evidence tends to suggest that plasma cholesterol and triglycerides are lower in patients on chronic HF than in patients on chronic HD [13]. Insofar as hyperlipidemia is a risk factor for the development of atherosclerosis, HF may have a role in patients with ESRD complicated by marked hyperlipidemia.

Both HF and HD are effective in controlling the metabolic acidosis observed in patients with ESRD. Studies by Bosch et al., comparing these two treatment modalities observed an increased pretreatment plasma HCO_3 in patients undergoing chronic HF [6]. This occurred despite the administration of similar quantities of base in both treatments. Presumably, factors other than the administration of base are responsible for the lower pretreatment plasma HCO_3 in HD. These authors have suggested that as red blood cells pass through the dialyzer, CO_2 is generated resulting in increasing acid production [14]. Whether the better control of acid-base balance during HF is of clinical significance is unclear at present.

In conclusion, HF is a suitable alternative to HD for the treatment of ESRD. Its greater expense has hampered its acceptance in the United States. HF appears to be particularly well suited for patients with vascular instability who are prone to large interdialytic weight gain. It also may be of value in maintaining ESRD patients with significant renal osteodystrophy.

We have identified groups of patients for whom HF might be the preferred modality for renal replacement therapy. These are the:

a) elderly,
b) patients presenting vascular instability with hypotensive reaction,
c) acidotic patients,
d) diabetics, and
e) hyperparathyroid patients.

While these particular patients might be best managed by HF, this does not mitigate against treating any or all renal failure patients with HF.

References

1. Maher JF, Schreiner GE (1965) Hazards and complications of dialysis. N Engl J Med 270: 370–377
2. Henderson LW (1980) Symptomatic hypotension during hemodialysis. Kidney Int 170: 571–576
3. Quellhorst EA, Schoenemann B (1979) A controlled study to compare hemodialysis and hemofiltration treatment in patients with chronic renal failure. In 12th annual contractors conference – Artifical kidney, chronic uremia program. National Institute of Arthritis, Metabolism and Digestive Disease, January 1979
4. Henderson LW, SanFilippo ML, Stone RA (1979) Comparison of hemodialysis and hemofiltration. In 12th annual contractors conference – Artificial kidney, chronic uremia program. National Institute of Arthritis, Metabolism and Digestive Disease, January 1979
5. Bosch JP, Ponti R, Glabman S, Lauer A (to be published) Sodium fluxes in hemodialysis.
6. Bosch JP, Glabman S, von Albertini B, Geronemus R, Kahn J, Goldstein MH, Kupfer S (1979) Comparison of hemofiltration and ultrafiltration plus hemodialysis to conventional hemodialysis. In 12th annual contractors conference – Artificial kidney, chronic uremia program. National Institute of Arthritis, Metabolism and Digestive Disease, January 1979
7. Jahn H, Schohn D, Gulberg C, Schmitt R (1982) Hemodynamic long-term effects of hemofiltration on dialysis and drug resistant hypertension. Contrib Nephrol 32: 61–68
8. Schaefer K, Herruth D, Gulberg CA, Asmus G, Hufler M, Offerman G, Cremer H, Heuch CC, Ritz E (1978) Chronic hemofiltration: A critical evaluation of a new method for the treatment of blood. J Soc Artif Organs 2: 386–394
9. Bosch JP, Glabman S, Geronemus R, Constantiner A, von Albertini B (1981) Effect of long-term hemodialysis and hemofiltration on intact PTH and C-Terminal PTH (Abstr). Am Soc Nephrol 37 A
10. DeFronzo R (1984) Glucose and insulin metabolism. In: Massry S, Glassock R (eds) Textbook of nephrology. Williams and Wilkins, Baltimore, pp 7.69–7.75
11. Kishimoto T, Ezuki K, Yamagumi S, Mackawa M (1982) Glucose tolerance and erythrocyte insulin receptors in undialyzed patients and patients on maintenance hemodialysis and hemofiltration. Contrib Nephrol 32: 97–110
12. Brunzell J, Goldberg A (1984) Hyperlipidemia. In: Massry S, Glassock R (eds) Textbook of nephrology. Williams and Wilkins, Baltimore, pp 7.75–7.78
13. Fuchs C, Armstrong VW, Cremer P, Henning HV, Wieland H, Quellhorst E, Seidel D (1982) An investigation of the lipoprotein profiles of patients on hemofiltration as compared to those on hemodialysis and intermittent peritoneal dialysis. Contrib Nephrol 32: 92–96
14. Bosch JP, Glabman S, Moutousis G, Belledonne M, von Albertini B, Kahn T (1984) Carbon dioxide removal in acetate hemodialysis: effect on acid-base balance. Kidney Int 25: 830–837

Angioaccess

A. J. FÜRSCH and C. A. BALDAMUS

Table of Contents

Introduction

Replacement of renal function by extracorporeal treatment has been common since satisfactory methods for angioaccess became available. Ideally, angioaccess should have the following features:

1) Adequate extracorporeal blood flow
2) Long survival of access
3) Painless connection to extracorporeal circuit
4) Highest possible integrity of the patient's vessels
5) No disturbance of peripheral limb perfusion
6) Little influence on cardiac output
7) Simple connection to extracorporeal blood flow

The most common method wich best realizes these requirements is the arteriovenous (AV) fistula, inaugurated by CIMINO and BRESCIA [8]. The artificial kidney era did not begin until adequate angioaccess of high longevity became available. While the methods for angioaccess with hemodialysis (HD) and hemofiltration (HF) are quite similar, differences exist because of treatment-specific requirements.

The main aims in chronic intermittent HF are to achieve small-solute clearance rates comparable to those in standard HD and to shorten treatment time. Today HF includes:

a) postdilution HF,
b) predilution HF, and
c) continuous arteriovenous hemofiltration (CAVH).

Postdilution HF is at present the usual method for chronic intermittent HF. Until replacement fluid of adequate i. v. quality becomes available, at low prices, predilution HF as the regular form of treatment will be the exception.

Effective postdilution HF depends on a high blood flow (Q_B) (see the chapter by OFSTHUN et al.). High blood flow is essential to achieve filtration rates of more than 100 ml/min. Extracorporeal blood flow should be at least 300 ml/min or higher.

Because the angioaccess should deliver a high extracorporeal blood flow, in the vast majority of cases a high AV shunt volume results. This high shunt volume is one factor that increases cardiac output. Renal failure itself increases cardiac output too, mainly resulting from renal anemia [5, 10, 13]. The degree of increase in cardiac output is proportional to the degree of anemia, as has also been demonstrated in nonuremic patients [14, 27]. The development of high output heart failure in severely anemic patients (Hb lower than 5 g/dl) is well documented. Raising the cardiac output further by an additional high fistula shunt volume should increase the incidence of such heart failures. The same occurs with other cardiac diseases, such as atherosclerotic and hypertensive heart disease; calcific cardiopathy with or without fluid overload is occurring more frequently. Hemodynamic studies show that the fistula blood flow may contribute to up to 28% of resting cardiac output [1, 2, 23]. In the majority of patients, however, an AV shunt delivering a Q_B of about 300 ml/min does not seriously alter cardiac function.

Methods Measuring Blood flow

Several methods have previously been proposed to measure fistula blood flow indirectly. Measurements of cardiac output with and without occluded fistula give only a rough estimate of AV fistula blood flow. Studies based on plethysmographic and dilution methods reflect the blood flow of the limb rather than that of the AV fistula itself. The bidimensional, pulsed Doppler method may become the method of choice for determination of peripheral arterial blood flow in man [4]. Using a Doppler-transducer probe, BOUTHIER et al. showed that it is possible to evaluate the angle between the ultrasound beam and the vessel axis with minor error. Thus, blood flow can be calculated from arterial diameter and blood flow velocity. In their study, they showed a mean radial AV fistula blood flow of 728 ml/min ± 53 ml/min, brachial AV fistula of 778 ml/min ± 152 ml/min. Blood flow of brachial artery bovine heterograft AV fistulas amounted to 1225 ml/min ± 125 ml/min. Somewhat lower values (440 ml/min ± 108 ml/min) were reported by HIRSCHL et al. [16] in 40 forearm CB fistulas. The measurement, however, is technically complicated and in practice seldom performed.

As experiences shows, a lot of common angioaccesses primarily created for HD are suitable for the performance of HF. In what follows, the common angioaccess methods are described.

Percutaneous Venous Access

SHALDON and coworkers (in 1963) developed a procedure placing two catheters into the femoral vein using SELDINGER technique. This angioaccess can be used for up to 4 weeks and even for months at low morbidity [12, 19, 30]. This type of access was later extended to puncture of the jugular and subclavian veins. Some researchers approach the vena cava superior via an external jugular vein puncture [26], while others prefer placing catheters directly into the right atrium [11]. Some speculate that access survival can be extended to 2–3 years [11].

The classical Shaldon catheter placed into the vena cava inferior via the femoral vein fits the needs for HD, but is not suited for HF. The SHALDON catheter has the disadvantages of length and small interior diameter, which according to the Hagen-Poiseuille law, are obstacles to high blood flow, the essential prerequisite for HF. In this regard, the access route via the subclavian or jugular vein into the vena cava offers the advantage of allowing short catheters to be used. Other advantages are the patient's mobility, and a diminished risk of infection when compared with femoral catheters. Indications for percutaneous venous access in HF are (a) the need for immediate availability in emergency situations, (b) the need to bridge the interval until an internal AV fistula has healed and developed, and (c) as a last-choice vascular access.

A single jugular or subclavian catheter might be used for single-needle HD or HF, but adequacy of HD could technically be improved by the double-lumen catheter introduced by ULDALL et al. [33]. However, its applicability for HF with obligatory high blood flows has yet to be proven. There are several dangers using this technique, such as local infection, thrombosis of the central vein, sepsis, and in only a few cases retroperitoneal hematoma [31] or hemomediastinum.

Internal AV Fistula

CIMINO and BRESCIA described (in 1966) the technique of arterializing the superficial forearm veins by side-to-side anastomosis of the radial artery with cephalic vein. An internal AV fistula seems to be the optimal angioaccess for HD and HF to date. In view of the high Q_B necessary for HF, the question might arise whether a forearm CIMINO-BRESCIA (CB) fistula, with its typical anastomosis between the radial artery and the cephalic vein, is adequate access or whether a fistula with guaranteed high blood flow should be created as the first access. Although midarm, cubital, and upper arm variations of CB fistulas deliver primarily high blood flow, one should be careful, in view of future needs for angioaccess, not to spoil precious access possibilities by creating any of these latter fistulas as first-choice accesses. As shown by BOUTHIER et al. [4] and HIRSCHL et al. [16], adequate Q_B can be drained from the majority of classical CB fistulas.

The kind of surgical anastomosis technique (side-to-side, end-to-side, or end-to-end) chosen will depend in practice on the local circumstances and habits and seems to have only minor effects on blood flow.

Complications

Hypotension decreasing peripheral blood flow can be one of the reasons for thrombosis. Thrombosis may also develop from mural thrombi caused by needle puncture. Aneurysms provoke thrombosis. Stenosis at either the venous or arterial site of the fistula may reduce blood flow and endanger shunt thrombosis.

In comparison with external prothetic devices, the low infection rate of AV fistula is its major advantage. Simple hygienic rules for access puncture minimize infections. However, when infection occurs it is a serious complication with high risk of thrombosis and recurrent bacteremia with sepsis.

Repetitive punctures at the same site of the fistula may weaken the wall of the arterialized vessel and cause an aneurysmal dilatation of this region. Clinical problems seldom arise.

In the case of high pressure syndrome, adequate blood flow for HF can rarely be achieved.

Disturbances of distal limb perfusion occur if an adequate arterial blood flow is channeled into a low-resistance venous system. This can be due to an excessively wide anastomosis or to an inappropriately increased resistance of the distal arterial bed.

External Prosthetic Access

To this group belong the QINTON-SCRIBNER shunt, THOMAS shunt, BUSELMEIER shunt, and Hemasite. QUINTON and SCRIBNER inaugurated their shunt principle in 1960; this was one of the major contributions in renal replacement therapy. Their later modifications is still in use [24, 25]. In HF special attention has to be given to inserting vessel tips of the largest possible diameter to achieve optimal blood flow. Straight and short silicone tubings serve the same purpose.

THOMAS [32] described a composite device to be used in the groin. A Dracon face plate which is connected with Silastic tubing is sutured to the femoral artery and vein. The tubing is brought through the skin and joined on the outside to construct the shunt. This kind of shunt provides large flows, and 50% will be functioning

Table 1. Multicenter experience of device-related complications [9]

	Thigh	Arm (graft)	Arm (graftless)
No. of implants	23	89	17
Infection	4	12	2
Thrombosis	4	24	4
Stenosis	4	11	3
Seroma	2	2	–
Steal syndrome	–	3	1
Jump graft	1	3	1
Congestive heart failure	1	2	1
Contact dermatitis	1	6	1
Device below skin	2	5	0

Data from March 1981 to March 1982

2 years later [20, 22]. The danger of infection and severe bleeding from the femoral artery outweighs the advantages.

The shunt described by BUSELMEIER [6], a short subcutaneous U-tube having two nipples projecting beyond the skin, is difficult to implant and has not gained extensive popularity.

In July 1980, a new access device, Hemasite (Renal Systems Inc.), was introduced. The first results with thigh implants showed good survival, but infection was a concern. In March 1981 the device was modified to improve septum life [9]. The Hemasite angioaccess is provided as a carbon-coated device body with or without 6-mm arterial and venous PTFE grafts (Gore-tex). The grafted device is either placed into the proximal anterior thigh or the upper arm, or spliced into an existing upper-arm PTFE graft. Graftless devices can be placed into the venous side of a simple forearm or upper-arm fistula or into an existing forearm bovine graft. Flow rate seems to be sufficient. The Hemasite placed in the upper arm between the brachial artery and the brachial vein showed a blood flow through the Hemasite device of 730 ± 91 ml/min (6 cases) and 1088 ± 235 ml/min (5 cases) [3]. In a multicenter clinical trial over a 1-year period, the survival of Hemasite devices calculated as cumulative survival was 19% at 11 months; 122 patients were investigated and 229 devices implanted. Table 1 shows the device-related complications [9]. The patient acceptance was very high because the painful puncture was eliminated. Another advantage is minimal blood loss.

Complications

Early postimplantation thrombosis of the external angioaccess devices described above is due to surgical technique. Loss of access is mostly related to infection and, in the very late period, to skin retraction around the carbon port. Although favorable survival data have been published for the Hemasite device, future large-scale clinical application will prove or disprove its long-term applicability [17].

Unnoted disconnection of external devices is a frightening complication, occasionally leading to exsanguination and death.

The THOMAS shunt involves the highest risk of initiating congestive heart failure because of its high and unpredictable shunt volume. A further complication arises from peripheral leg ischemia.

Graft AV Fistulas

Angioaccess using graft material is generally a method of secondary choice. Graft materials include an

- autologous vein (vena saphena magna)
- homologous (vena saphena magna) and umbilical veins (placental),
- heterologous tubes of collagen grafts or bovine carotid artery, and
- alloplastic material (Dacron, velour, PTFE).

The autologous saphenous vein is not the ideal graft material [21]. Autologous and allogenic material is seldom used. Although bovine carotid artery has been implanted frequently, it is being increasingly replaced by synthetic prosthesis.

The graft material most often used today is alloplastic material like Dacron and PTFE. PTFE grafts like Impra, (one-layer prosthesis), or Gore-tex (a two-layer prosthesis) are very commonly used in practice. Although the majority of PTFE grafts guarantee adequate blood flow for HF, the posttreatment bleeding time, especially when using large bore needles for HF, is prolonged because synthetic graft do not contract as natural vessel walls do.

Complications

Often myoepithelial elements of the intima proliferate at the site of the graft-to-vein junction with progressive narrowing of the lumen of the vein, and this leads to thrombosis. About 50% of thromboses occur because of poor venous run-off [7].

Due to the extensive operation, wound infection is a major risk. In some cases infection can only be cured by removal of the graft.

The kind of angioaccess chosen depends on the patient's circumstances. First, a subcutaneous AV fistula should be tried in the nondominant forearm. If this is not successful, the other possibilities should be chosen bearing in mind that a patient's survival is largely dependent on angioaccess using renal replacement therapy.

Continuous Arteriovenous Hemofiltration

The physical principle of continuous arteriovenous hemofiltration (CAVH) takes advantage of the AV pressure gradient and uses it as the driving force for the extracorporeal circuit. This is only possible with direct vascular access to a main artery or vein. For the technical variation of a pump-driven continuous HF, any of the above-discussed vascular accesses can be used. In some patients, this latter form of continuous treatment can even be applied by puncturing two peripheral veins because only low blood-flow rates are necessary.

To date, continuous HF is limited to acute renal failure patients and of these especially to the most severely ill multiorgan failure patients in intensive care units (see the chapter by Bosch on CAVH). This special form of treatment requires different extracorporeal circulation than is the case with patients on intermittent HF. Intensive care patients with renal failure quite frequently suffer from cardiovascular complications resulting in low systemic blood pressure. Therefore, it is mandatory with CAVH to use extracorporeal circulation material with low flow resistance. The SCRIBNER shunt is frequently used for CAVH.

KRAMER, who in 1977 first described CAVH, gave preference to access to the femoral artery and vein [18]. The puncture set, which his group suggested, contains

- an insertion needle,
- a guide wire with a 4-cm flexible tip,
- a dilating catheter,
- and a permanent catheter.

The material used as permanent catheter is Teflon mixed with polypropylene. This catheter, with a length of 11 cm (conncetions not included), has only a one-tip orifice and a diameter of 8-10 ch, to obtain high blood flow at low internal flow resistance. The technique of puncturing the femoral artery and vein is based on SELDINGER's method [28].

KRAMER et al., who have the most and longest experience with this technique, reported a low rate of puncture-related complications. Two patients from a population of 150 [15] had major bleeding complications.

In an analysis of the autopsy reports of 16 patients who died of causes unrelated to CAVH, Kramer's group found various large thrombi within the catheter lumen in all the cases. The size of thrombi was not dependent on the amount of time that the catheter had been in place. Lung embolization, possibly deriving from the venous site, could not be found. In one patient, the popliteal artery was embolized as a consequence of the arterial catheter. No infection of the catheter site was detected in these patients.

The authors discussed the following as possible complications of CAVH:

1) Thrombosis
2) Thrombophlebitis
3) Embolism of peripheral arteries and of lung
4) Sepsis

5) Bleeding
6) Aneurysm of artery
7) Development of a local AV-shunt
8) Damage to the nerve

The very optimistic experience reported by Gröne and Kramer in this rather small patient population will be challenged in the future as CAVH following Kramer's technique becomes more widely practiced.

A permanent external angioaccess with long survival would help to realize the dream of continuous HF in chronic renal failure patients as was suggested by Shaldon [29].

References

1. Ahearn DJ, Maher JF (1972) Heart failure as a complication of hemodialysis arteriovenous fistula. Ann Intern Med 77: 201
2. Anderson CB, Codd JR, Craff GM, Harter HR, Newton WT (1976) Cardiac failure and upper extremity arteriovenous dialysis fistulas. Arch Intern Med 136: 292
3. Bonalumi U, Simoni GA, Friedman D, Borzone E, Griffanti F (1984) Initial experience with hemasite vascular access device %HD < for maintenance hemodialysis. Kidney Int 26: 540
4. Bouthier JD, Levenson JA, Simon AC, Bariety JM, Bourquelot PE, Safar ME (1983) A noninvasive determination of fistula blood flow in dialysis patients. Artif Organs 7: 404
5. Bower JD, Coleman TG (1969) Circulatory function during chronic hemodialysis. Trans Am Soc Artif Intern Organs 15: 373
6. Buselmeier TJ, Simmons RL, Najarian JS, Ducean DA, von Hartitsch B, Kjellstrand CM (1973) The clinical application of a new prothetic arteriovenous shunt. Nephron 12: 22
7. Butt KMH (1978) Bovine heterograft for arteriovenous fistulas. In: Sawyer PN (ed) Vascular grafts. Appleton-Century-Crofts, New York, p 278
8. Brescia MJ, Cimino JE, Appel K, Hurwich BJ (1966) Chronic hemodialysis using venipuncture and a surgically created arteriovenous fistula. N Engl J Med 275: 1089
9. Collins AJ, Shapiro FL, Keshaviah P, Ilstrup K, Andersen R, O'Brien T, Costentino LC (1983) Multicentre clinical experience with the hemasite blood access device. In: Kootstra G (ed) Access surgery. MTP Press, Lancaster, p 297
10. De Fazio V, Christensen RC, Regan TJ, Baer LJ, Morita Y, Hellems HK (1959) Circulatory changes in acute glomerulonephritis. Circulation 20: 190
11. Francis DMA, Hoenich NA, Taylor RMR, Ward MK, Kerr DNS (1983) An indwelling right atrial catheter for long-term hemodialysis. Trans Am Soc Artif Intern Organs 29: 348
12. Friedman EA, Butt KMH, Pascua LJ, Hardy MA, Lawton RL, Uldall PR (1979) Vascular access update. Trans Am Soc Artif Intern Organs 25: 526
13. Goss JE, Alfrey AC, Vogel JHK, Holmes JH (1967) Hemodynamic changes during hemodialysis. Trans Am Soc Artif Intern Organs 13: 68
14. Graettinger JS, Parsons RL, Campbell JA (1963) Correlation of clinical and hemodynamic studies in patients with mild and severe anemia with and without congestive failure. Ann Intern Med 58: 617
15. Gröne HJ, Kramer P (1982) Punktion und Langzeitkanülierung der Arteria - und Vena femoralis beim Erwachsenen. In: Kramer P (ed) Arteriovenöse Hämofiltration. Vandenhoeck and Ruprecht, Göttingen
16. Hirschl M, Ehringer H, Marosi L, Minar E, Schmidt P, Zazgornik J (1984) Perkutane quantitative Shuntflußmessung an großen Transportarterien bei chronischen Dialysepatienten (Percutaneous quantitative shunt flow measurement and flow measurement of large transport arteries in chronic dialysis patients). Vasa 13: 159
17. Kaplan AA, Grant J, Galler M, Galen MA, Longnecker RE (1983) Regional experience with the Hemasite no-needle access device. Trans Am Soc Artif Intern Organs 29: 369

18. Kramer P, Wigger W, Rieger D, Matthaei D, Scheler F (1977) Arterio-venous hemofiltration: a new and simple method for treatment of over-hydrated patients resistant to diuretics. Klin Wochenschr 55: 1121
19. Kjellstrand CM, Merino GE, Mauer SM, Casali R, Buselmeier TJ (1975) Complications of percutaneous femoral vein chatheterization for hemodialysis. Clin Nephrol 4: 37
20. May J, Johnson JR, Evans R, Sheil AGR (1969) Experience with large vessel applique (Thomas) shunts for hemodialysis. Med J Aust 2: 77
21. May J, Harris J, Fletcher J (1980) Long-term results of saphenous vein graft arteriovenous fistulas. Am J Surg 140: 387
22. Morgan AP, Knight DC, Tilney NL, Lazarus JM (1980) Femoral triangle sepsis in dialysis patients; frequency, management and outcome. Ann Surg 191: 460
23. Payne RM, Soderblom RE, Lobstein PH, Hull AR, Mullins CB (1972) Exercise-induced hemodynamic effects of arteriovenous fistulas used for hemodialysis. Kidney Int 2: 344
24. Quinton WE, Dillard DH, Scribner BH (1960) Cannulation of blood vessels for prolonged hemodialysis. Trans Am Soc Artif Intern Organs 6: 104
25. Quinton WE, Dillard DH, Cole JJ, Scribner BH (1962) Eight month's experience with Silastic-Teflon cannulas. Trans Am Soc Artif Intern Organs 8: 236
26. Reed WP, Light PD, Sadler JH (1934) Access for hemodialysis by means of long-term central venous catheters. Kidney Int 25: 838
27. Richardson TQ, Guyton AC (1959) Effects of polycythemia and anemia on cardiac output and other circulatory factors. Am J Physiol 197: 1167
28. Seldinger SJ (1953) Catheter replacement of needle in percutaneous arteriography new technique. Acta Radiol 39: 368
29. Shaldon S, Beau MC, Deschodt G, Lysaght MJ, Ramperez P (1980) Contineous ambulatory hemofiltration. Trans Am Soc Artif Intern Organs 26: 210
30. Shaldon S, Silva H, Pomeroy J, Rae AJ, Rosen SM (1964) Percutaneous femoral venous catheterization and reusable dialyzers in the treatment of acute renal failure. Trans Am Soc Artif Intern Organs 10: 133
31. Sharp KW, Spees EK, Selby LR, Zachary JB, Ernst CB (1984) Diagnosis and management of retroperitoneal hematoma after femoral vein cannulation for hemodialysis. Surgery 95: 90
32. Thomas GJ (1969) A large-vessel applique a-v shunt for hemodialysis. Trans Am Soc Artif Intern Organs 15: 288
33. Uldall PR, Woods F, Merchant N, Crichton E, Carter H (1980) A double-lumen subcalvian cannula (DLSC) for temporary hemodialysis access. Trans Am Soc Artif Intern Organs 26: 93

Quantitation and Prescription of Therapy

L. W. Henderson and J. K. Leypoldt

Table of Contents

Introduction

Since the inception of artificial kidney treatment, the renal clinician/researcher has been faced with the need to determine an adequate amount of therapy for the patient. As the artificial kidney attempts to replace the excretory function of the native kidney, determination of solute removal rates by the artificial kidney provides an important element necessary for quantitation of therapy. The classic work of Wolf et al. [1], who introduced the term dialysance to describe solute transport by hemodialyzers in analogy to renal clearance as defined by Van Slyke [2], was a major contribution and facilitated comparison of solute removal by the artificial kidney with that of the native kidney. Additional studies [3–5] provided the functional dependence of solute removal by the artificial kidney on clinical operating conditions, such as blood flow rate, dialyzer flow rate, membrane area, and membranes with different permeability spectra. While such studies contributed materially toward greater understanding of the impact of these variables on solute removal by the artificial kidney, they helped little, in the absence of good quality clinical correlations, to decide what an adequate amount of therapy should be for a given patient.

Based upon a qualitative understanding of artificial kidney performance, general working guidelines for an adequate prescription have been empirically established from an enormous body of clinical experience in the treatment of end stage renal failure (ESRF) patients with hemodialysis (HD). Notable advances in this highly empirical state of affairs were made in the past decade by researchers using different approaches. BABB, SCRIBNER and coworkers have promoted the concept of prescribing treatment by square meter-hour [6] and the dialysis index [7]. For example, the dialysis index prescribes an equivalent removal of solutes with a molecular size equivalent to vitamin B_{12} as that for a standard treatment with a D-1 Kiil hemodialyzer. The strength underlying these concepts lies in extensive experience with different clinical dialysis treatment techniques which assured a satisfactory "state of the art" best clinical result. The weakness of this approach is the uncertain identity of and inability to measure the solute (or solutes) that must be removed to assure adequate correction of uremia. Thus, the initial focus on such small molecular weight solutes as water, potassium, urea, and creatinine was redirected by SCRIBNER to concerns about middle molecules [8], solutes with molecular weights between the above mentioned small molecular weight solutes (less than 500 daltons) and large solutes the size of proteins (greater than 60000 daltons). Another approach to the prescription of HD therapy that was formulated during the past decade was urea kinetic modeling, as popularized by SARGENT and GOTCH [9, 10]. By focusing on the readily measured solute urea, the quantitation of therapy was more concrete and provided the opportunity for individualized prescription. This approach demonstrated the importance of uremic solute generation or accumulation rates and returned attention to and gave a quantitative frame of reference for what was empirically known about small molecular weight toxicity.

The following review is an effort to clarify the role of kinetic modeling of solutes in HD as a means to provide quantitation of therapy, to examine its contributions and limitations in the prescription of HD therapy, and to apply this knowledge to the quantitation and prescription of HF therapy.

Quantitation and Prescription of Hemodialysis Therapy

Urea Kinetic Modeling

At present, kinetic modeling of urea using a variable volume, single pool model for the quantitation of HD therapy has the soundest clinical base to judge its contribution. Although other more complicated models where two or more pools are employed have lent insight into the dynamics of urea concentrations with time [11, 12], they are generally perceived as too complex to be used in the clinic. The single pool urea model is conceptually simple, but the mathematical details are relatively complex and are described in the Appendix. It is noted that although this discussion is concerned with kinetic modeling of urea, it also applies to other solutes that can be assumed to be adequately described by a single pool model.

To apply urea kinetic modeling for the quantitation of therapy, it is necessary to measure the concentration of urea prior to treatment (C_{o1}), at the conclusion of treatment (C_{t1}), and prior to the next treatment (C_{o2}). With careful timing of the duration of dialysis t_d and the interval between treatments Θ, coupled with knowledge of the dialyzer clearance for urea K_d, the volume of distribution for urea V and, more importantly, the generation or accumulation rate for urea G can both be calculated. The values of V and G are obtained by solving the following two simultaneous equations iteratively (on a digital computer or hand calculator [13]):

$$V = \frac{K_d t_d}{\ln\left[\dfrac{C_{o1} - G/K_d}{C_{t1} - G/K_d}\right]} \tag{1}$$

$$G = \frac{(C_{o2} - C_{t1})V}{\Theta} \tag{2}$$

In this example, we have neglected the residual renal clearance of urea K_r and the changes in urea distribution volume that may result from ultrafiltration during the dialysis procedure. The addition of these variables does not result in any conceptual differences in this approach, but may be necessary for certain clinical applications (see Appendix).

To use the computed values of V and G for the prescription of HD therapy, it is necessary to understand how they relate to clinical parameters. BORAH and coworkers [14] have shown that the generation of urea is directly related to the protein catabolic rate (PCR) and is similar for both normal individuals and ESRF patients. A recent modification of this relationship between the PCR and G is given by the following [15]:

$$PCR = 9.35G + 0.294V \tag{3}$$

where the units of PCR, G, and V are g/day, mg/min, and liters, respectively. For patients that are maintained in nitrogen balance, the protein catabolic rate is approximately equal to the dietary protein intake (DPI). The value of V approximates the volume of total body water [16], approximately 60% of body weight.

The prescribed amount of therapy, cast in terms of the volume of urea cleared $K_d t_d$ to achieve a desired blood urea concentration, can be calculated for the patient with a stable DPI and body weight (or values of G and V) from the above equations. The procedures for such calculations are complex and have been described by others elsewhere [9, 17]. Much of this complexity results from the nonuniform interdialytic times that apply to patients treated on Mondays, Wednesdays, and Fridays. It is, however, instructive to illustrate these calculations with certain simplifying assumptions as described recently by LOWRIE and TEEHAN [18]. By assuming constant interdialytic time intervals and neglecting the generation of urea when the patient is on dialysis, LOWRIE and TEEHAN have shown that the prescribed amount of treatment can be approximately calculated by the following:

$$K_d t_d = - V \ln (1 - G\bar{\Theta}/VC_o) \tag{4}$$

where C_o is the target midweek pretreatment urea concentration and $\bar{\Theta}$ is the mean interdialytic interval. Because of recent clinical studies (see below), it is also of interest to express this result in terms of the time averaged urea concentration (TAC_{urea}) that can be approximated by

$$TAC_{urea} = (C_o + C_t)/2 \qquad (5)$$

The midweek pretreatment and posttreatment urea concentrations will provide a simple estimate of TAC_{urea}. The prescription formula is then given by

$$K_d t_d = V \ln \left[\frac{1 + G\bar{\Theta}/2V\,TAC_{urea}}{1 - G\bar{\Theta}/2V\,TAC_{urea}} \right] \qquad (6)$$

The use of either Eq. (4) or (6) allows one to determine the quantity of therapy to achieve the desired midweek pretreatment urea concentration C_o or time averaged urea concentration TAC_{urea} with predetermined values of G and V. The quantity of therapy can be varied by either altering the treatment time for a dialyzer with a given urea clearance or by altering the dialyzer clearance for a given treatment time. The desired urea clearance can be obtained clinically by using dialyzers with different membrane areas or by altering the blood and/or dialysate flow rates. It is notable that this formulation is very flexible and allows the dialysis prescription to be individualized to each patient. Moreover, the dialysis prescription can be easily altered with changes in patient DPI, since a new estimate of the value of G can be calculated with Eq. (3). More details of the application of urea kinetic modeling for the prescription of HD therapy are described elsewhere by others [9, 15–18].

There are several fundamental assumptions involved in this model that require elucidation. First, urea is assumed to be equally distributed throughout a single body compartment. Urea is generally believed to be distributed in total body water, and the volume of distribution for urea as calculated by urea kinetic modeling yields values that are often in good agreement with estimates of total body water. This suggests that the urea mass transfer coefficient across both the cell wall and the capillary vascular wall greatly exceeds the urea clearance of the dialyzer employed. While it is likely true that urea transport across the capillary wall is sufficiently fast to allow rapid equilibration [12], transport rates across the cell wall may be limiting. This slow movement of urea across the cell wall may result in the well known rebound of urea concentration in the hour following dialysis, in addition to the concern about dialysis disequilibrium syndrome when large surface area, high clearance dialyzers are used in patients with high starting urea concentrations. The rebound of urea concentration following dialysis may also result from a violation of a different assumption of this model. The generation rate for urea (and also dialyzer clearance) is assumed to be independent of time. Others have shown, however, that generation of urea is greater on days on dialysis than on days off dialysis [16, 19, 20]. As a result of these studies, HD has been described as a catabolic process, yet the mechanisms resulting in this phenomenon are not well understood. Several possible mechanisms may stimulate protein breakdown, such as the loss during dialysis therapy of amino acids and polypeptides or the rapid fall in urea concentration [20]. Glucose loss has, however, been shown [19, 20] not to influence this increase in protein catabolic rate. An additional possible mechanism for increased protein breakdown during dialysis with cellulosic membranes is the catabolic action of interleu-kin-1 [21, 22] that is released as a result of complement activation.

Although the above assumptions are necessary for the accurate quantitation of therapy using urea kinetic modeling, the fundamental assumption of urea kinetic modeling for prescription of therapy is that either urea is a toxic solute or urea concentration bears a relationship to the concentration of the most toxic uremic solutes. JOHNSON et al. [23] have shown that adding urea to the dialysate solution, resulting in relatively large blood urea concentrations (up to 300 mg/dl), does not produce any acutely demonstrable toxic symptoms. The success of a therapeutic prescription for HD using urea kinetic modeling does not identify the toxic solute or the toxic solute molecular weight, but only requires that it bear a relationship to urea and result from protein catabolism.

Other Considerations and Constraints

Application of urea kinetic modeling for the prescription of therapy with techniques other than HD has not yet been clinically qualified and as such may not be appropriate. If urea is not the only toxic solute, but rather merely a surrogate for other toxins of different molecular weight, then its surrogate status could be altered by phenomena specific to the treatment and not accounted for by urea kinetic modeling. For example, urea kinetic modeling suggests that only the quantity of therapy (the product $K_d t_d$) is important and that therapy prescription is independent of the duration of dialysis treatment. The clinical observations by SCRIBNER [8] and, subsequently, but independently, by SHALDON [24] that certain uremic symptoms, such as uremic neuropathy, were less with longer dialysis times suggest that the duration of dialysis treatment is an important independent prescription variable. This basic observation has recently been reaffirmed by the National Cooperative Dialysis Study (NCDS), as discussed below. The above clinical observations led to the concern that molecules of larger molecular weight contributed significantly to uremic morbidity. As plasma levels of a uremic toxin show an exponential fall with time on dialysis, with small solutes more swiftly removed than large ones, it follows that the driving force for the diffusional transport of small solutes deteriorates more rapidly than for large ones. Adding an additional hour to the treatment time results in an increase in the relative loss of large solutes compared with small ones. This concept is obscured when cast in terms of clearance which by the nature of its definition is relatively constant throughout the treatment. Duration of therapy is then one potential factor that can alter the relation between urea and its surrogate toxins. Consideration of treatment time, therefore, needs to be addressed when urea kinetic modeling is used to guide HD therapy.

A second means for altering the relationship between the concentration of urea and its surrogate toxins involves the difference in the solute clearance profile of the separating membrane. At least two areas of concern bear on this second potential limitation in guiding treatment solely on urea kinetic modeling. Membranes with significantly different permeability spectra, while removing equivalent amounts of urea, will remove considerably different amounts of other solutes. An extreme case of this would be the peritoneal membrane where the relative dialysance of urea to inulin is tenfold greater than with a Cuprophan HD membrane [25]. This line of reasoning is of importance when contrasting HD and HF membranes. Second, residual renal function, even at very low levels, is a convective process and can make a major impact on solute removed, since its permeability spectrum is dramatically different from that of the artificial kidney treatment employed. This point contributed materially to SCRIBNER's early thinking about middle molecules [26]. For example, a residual glomerular filtration rate of 5 ml/min will clear 10 l/week of both urea and inulin; whereas, 1 m^2 Cuprophan HD treatment with three 5-h treatments will clear only 4.5 l/week of inulin, but 40-50 l/week of urea.

Clinical Implications of the National Cooperative Dialysis Study

The National Cooperative Dialysis Study (NCDS) was designed to test whether urea kinetic modeling could provide a quantitative approach to the prescription of HD. The NCDS was a large-scale, carefully controlled study that included 160 patients from nine different dialysis centers in the United States who had protein catabolic rates between 0.8 and 1.4 g/day/kg body weight. These patients were without significant residual renal function and were treated three times a week with either Cuprophan or cellulose acetate dialyzers. After completing a control phase of the study, each patient was randomly assigned to one of four experimental groups that differed in time duration of treatment and blood concentrations of urea. As the time duration of dialysis treatment was fixed for each experimental group, urea blood concentrations were maintained by altering the urea clearance of the dialyzer guided by the urea kinetic model. Clinical outcome of each experimental group was extensively monitored, and detailed reports of these study variables have recently been published [27].

The most forceful message that comes from the NCDS is the strong correlation between TAC$_{urea}$ and patient morbidity. Simply stated, this study suggests that urea and the toxins for which it is surrogate have important etiologic roles in the morbid events occurring in the maintenance dialysis population. Figure 1 shows the probability of failure for each of the experimental groups as a function of the protein catabolic rate normalized by body weight as predicted by a statistical model of the study results [28]. Failure was defined here as death, withdrawal of the experimental dialysis prescription for medical reasons, or the occurrence of a morbid event that required hospitalization. For each experimental group, the probability of failure decreased with increasing values of the normalized PCR, indicating that a low dietary protein intake is clearly associated with greater morbidity. This analysis also permits selecting out the separate effects of different time averaged urea concentrations (low TAC$_{urea}$ of 53 mg/ml, high TAC$_{urea}$ of 88 mg/ml) and different treatment times (long t_d of 4.5 h, short t_d of 3.2 h). For a fixed protein catabolic rate of 1 g/day/kg body weight, the graphs can be read from left to right showing that a high TAC$_{urea}$ in patients on long treatment time increases the probability of failure from 10% to

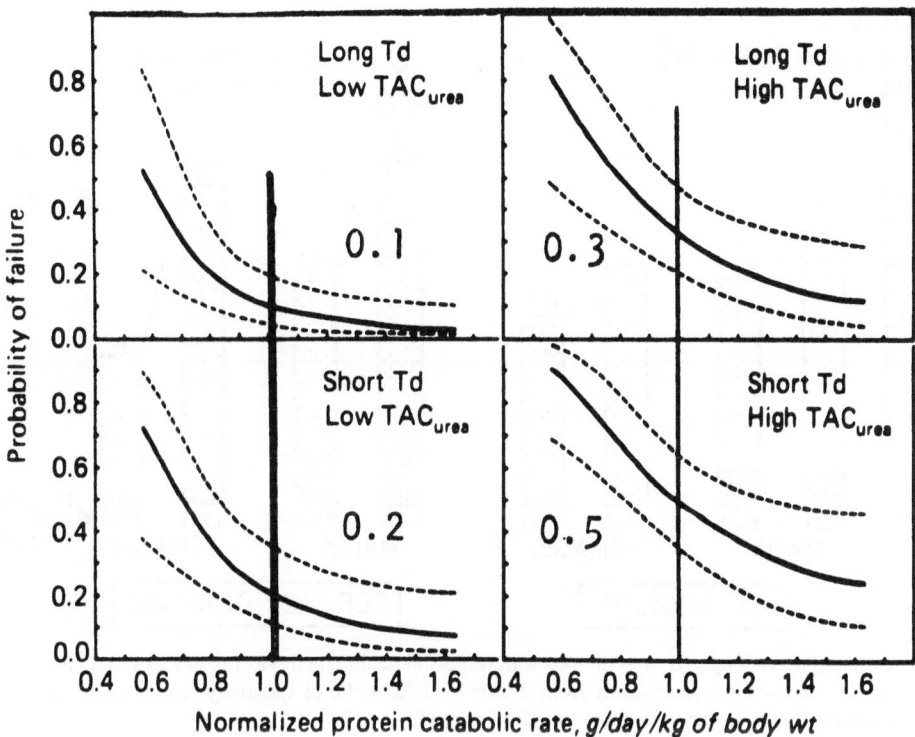

Fig. 1. The probability of failure (see text for definition) plotted as a function of normalized protein catabolic rate. *Dotted lines* represent the 95% confidence limits. *Vertical lines* at a normalized PCR of 1 g/day/kg body weight are taken for arbitrary comparison of the two investigative strategies. Modified from LAIRD et al. [28]

30%. For short treatment time, the failure rate rises from 20% to 50%, when a high TAC$_{urea}$ is allowed. Urea or the toxins for which it is surrogate correlate strongly with important clinical measures of bad outcome.

The vertical reading of Fig. 1, also at a fixed protein catabolic rate of 1 g/day/kg body weight, offers similar information about the influence of treatment time t_d. Shorter treatment time protocols show an approximate doubling of the failure rate as well, from 10% to 20% for the low TAC$_{urea}$ group and from 30% to 50% for the high TAC$_{urea}$ group. As noted above, the duration of dialysis treatment may be regarded as surrogate for toxins that are larger in molecular weight than urea. The design of this study called for the adjustment of urea clearance by either altering blood flow rate, dialysate flow rate, or membrane area. For example, to achieve a short treatment time and a low TAC$_{urea}$, a large area membrane might be selected. In like fashion, to achieve a long treatment time with a high TAC$_{urea}$, a small area membrane would be selected. Therefore, although the duration of treatment was decreased by one-third, the decrease of the product of treatment duration times membrane area, a better measure of the removal of larger molecules [6], was much less. These two opposing effects would be expected to minimize the influence of larger molecular weight toxins on the study results. A statistically significant decrease in morbidity with longer time on dialysis was nevertheless found, not surprisingly at a

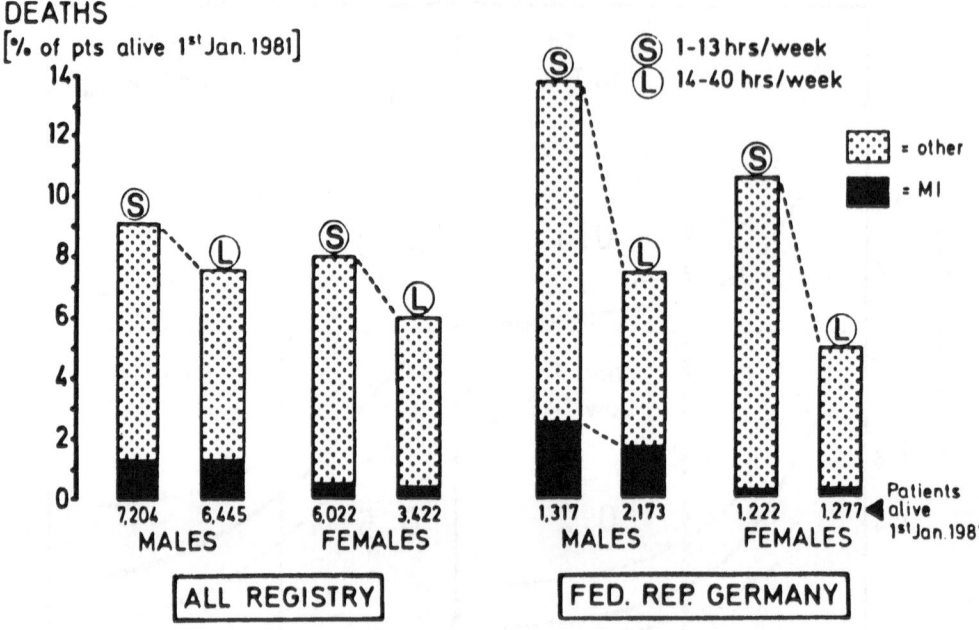

Fig. 2. Comparison of long and short dialysis with respect to death rate by sex for all registered patients and a more homogeneous subset from the Federal Republic of Germany. The fraction of
deaths resulting from myocardial infarction *(MI)* is noted [29]

lower level of significance. We must conclude, then, that given the experimental design, the contributions to morbid events made by variation in treatment time in the
NCDS must be considered to be minimum values and supportive of the pathophysiological importance of molecules of larger molecular weight than conventional
uremic toxins.

The importance of treatment time has also been previously shown to be a significant variable of the dialysis prescription in other less well controlled, retrospective
clinical reports. The 1981 report on regular dialysis and transplantation in Europe
as prepared by the European Dialysis and Transplantation Association [29] compared the death rate for short dialysis (1-13 h/week) with long dialysis (14-40 h/
week). Figure 2 (from this work) shows that for both male and female patients, the
death rate was lower for long dialysis. In addition, for patients from the Federal Republic of Germany (this population had the highest incidence of HD patients who
had never received a renal allograft), survival on long dialysis was even more striking than for all registry patients. These findings are again best explained by the presence and pathophysiological importance of solutes with larger molecular weights
than urea.

In summary, the NCDS has shown that HD therapy can be quantified and applied to individual patients in a manner that lowers patient morbidity in comparison with other, more empirical, treatment schedules. The prescription for HD therapy using Cuprophan or cellulose acetate dialyzers should include both an adequate
dietary protein intake (greater than 1 g/day/kg body weight) as well as sufficient dialysis to maintain a TAC_{urea} at or below 60 mg/dl maintaining the level of urea and

its surrogates at safe concentrations. This prescription is, however, not independent of treatment time and cannot be extrapolated beyond the limits of the study or cavalierly applied to other artificial kidney treatment modalities such as HD with membranes of different permeability spectra, peritoneal dialysis, or HF.

Quantitation and Prescription of Hemofiltration Therapy

At present, the guidelines for adequate HF therapy are not well developed. The amount of HF treatment is commonly cast in terms of the amount of liters of plasma water exchanged per treatment (or per week). Certain, more recent, prescriptions have accounted for differences in patient size by altering the amount of plasma water exchanged as a percentage of patient body weight. While this designation may have clinical utility for a specific patient/membrane combination, it loses force when comparisons are made between patients with different nutritional needs or with hemofilters that have different solute transport characteristics.

Urea Kinetic Modeling

The application of urea kinetic modeling for the quantitation of HF therapy can be performed by analogous extrapolation from the extensive studies with HD. Assuming a urea sieving coefficient of unity, urea kinetic modeling for postdilution HF is identical to that for HD if the ultrafiltration flow rate is substituted for the urea dialyzer clearance. Indeed, several recent reports [30, 31] have applied urea kinetic modeling to HF and demonstrated the need for individualization of therapy. It has also been reported [32] that postdilution HF like HD is a catabolic process with generation rates for urea greater on HF than when the treatment is not applied. In all reported aspects, urea kinetic modeling for the quantitation of HF therapy is similar to HD.

The recent study by Bosch and coworkers [30] has applied a more simple approach to the prescription of HF therapy that also accounts for differences in patient dietary protein intake. They studied ten patients on both HD and HF, applying urea kinetic modeling as described above to quantitate the patient urea generation rate G and urea distribution volume V. The reported values of G and V were similar whether patients were on either HD or HF. Furthermore, they suggested the following simple formula for the prescription of HF therapy [30]:

$$\text{Ultrafiltrate} = \frac{\text{DPI} \times 0.12 \times 7}{0.70} \tag{7}$$

where ultrafiltrate is the number of liters per week required to achieve a mean urea nitrogen concentration of 0.70 g/l. The value of DPI is the dietary protein intake (g/day) based upon dietary interviews. This equation is based upon a simple weekly urea mass balance, since the amount of urea removed per week (ultrafiltrate $\times$ 0.70 g/l) is equated to the amount generated [DPI $\times$ 0.12 (the amount of nitrogen recovered per g of protein ingested)[1] $\times$ 7 (the number of days in a week)]. It is notable that this prescription formula is independent of the volume of distribution for urea. As stated by these workers [30], this formula requires a stable patient and a residual renal function not greater than 1.4 ml/min. These workers report that Eq. (7) provides for more individualized therapy (that accounts for differences in urea generation rate) than does the alternative of simply using a constant number of liters per treatment or an amount that depends upon a fraction of body weight. It should be emphasized that although these recent studies have shown that HF therapy can be quantified and therapy can be prescribed using urea kinetic modeling, the adequacy of the therapy prescription has not been sufficiently addressed. Extensive prospective clinical qualifying studies will be required before the amount of treatment may properly be prescribed using urea kinetic modeling; to date, no such qualification is available.

Nonetheless, the formula introduced by BOSCH and coworkers is sufficiently simple and interesting that it requires further comment. The extension of this approach to situations where residual renal function is important is straightforward. Expressed in terms of traditional urea kinetic modeling parameters, this extended version of Eq. (7) is simply

$$K_d T_d = T \left[\frac{G}{\text{TAC}_{\text{urea}}} - K_r \right] \tag{8}$$

where the values of T_d and T are the weekly duration of treatment and the total elapsed time (i. e., hours in a week), respectively. This weekly version of the urea kinetic modeling equations can provide a more simple approach to quantitation of therapy than that previously described by others. First, the volume of distribution of urea is not an important parameter in patient morbidity and does not appear in the prescription formula. Second, this equation shows directly the interrelationship between the parameters and does not require a computer for calculations. Third, it emphasizes the relationship between the amount of therapy and the urea generation rate, an important parameter determining patient morbidity. Finally, it can be applied to HD as well as HF.

The application of Eq. (8) for prescribing therapy is simple once the generation rate for urea is known. The clinician/researcher chooses the desired TAC_{urea} and simply computes the weekly amount of urea clearance required (for postdilution HF $K_d T_d$ is simply the weekly exchange volume). Equation (8) can also be used for estimating the patient generation rate of urea. The value of TAC_{urea} can be approximated by the average of the pretreatment and posttreatment midweek urea concentrations (Eq. (5)). By accurate measurement of the total weekly exchange volume $K_d T_d$, the generation rate for urea is given by rearrangement of Eq. (8) to

---

1 While 0.16 is the commonly cited factor for determining the nitrogen content of protein, both the quality of the ingested protein and the nutritional status of the subject injesting the protein can affect the relationship of urea nitrogen appearance in the blood to dietary protein intake [33]. The given value of 0.12 is a reasonable estimate of the appearance rate.

$$G = \left[\frac{K_d T_d}{T} + K_r \right] (C_o + C_t)/2 \tag{9}$$

Note also that Eq. (8) and (9) are flexible and can be applied over a 2-week period or a monthly interval.

Equation (8) can be used to assess the empirical approach for prescribing HF therapy as applied today by Clinician-Researchers as compared with the recommendations from the NCDS. For example, QUELLHORST et al., who have the largest single population on maintenance HF, have recently published a summary of morbidity and mortality for these patients [34]. The amount of therapy was initially guided by offering a 20 l exchange per treatment that gave way to a formula that resulted in one-third of the body weight being exchanged per treatment. This prescription resulted in blood urea and creatinine concentrations that are similar to those achieved by routine HD. A comparison of this amount of therapy with that suggested by the NCDS for HD can be calculated using Eq. (8). Neglecting residual renal clearance and assuming the recommended TAC_{urea} of 60 mg/ml with a PCR of at least 1 g/day/kg body weight, Eq. (8) suggests that $K_d T_d$ should be at a minimum of 180% of body weight or $K_d t_d$ should be 60% of body weight for each of the three weekly treatments. Thus, the adequacy of therapy as guided by urea kinetic modeling and the recommendations of the NCDS for HD suggest that these patients on HF should be at risk. In a retrospective examination of other, earlier HF studies, GOTCH [35] has similarly reasoned that patients on HF may have lower protein catabolic rates than those on HD because of decreased urea clearance putting these patients at nutritional risk. QUELLHORST and coworkers have, however, found [34] no difference in morbidity and mortality between maintenance HD ($N = 132$) and HF ($N = 115$) using this prescription in "standard" populations (patients aged 15–60 years old with no serious complication such as diabetes mellitus, malignant tumors, systemic or severe cardiovascular or cerebrovascular disease). These extensive clinical observations suggest that the recommendations of the NCDS for HD cannot be directly applied to HF and that other mechanisms must be at work to compensate for the additional risks involved in allowing high blood urea concentrations and low protein catabolic rates. It is of interest to note that patients on chronic ambulatory peritoneal dialysis (CAPD) also have low protein catabolic rates [36, 37] that fall below the nutritional recommendations of the NCDS.

Other Considerations

Although there are other clinical advantages to HF over HD, such as improved tolerance to ultrafiltration and perhaps better control of blood pressure that could compensate for this increased risk with high TAC_{urea}, a most interesting explanation, especially in light of the significant effect of duration of treatment as reported by the NCDS, is the difference in the properties of the membranes employed during HF. One feature of HF therapy is the increased removal of larger molecular weight solutes and this increased removal of larger molecular weight solutes may "compensate" for the high blood urea concentrations. If the removal of large molecular

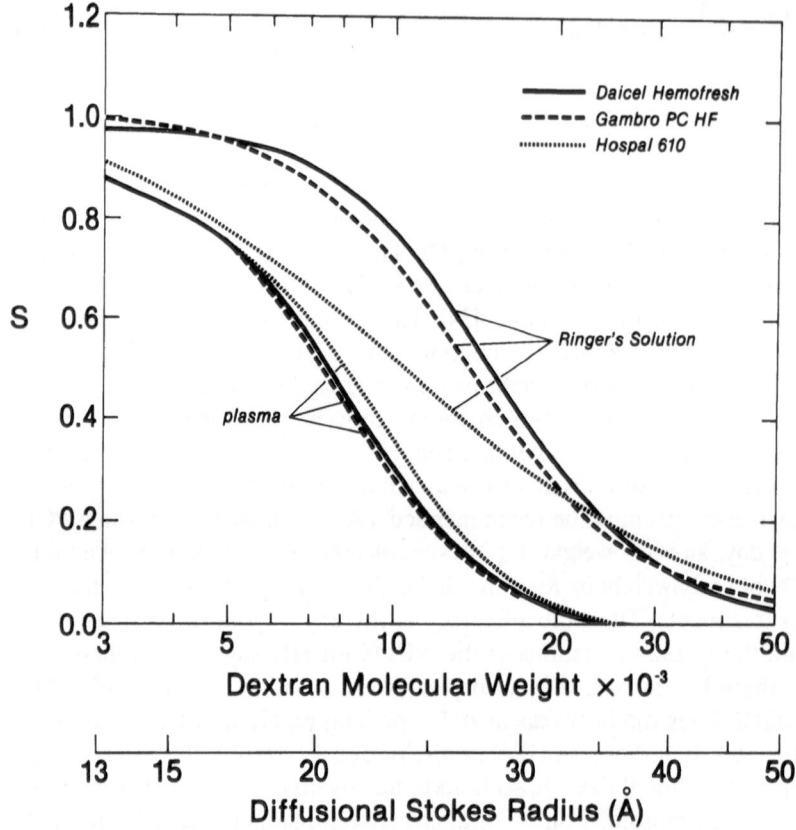

Fig. 3. Sieving coefficient S of dextran plotted as a function of molecular weight and diffusional Stokes radius. Inulin would fall at approximately 14 Å and albumin at 35 Å. Hemofilters in sheet membrane format were tested in both RINGER's solution and plasma [38]

weight solutes is indeed the compensatory mechanism, it follows that therapy prescription will differ depending on the efficiency of solute transport with different membranes. For example, Fig. 3 and 4 show sieving coefficients for some commonly employed membrane devices used for HF therapy in hollow-fiber and sheet format, respectively [38]. Note the striking difference in sieving coefficients that are observed for different HF membranes. These observations suggest that prescription of therapy may depend greatly on the HF membrane employed.

The importance of membrane properties was illustrated by the recent study of HD with Cuprophan and polyacrylonitrile membranes by CHANNARD and coworkers [39]. They prescribed therapy for each membrane by requiring equivalent removal of solutes with a molecular size similar to vitamin B_{12}, resulting in different treatment times. For the patients studied with the different membranes, the weekly vitamin B_{12} clearance was the same, but the blood urea concentrations for the patients treated with the polyacrylonitrile membrane had slightly but significantly higher pretreatment concentrations of urea. They have shown that using a polyacrylonitrile membrane and a treatment time of 9.3 ± 0.2 h/week compared with a Cuprophan membrane and a treatment time of 16.2 ± 0.3 h/week, the number of days

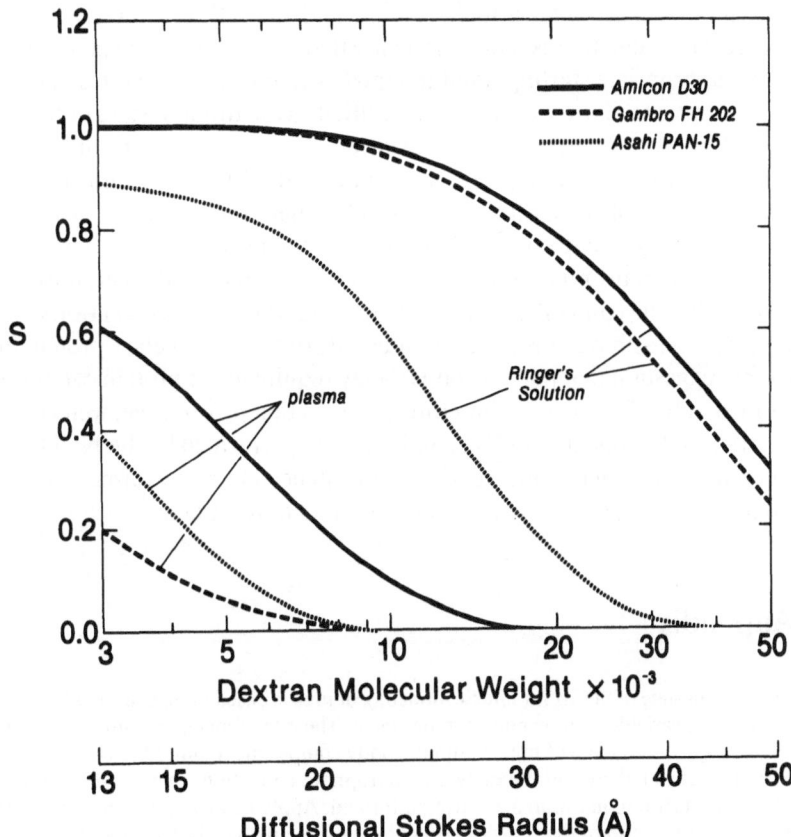

Fig. 4. A comparable plot to Fig. 3, studying hemofilters in hollow-fiber format [38]

of hospitalization for the polyacrylonitrile group ($N=31$) was considerably shorter at 2.1 ± 0.5 days/year compared with 6.0 ± 1.1 days/year for the Cuprophan group ($N=31$). This study demonstrates that a decrease in treatment time accompanied by an equivalent removal of larger molecular weight solutes does not result in an increase in patient morbidity. Information on dietary protein intake for the two study groups was, however, not reported, but it does not seem possible that nutritional considerations could result in the increased hospitalization of the patients studied with Cuprophan membranes. Since the urea concentrations for both treatment groups were similar and within the recommendations of the NCDS, the decreased removal of urea with the polyacrylonitrile membrane (caused by the decreased treatment time) suggests that the polyacrylonitrile study group had a lower protein catabolic rate and would be more likely to be at nutritional risk. In addition, it is unclear whether serial activation of complement that occurs with Cuprophan and not with polyacrylonitrile membranes plays a role in longterm patient morbidity. Nevertheless, this study by CHANNARD and coworkers [39] demonstrates the importance of membrane properties on the prescription of therapy.

What position may the clinician/researcher employ today for guiding treatment? A conservative approach would be to prescribe therapy based on the lessons learned from the NCDS for HD based on urea kinetic modeling. Recognizing the toxicity associated with a high TAC_{urea} and that HF membranes will clear larger molecular weight toxins more efficiently than Cuprophan HD membranes, it would be an appropriate starting point to equate protein catabolic rates and pretreatment concentrations of urea with those identified as the result of state of the art treatment with HD. As discussed above, however, this would require at least double the amount of treatment that is presently employed. Either a doubling of treatment time on HF or use of hemodiafiltration (HDF) that employs large clearances for both small and large solutes will be required to reach such a goal. To arbitrarily fall below this standard raises the concern, but by no means the certainty, of increased morbidity. The eminent success of clinical treatments by QUELLHORST and coworkers [34], noted above, albeit with limited information on dietary protein intake, leads to the suggestion that patients on HF may require lower protein catabolic rates than those on HD. This review, therefore, suggests that prospective, well controlled clinical trials of treatment with HF, similar to that performed by the NCDS, with special reference to the dietary intake of protein will need to be performed in order to determine the necessary levels of adequate treatment for maintenance HF.

Appendix

The present state of the art for kinetic modeling of urea is based upon conservation of mass within a single-pool, variable-volume body compartment. The rate of increase in urea mass is simply equated to the generation rate of urea within the body compartment minus the clearance rate of urea by both the native kidney and the dialyzer. Appropriate corrections to account for the change in the volume of distribution for urea are also performed. Applying these principles, the following differential equations govern the concentration of urea when dialysis is performed:

$$\frac{d\,(CV)}{dt} = G - K_T C \tag{A1}$$

$$\frac{dV}{dt} = - K_{UF} \tag{A2}$$

where C denotes the concentration of urea, V the urea volume of distribution, G the generation rate of urea, t the time from the start of dialysis, and K_T the clearance of urea during dialysis that consists of the sum of renal clearance K_r and dialyzer clearance K_d. The value of K_{UF} denotes the rate that the urea volume of distribution decreases as a result of fluid loss. Note that the value of K_{UF} is the ultrafiltration flow rate across the artificial kidney only for HD. For HF, the value of K_{UF} is equal to the ultrafiltration flow rate minus the substitution fluid flow rate.

Assuming all parameters are constant with time, the concentration of urea as a function of time during treatment is given by

$$C(t) = \left[C_0 - \frac{G}{K_T - K_{UF}} \right] \left[\frac{V_0 - K_{UF}t}{V_0} \right]^{(K_T - K_{UF})/K_{UF}} + \frac{G}{K_T - K_{UF}} \tag{A3}$$

and

$$V(t) = V_0 - K_{UF}t \tag{A4}$$

where C_0 and V_0 denote the urea concentration and volume of distribution at the initiation of dialysis.

The governing equations when the patient is off dialysis are similar and are given by

$$\frac{d(CV)}{dt} = G - K_r C \tag{A5}$$

$$\frac{dV}{dt} = K_{WG} \tag{A6}$$

Equation (A5) is identical to Eq. (A1) except for a zero dialyzer clearance, and Eq. (A6) differs from Eq. (A2) in that the urea volume of distribution increases at a rate equal to the average weight gain of the patient for the interdialytic interval K_{WG}. The solutions of these equations are given by

$$C(t) = \left[C_t - \frac{G}{K_r + K_{WG}} \right] \left[\frac{V_{DW} + K_{WG}t}{V_{DW}} \right]^{-(K_r + K_{WG})/K_{WG}} + \frac{G}{K_r + K_{WG}} \tag{A7}$$

and

$$V(t) = V_{DW} + K_{WG}t \tag{A8}$$

where C_t and V_{DW} denote the urea concentration and volume of distribution at the beginning of the interdialytic interval. The urea volume of distribution at the start of the interdialytic period is also known as the distribution volume at dry weight. Note that t in these equations denotes the time from the start of the interdialytic interval and not from the start of the previous dialysis period.

For the stable chronic renal failure patient, it is of interest to compute the generation rate G and the volume of distribution at dry weight V_{DW}. It is first assumed that the patient is maintained at a constant dry weight, with the fluid gained during the interdialytic period equal to the fluid removed by the previous dialysis period. Stated mathematically, this assumption is

$$K_{WG} = K_{UF}t_d / \Theta \tag{A9}$$

where t_d and Θ denote the time of the dialysis period and time of the interdialytic period, respectively. By measurement of the urea concentrations at the start of a dialysis period C_{o1}, at the start of the interdialytic period (also the end of the dialysis period) C_{t1}, and at the start of the following dialysis period C_{o2}, Eq. (A3), (A4), (A7), and (A8) can be solved simultaneously to yield the following:

$$V_{DW} = \frac{K_{UF}t_d}{\left[\dfrac{C_{o1} - G/(K_T - K_{UF})}{C_{t1} - G/(K_T - K_{UF})} \right]^{K_{UF}/(K_T - K_{UF})} - 1} \tag{A10}$$

$$G = \frac{(K_r + K_{WG})[C_{o2} - C_{t1} \,[1 + K_{WG}\Theta/V_{DW}] - (K_r + K_{WG})/K_{WG}]}{1 - [1 + K_{WG}\Theta/V_{DW}] - (K_r + K_{WG})/K_{WG}} \tag{A11}$$

When K_r, K_{UF}, and K_{WG} are equal to zero, Eq. (1) and (2) are the result.

References

1. Wolf AV, Remp DG, Kiley JE, Currie GD (1951) Artificial kidney function: kinetics of hemodialysis. J Clin Invest 30: 1062–1070
2. Van Slyke DD, Hiller A, Miller BF (1935) The distribution of ferrocyanide, inulin, creatinine and urea in the blood and its effect on the significance of their extraction percentages. Am J Physiol 113: 629–641

3. Michaels AS (1966) Operating parameters and performance criteria for hemodialyzers and other membrane-separation devices. Trans Am Soc Artif Intern Organs 12: 387–392
4. Colton CK, Smith KA, Merrill EW, Farrell PC (1971) Permeability studies with cellulosic membranes. J Biomed Mater Res 5: 459–488
5. Colton CK, Lowrie EG (1981) Hemodialysis: Physical principles and technical considerations. In: Brenner BM, Rector FC Jr (eds) The kidney, chap 47. Saunders, Philadelphia, pp 2425–2489
6. Babb AL, Popovich RP, Christopher TG, Scribner BH (1971) The genesis of the square meter-hour hypothesis. Trans Am Soc Artif Intern Organs 17: 81–91 1971
7. Babb AL, Strand MJ, Uvelli DA, Milutinovic J, Scribner BH (1975) Quantitative description of dialysis treatment: a dialysis index. Kidney Int 7 [Suppl 2]: S-23–S-29
8. Scribner BH (1965) Discussion. Trans Am Soc Artif Intern Organs 11: 29
9. Sargent JA, Gotch FA (1975) The analysis of concentration dependence of uremic lesions in clinical studies. Kidney Int 7 [Suppl 2]: S-35–S-44
10. Gotch FA, Sargent JA, Keen M, Lam M, Prowitt M, Grady M (1976) Clinical results of intermittent dialysis therapy guided by ongoing kinetic analysis of urea metabolism. Trans Am Soc Artif Intern Organs 22: 175–188
11. Popovich RP, Hlavinka DJ, Bomar JB, Moncrief JW, Decherd JF (1975) The consequences of physiological resistances on metabolite removal from the patient-artificial kidney system. Trans Am Soc Artif Intern Organs 21: 108–115
12. Frost TH, Kerr DNS (1977) Kinetics of hemodialysis: A theoretical study of the removal of solutes in chronic renal failure compared to normal health. Kidney Int 12: 41–50
13. Sanfellipo ML, Hall DA, Walker WE, Swenson RS (1975) Quantitative evaluation of hemodialysis therapy using a simple mathematical model and a programmable pocket calculator. Trans Am Soc Artif Intern Organs 21: 125–130
14. Borah MF, Schoenfeld PY, Gotch FA, Sargent JA, Wolfson M, Humphreys MH (1978) Nitrogen balance during intermittent dialysis therapy of uremia. Kidney Int 14: 491–500
15. Sargent JA (1983) Control of dialysis by single-pool urea model: the National Cooperative Dialysis Study. Kidney Int 23 [Suppl 13]: S-19–S-25
16. Sargent J, Gotch F, Borah M, Piercy L, Spinozzi N, Schoenfeld P, Humphreys M (1978) Urea kinetics: a guide to nutritional management of renal failure. Am J Clin Nutr 31: 1696–1702
17. Lowrie EG, Sargent JA (1980) Clinical example of pharmacokinetic and metabolic modeling: quantitative and individualized prescription of dialysis therapy. Kidney Int 18 [Suppl 10]: S-11–S-16
18. Lowrie EG, Teehan BP (1983) Principles of prescribing dialysis therapy: Implementing recommendations from the National Cooperative Dialysis Study. Kidney Int 23 [Suppl 13]: S-113–S-122
19. Ward RA, Shirlow MJ, Hayes JM, Chapman GV, Farrell PC (1979) Protein catabolism during hemodialysis. Am J Clin Nutr 32: 2443–2449
20. Farrell PC, Hone PW (1980) Dialysis-induced catabolism. Am J Clin Nutr 33: 1417–1422
21. Henderson LW, Koch KM, Dinarello CA, Shaldon S (1983) Hemodialysis hypotension: The interleukin hypothesis. Blood Purif 1: 3–8
22. Dinarello CA (1983) The biology of interleukin-1 and its relevance to hemodialysis. Blood Purif 1: 197–224
23. Johnson WJ, Hagge WW, Wagoner RD, Dinapoli RP, Rosevear JW (1972) Effects of urea loading in patients with far-advanced renal failure. Mayo Clin Proc 47: 21–29
24. Shaldon S (1966) Haemodialysis in chronic renal failure. Postgrad Med J 42: 669–695
25. Henderson LW (1973) The problem of peritoneal membrane area and permeability. Kidney Int 3: 409–410
26. Babb AL, Farrell PC, Strand MJ, Uvelli DA, Milutinovic J, Scribner BH (1972) Residual renal function and chronic hemodialysis therapy. Proc Dial Transplant Forum 2: 142–148
27. Lowrie EG, Lard NM (1983) Cooperative dialysis study. Kidney Int 23 [Suppl 13]: S-1–S-122
28. Laird NM, Berkey CS, Lowrie EG (1983) Modeling success or failure of dialysis therapy: the National Cooperative Dialysis Study. Kidney Int 23 [Suppl 13]: S-101–S-106
29. Wing AJ, Broyer M, Brunner FP, Brynger H, Donckerwolcke RA, Jacobs C, Kramer P, Selwood NH (1981) Combined report on regular dialysis and transplantation in Europe. 19th Proceedings of the European Dialysis and Transplant Association

30. Bosch JP, von Albertini B, Glabman S (1982) Prescription for hemofiltration. Contrib Nephrol 32: 137-145
31. Canaud B, Mayr H, Garred LJ, Farrell PC, Mion C (1983) Urea kinetic model for hemofiltration. Blood Purif 1: 42 (Abstract)
32. Canaud B, Mayr H, Araujo A, Garred LJ, Farrel PC, Mion C (1983) Protein catabolic changes induced by postdilution hemofiltration. Blood Purif 1: 42 (Abstract)
33. Walser (1981) Conservative management of the uremic patient. In: Brenner BM, Rector FC Jr (eds) The kidney, chap 46. Saunders, Philadelphia, pp 2383-2424
34. Quellhorst EA, Schuenemann B, Hildebrand U (1983) Morbidity and mortality in long-term hemofiltration. asaio J 6: 185-191
35. Gotch FA (1980) A quantitative evaluation of small and middle molecule toxicity in therapy of uremia. Dial Transpl 10 (3): 184-194
36. Blumenkrantz MJ, Kopple JD, Moran JK, Grodstein GP, Coburn JW (1981) Nitrogen and urea metabolism during continuous ambulatory peritoneal dialysis. Kidney Int 20: 78-82
37. Randerson DH, Chapman GV, Farrell PC (1981) Amino acid and dietary status in CAPD patients. In: Atkins RC, Thomson NM, Farrell PC (eds) Peritoneal dialysis. Churchill Livingstone, New York, pp 179-191
38. Leypoldt JK, Frigon RP, Henderson LW (1983) Sieving coefficients of hemofiltration membranes. Trans Am Soc Artif Intern Organs 29: 678-683
39. Channard J, Brunois JP, Melin JP, Lavaud S, Toupance O (1982) Long-term results of dialysis therapy with a highly permeable membrane. Artif Organs 6: 261-266

Acid-Base Balance in Hemofiltration

J. P. BOSCH and A. LAUER

Table of Contents

Acid-Base Balance in Chronic Renal Failure

Dietary intake and metabolism provide a number of potential sources of acid. Sulfur in the sulfur-containing amino acids is oxidized to sulfuric acid, phosphorus in proteins and phospholipids is converted to phosphoric acid, and organic acids may be produced in excess of the capacity to metabolize them. Since none of these products can exist in the body fluids as free dissociated acid, the hydrogen must react with the buffers of the body. Most of the extracellular buffering occurs by reaction of the acid with bicarbonate to yield the corresponding sodium salt and carbonic acid. The carbonic acid is then converted to water and carbon dioxide, the latter being excreted in the lungs. The net result is the replacement in the extracellular fluid of one equivalent of bicarbonate by one anion equivalent of the acid [1]. The buffer capacity of the extracellular fluid can be restored if bicarbonate is regenerated. In healthy people, this is accomplished by the Kidney. In patients with chronic renal failure (CRF) on maintenance therapy, bicarbonate regeneration must be achieved by the treatment technique.

In estimating the contribution of any treatment technique to the acid-base balance of these patients, it is useful to calculate the net base gain (NBG) during the procedure, i.e., the sum of base administered (acetate, lactate, bicarbonate, etc.) less the base lost from the blood to the dialysate, or to the ultrafiltrate (bicarbonate plus acetate). Organic anions wasted during the treatment must be considered base equivalent and, therefore, added to the bicarbonate loss [2]. Since the base administered is aquantitatively related to the generation of bicarbonate, the net base retained during the treatment is analogous to bicarbonate regeneration. In order to maintein body buffers, the bicarbonate dissipated by hydrogen ions produced during the interdialytic period must be completely replaced during the treatment. Assuming an adequate protein intake (1.0–1.5 g/kg/day) and a steady state in a patient treated three times a week, 160–200 mEq of net base per treatment should be sufficient to maintain body buffers [3].

Hemofiltration

Net Base Gain in Hemofiltration

In hemofiltration (HF), the most common base used in the substitution fluid is sodium acetate. This choice has been one of convenience, while other buffers have also been used [4].

The NBG during HF will be equal to Base gain − Base loss during the treatment.

Base Gain.
Total acetate (Ac) administered in the substitution fluid (S) × will be equal to vol. (l) of S administered × Ac (mEq/1).

Base Loss

A sum of the following will give the base loss:

1) Total bicarbonate (HCO_3) loss in the ultrafiltrate (Uf), which can be expressed as
   Total HCO_3 loss (mEq) = vol. Uf (1) × [HCO_3] Uf (mEq/1)
2) Total Ac loss in the ultrafiltrate, which can be expressed as
   Total Ac loss (mEq) = vol. Uf (1) × [Ac] Uf (mEq/1)
3) Total organic anions (O An) loss in the ultrafiltrate, which can be expressed as
   Total O An loss (mEq) = vol. Uf (1) × [O An] Uf (mEq/1)

The organic anions important during the procedure, in addition to acetate, are pyruvate, lactate, and citrate. Their contribution should be calculated separately and added.

Table 1 shows the measurements from four patients during postdilution HF and the calculation of the NBG. For these studies the following measurements and calculations were made:

a) Volume of ultrafiltrate (V Uf) was measured directly using a graduated container.
b) Volume of substitution fluid was calculated from V Uf minus the weight loss.
c) Plasma and ultrafiltrate bicarbonate concentrations were mearured using the Natelson Microgasometer [5].

Table 1. Base balance during postdilution hemofiltration at midweek treatment (mean values for four patients)

A. Fluid balance

	Ultra filtrate (ml)	Ultrafiltration rate (ml/min)	Substitution fluid (ml)	weight loss (ml)
1st Hour	5000	83	4500	500
2nd Hour	5230	87	4630	600
3rd Hour	5280	88	4450	830
4th Hour	4750	79	4450	300
5th Hour	5100	85	5000	100
Total	25360		23060	2330

B. Plasma and ultrafiltrate concentrations (mEq/l)

	P $[CO_2]$	Uf $[CO_2]$	P $[Ac]$	Uf $[Ac]$	P $[Lac]$	Uf $[Lac]$	P $[Pyr]$	Uf $[Pyr]$
Initial	21.0		0.87		1.10		0.02	
1st Hour	23.3	25.6	1.92	2.11	1.10	1.20	0.03	0.00
2nd Hour	24.5	27.0	2.66	2.93	1.00	1.08	0.04	0.05
3rd Hour	26.0	28.6	2.42	2.66	0.90	0.99	0.02	0.03
4th Hour	27.0	29.7	2.43	2.67	1.05	1.05	0.05	0.04
5th Hour	28.0	30.8	2.30	2.53	1.09	1.09	0.04	0.05

C. Net base gain (Base administered in substitution fluid less base lost in ultrafiltrate measured in mEq)

	CO_2	Acetate	Lactate	Pyruvate	Acetate administered	Net Base Gain
1st Hour	128.2	10.6	6.0	0.0	184.5	39.8
2nd Hour	141.0	15.3	5.7	0.3	189.9	27.7
3rd Hour	151.0	14.1	5.2	0.2	169.6	13.2
4th Hour	141.1	12.7	5.0	0.2	169.8	23.5
5th Hour	157.1	12.9	5.6	0.3	205.0	29.3
Total	718.3	65.5	27.4	1.0	945.5	133.4

D. Urea nitrogen balance during the treatment

	P [UN] (mg/ml)	Uf [UN] (mg/ml)	UN Removed (g)
Initial	1.01		
1st Hour	0.89	0.99	4.95
2nd Hour	0.82	0.86	4.50
3rd Hour	0.75	0.80	4.22
4th Hour	0.70	0.73	3.47
5th Hour	0.67	0.68	3.47
Total			20.61

d) Plasma and ultrafiltrate acetate, lactate, and pyruvate concentrations were measured using an enzymatic method [6].

Three factors determine the magnitude of the NBG during postdilution HF:

1) The concentration of base in the substitution fluid. The Ac concentration used in the studies reported in Table 1 was 41 mEq/l. Other authors have used smaller [4] or higher [8] concentrations. More important than the actual concentration of base in the substitution fluid is the effective base concentration.

- Effective base [ ] mEq/l = S [Base] − Uf [Base]
- S [Base] = S [Ac]
- Uf [Base] = Uf [CO$_2$] + Uf [Ac] + Uf [O An]

The NBG during the treatment is directly related to this value. The effective base concentration is not constant throughout the treatment. In the experiments shown in Table 1, the effective base concentration averaged 12.1 mEq/l in the first hour of the treatment. In the last hour of the procedure it averaged 6.5 mEq/l. These changes are the result of the rise in plasma bicarbonate as well as small increments in acetate and organic anions in the plasma during the treatment. An important factor in determining the effective base concentration is the rate of fluid exchange. In those treatments where the ultrafiltration rate is excess of 120 ml/min and thus the administration of substitution fluid is greater than 7.5 l/h, the amount of acetate administered may be greater than the capacity of the body to metabolize it. If more than 300 mEq/h acetate are given, plasma acetate concentration will rise and plasma bicarbonate will decrease [7]. These changes will result in metabolic acidosis and a decrease in the effective base concentration in the substitution fluid.

2) The amount of substitution fluid used. The NBG during the treatment is directly related to the amount of substitution fluid used in the procedure.
3) The negative fluid balance. The amount of ultrafiltrate not replaced by substitution fluid (weight loss) is inversely related to the NBG in the treatment.

Acid-Base Balance in Hemofiltration

To maintain body buffers, the bicarbonate dissipated by the hydrogen ions produced during the interdialytic period must be completely replaced during the treatment. In patients in steady state, the hydrogen generation (HG) can be estimated from the dietary protein intake (DPI) [9]. The latter can be derived from the urea nitrogen (UN) produced [9]:

- DPI = UN g/day/0.12 [11]
- HG = DPI × 0.77 [9]

In the patients studied and reported in Table 1, the DPI calculated was 85.8 g/day or 1.2 g/kg/day (UN = 10.3 g/day). Calculated, from the DPI, the HG averaged

66.1 mEq/day. The NBG (Table 1) averaged 133.4 mEq per treatment; thus, the amount of base administered during HF was sufficient to replace the bicarbonate consumed in the interdialytic period (daily $HG \times 2 = 132.2$ mEq). The values used for these calculations represent (midweek parameters in patients in an assumed steady state. These calculations cannot be extrapolated to daily values. For example, in these patients the weekly HG would average 462.7 mEq (66.1 mEq/day $\times$ 7 days). The weekly NBG would be 400.2 mEq (133.4 mEq/treatment $\times$ 3). It would appear that the quantity of base administered in the treatment given here was insufficient. However, this is not the case, since the treatment that follows the longest interdialytic period will be different from the midweek results. Plasma bicarbonate will be lower, the effective base concentration in the substitution fluid higher and hence the NBG higher. In patients with acute renal failure (ARF) and/or patients with negative nitrogen balance, for example, a comparable situation will occur and the treatment, at equal volumes of substitution fluid will deliver a higher NBG per treatment.

Blood Gases During Hemofiltration

Figures 1-4 show the results obtained from hourly measurements of the blood gases during HF and HD. These results, obtained simultaneously with those depicted in Table 1, do not differ from those reported in the literature [10, 11].

In HF, the changes in partial pressure of oxygen (pO_2) and in the partial pressure of carbon dioxide (pCO_2), were not different from those observed in HD. Plasma bicarbonate and plasma pH were significantly higher in HF than in HD.

The mechanisms involved in the pathogenesis of the hypoxemia of HD have

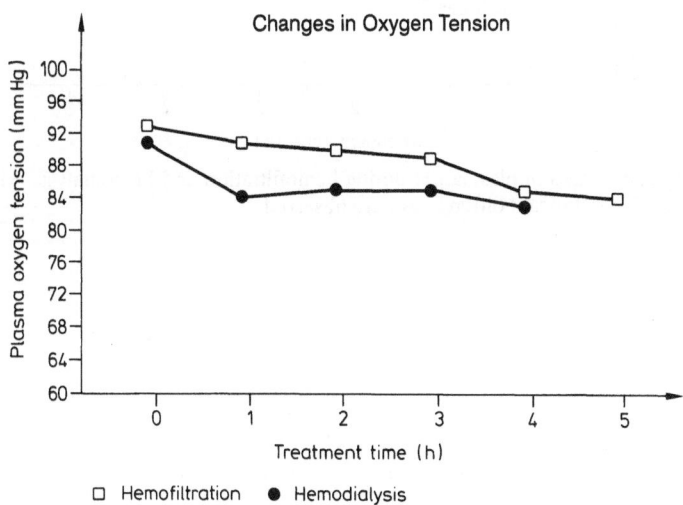

Fig. 1. Changes in arterial oxygen tension during hemofiltration and hemodialysis. Mean values in four patients. No significant statistical differences were demonstrated between the two treatments. In both treatments pO_2 was significantly different from 0 one hour after initiation of therapy

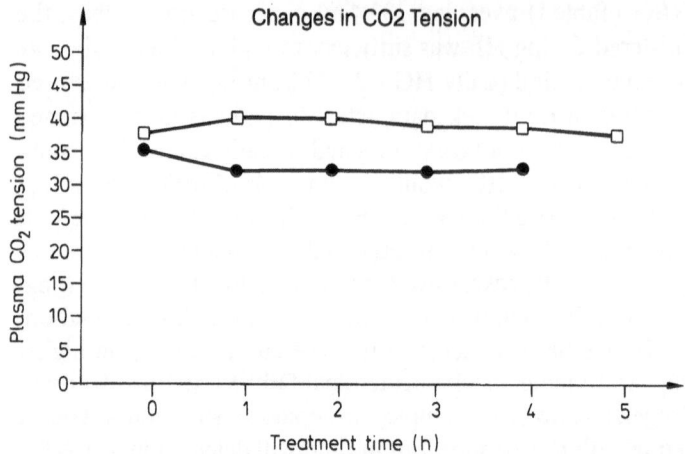

Fig. 2. Changes in arterial carbon dioxide tension during hemofiltration and hemodialysis. Mean values in four patients. No significant differences were demonstrated in either treatment between beginning and end. At all times values were significantly different between hemofiltration and hemodialysis

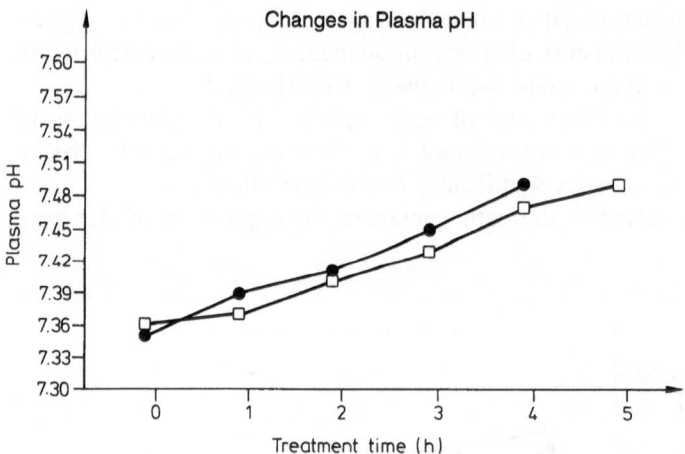

Fig. 3. Changes in plasma pH during hemofiltration and hemodialysis. Mean values in four patients. No significant differences were observed

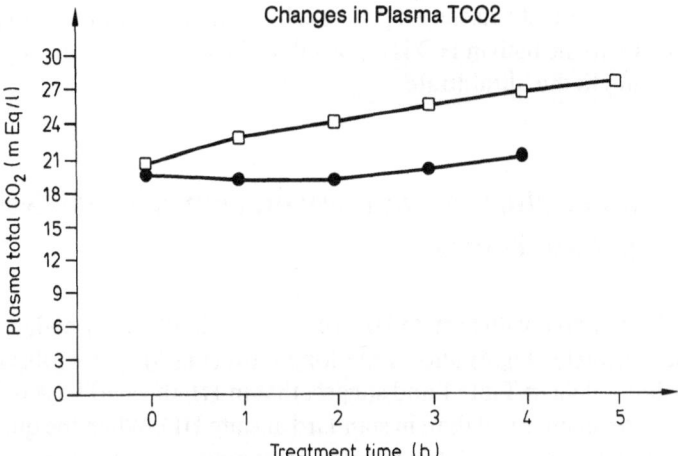

Fig. 4. Changes in plasma total CO_2 during hemofiltration and hemodialysis. Mean values in four patients. Values were statistically different at all times. (Results for all figures were statistically significant, with $P < 0.05$ using paired analysis.)

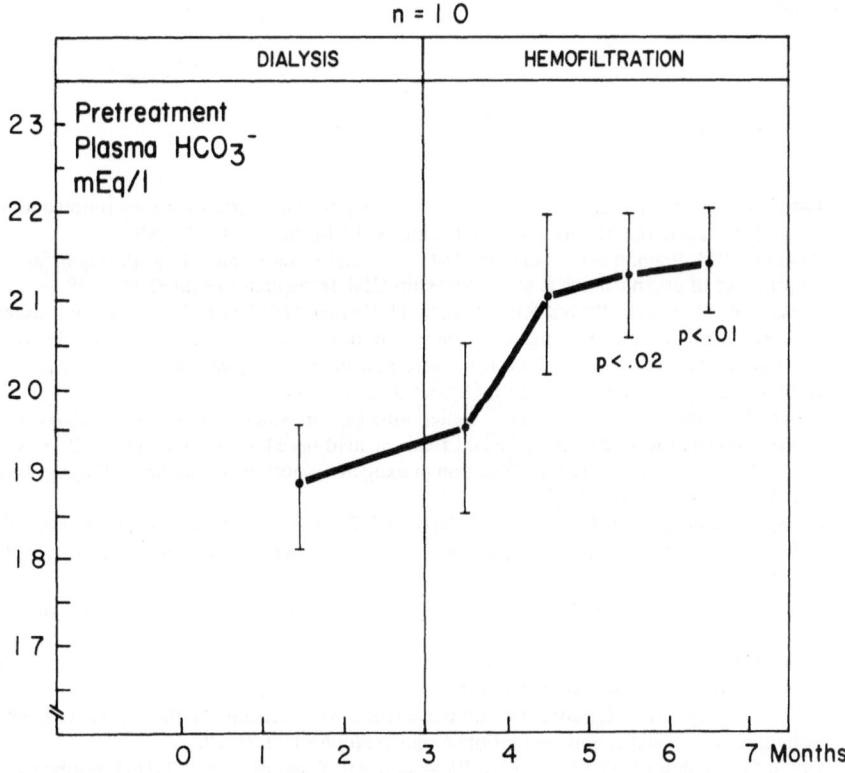

Fig. 5. Chronic changes in pretreatment plasma TCO_2. Mean values for 10 patients

been extensively discussed [11]. It is likely that similar factors apply to HF. The loss of CO_2 to the bath in HD is replaced by the loss of CO_2 (mainly in the form of bicarbonate) to the ultrafiltrate.

Hemofiltration in Comparison with Hemodialysis: Long-Term Effects

HF compared with acetate HD, results in a significantly higher plasma bicarbonate, both acutely (Fig. 4) and in the long term (Fig. 5). These observations support the balance data in Table 1 and suggest that in HF the acid-base balance of the patients is better maintained than in standard acetate HD. When the quantity of base administered during one HF treatment is compared with the amount of base administered during one acetate HD treatment, no significant differences can be demonstrated. In both treatments sufficient base is given to regenerate the bicarbonate dissipated during the intertreatment period. The failure of acetate HD to maintain a normal pretreatment plasma bicarbonate has been reviewed elsewhere [5]. HF appears better able than HD to restore pretreatment plasma bicarbonate to values closer to the normal range.

References

1. Goodman AD, Lemmann J Jr, Lennon EJ, Relman AS (1965) Production, excretion and net balance of fixed acid in patients with renal acidosis. J Clin Invest 44: 495–506
2. Assomull VM, Vreman HJ, Weiner MW Mass balance of base equivalents during hemodialysis: Importance of organic acids anions. Proc Clin Dial Transplant Forum 8: 137–140
3. Kaiser BA, Potter DE, Bryant RE, Vreman HJ, Weiner MW (1981) Acid-base and acetate metabolism during routine and high efficiency hemodialysis in children. Kidney Int 19: 70–70
4. Shaldon S, Beau MC, Deschodt G, Ramperez P, Mion C (1980) Vascular stability during hemofiltration. Trans Am Soc Artif Intern Organs 26: 391–393
5. Bosch JP, Glabman S, Moutoussis G, Belledonne M, von Albertini B, Kahn T (1984) Carbon dioxide removal in acetate hemodialysis: Effects on acid-base balance. Kidney Int 25: 830–837
6. Kveim M, Nebaskken R (1975) Utilization of exogenous acetate during hemodialysis. Trans Am Soc Artif Intern Organs 21: 138–140
7. Graefe U, Milutinovich J, Follette WC, Vizzo JE, Babb AL, Scribmer BH (1978) Less dialysis-induced morbidity and vascular instability with bicarbonate in dialysate. Ann Intern Med 88: 332–336
8. Bosch JP, von Albertini B, Glabman S (1982) Prescription for hemofiltration. Contrib Nephrol 32: 137–145
9. Gotch FA (1976) Hemodialysis: Technical and kinetic considerations. In: Brenner BM, Rector FC (eds) The kidney. Saunders, Philadelphia
10. Schaefer K, Ryzlewicz T, Sandri M, von Bernewitz S, von Herrath D (1982) Effect of hemofiltration on acid-base status and ventilation. Contrib Nephrol 32: 69–76
11. Dolan MJ, Whipp BJ, Davidson WD, Weitzman RE, Wasserman K (1981) Hypopnea associated with acetate hemodialysis: Carbon dioxide-flow-dependent ventilation. N Engl J Med 305: 72–75

Hemodynamics in Hemofiltration

C. A. BALDAMUS

Table of Contents

Introduction

Hemodynamic disturbances during end-stage renal disease (ESRD) treatment are clinically observable as changes in blood pressure, predominantly hypotension. The incidence of symptomatic hypotension during hemodialysis has increased in recent years in spite of the fact that dialysis regimes have been altered to three times weekly. The French dialysis registry reports a rise in the incidence of symptomatic hypotension from 15% in 1973 to 25% in 1979 [1–3]. This increased risk of hypotension is due to several independent factors, of which rapid fluid withdrawal during shortened treatment time seems to be the most important, but increasing age and multimorbidity of the dialysis population also seem to contribute. In fact from 1973 to 1970, patients' mean age increased from 41 to 48 years, and mean treatment time decreased from 19 to 12 h a week [4, 5]. Increasing frequency of transplantation, mainly among the uncomplicated ESRD patient pool, constitutes an additional factor.

In the mid-1970s, when other treatment modalities with improved vascular stability became available, such as hemofiltration, scientific interest started to focus on hemodynamics in hemodialysis and on alternative regimes. However, before analyzing these different treatment modalities and discussing the various mechanisms proposed, the physiology of blood pressure maintenance has to be reviewed. According to Ohm's law, blood pressure is the resultant product of total peripheral vascular resistance and cardiac output, which is determined by stroke volume and heart rate. Stroke volume is dependent on myocardial contractility and vascular volume.

Maintenance of blood pressure is such a vital function that it is maintained even at the expense of other organ perfusion and function, which are sacrificed in order of importance.

The circulatory control of blood pressure is regulated by about 400 basic physiologic phenomena and their interdependence, a fact identified by GUYTON et al. [6] in a classic paper on circulatory control. Several mechanisms, largely neural and humoral, have the capacity to modulate vascular resistance independently of local control and to influence the mechanisms by which vascular resistance is adjusted to meet peripheral metabolic demands. Cardiac output itself is strongly determined by peripheral vascular resistance. Cardiac output will increase and remain elevated if total peripheral resistance (TPR) decreases, as occurs, for instance, with the creation of an arteriovenous (AV) fistula for vascular access in dialysis. The second determinant of cardiac output is venous return. This is related to blood volume and to the capacitance of the systemic venous system. Cardiac output may drop, owing to either a decrease in total blood volume or a reduction in venous tone, thereby increasing the capacitance of the systemic venous bed.

The time course of blood pressure regulation varies from seconds to days (Fig. 1). Of the regulatory systems shown, the neural and humoral mechanisms respond within seconds or minutes [7]. Only aldosterone secretion occurs late and can be left out of consideration when discussing blood pressure regulation during intermittent dialysis and hemofiltration.

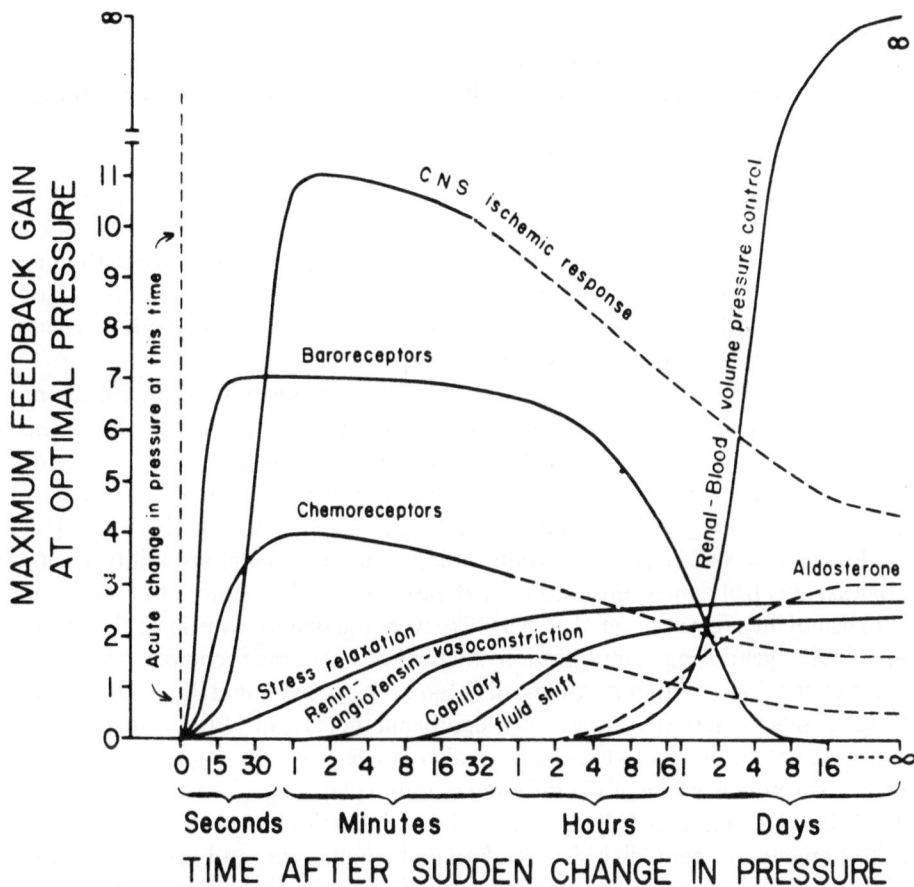

Fig. 1. Degree of activation, expressed in terms of feedback gain, of different pressure control mechanisms following a sudden change in arterial pressure. Note the rapid activation of nervous mechanisms, followed within minutes by hormonal reactions (From [7])

Literature Review

A literature review of blood pressure regulation during hemodialysis and related therapies is complicated by the fact that it is difficult to maintain comparability of the operating conditions of the various renal replacement therapies. But even when investigating in a single form of treatment the change in one response in reaction to one test parameter, additional variables have seldom been maintained constant. There are a great number of publications reporting only on the incidence of decreases in blood pressure during treatment, but these reports do not sufficiently describe hemodynamic regulation of blood pressure during treatment. To obtain a deeper insight it is necessary to measure blood pressure, cardiac output, and heart rate, which makes it possible to calculate TPR. There are only a few publications available in which, in addition to hemodynamic parameters, hormonal or other responses are reported.

The observation that ultrafiltration only rarely causes symptomatic hypotension was first reported by KOBAYASHI et al. [8] in 1972 and was later confirmed by ING et al. [9] in 1975. It was BERGSTRÖM et al. [10] who in 1976 compared ultrafiltration with hemodialysis and found that ultrafiltration was hemodynamically well tolerated on its own, but not when combined with diffusive solute transport. They used acetate as a dialysate buffer. At the same meeting QUELLHORST et al. [11] reported their first clinical experience with postdilution hemofiltration using lactate as a buffer substance. Beside other benefits they found an excellent tolerance to fluid removal of up to 5 kg/4 h without hypotension or muscle cramps. This improved tolerance to fluid withdrawal during hemofiltration as compared to hemodialysis was confirmed by several other investigators [12–17].

In 1977 GRAEFE et al. [18] observed a reduced intratreatment morbidity when replacing the acetate dialysate buffer with bicarbonate. In a systematic study this group then substantiated their initial observation by showing that in a given period of time more fluid can be withdrawn without symptomatic hypotension during bicarbonate than during acetate hemodialysis [19]. In view of BERGSTRÖM's data [10], they discussed acetate as one main contributing factor in vascular instability, whereas BERGSTRÖM [20] denied this and related vascular instability more to changes in serum osmolality. SHALDON et al. [17] in 1979 were the first to investigate the hemodynamic changes during hemofiltration and hemodialysis under comparable conditions. At a maximal drop in mean arterial blood pressure of 5 mmHg, in contrast to 32 mmHg in hemodialysis, they found a significant increase in TPR during hemofiltration, but not during hemodialysis. They also showed that the change in serum osmolality was not the cause of the differences found [27].

In 1980 BALDAMUS et al. [12] reported on hemodynamics in a study comparing ultrafiltration, acetate hemodialysis, bicarbonate hemodialysis, and acetate hemofiltration. They also measured intratreatment changes in catecholamines. Other operating conditions like weight loss, treatment time, small-solute removal rates, and constitution of dialysate and hemofiltration replacement fluid were kept constant in order to achieve comparable experimental conditions. Blood pressure (Fig. 2 a, b) remained stable during ultrafiltration and hemofiltration, but fell significantly during acetate dialysis and also during bicarbonate hemodialysis, although to a lesser degree in the latter. Heart rate (Fig. 2 c, d) increased in acetate hemodialysis and bicarbonate hemodialysis, but not during ultrafiltration and hemofiltration. Cardiac output (Fig. 3 a, b) fell during ultrafiltration and hemofiltration, but less during bicarbonate hemodialysis. The drop during acetate hemodialysis was not significantly different from that in all other three treatments. TPR (Fig. 3 c, d) increased during ultrafiltration and hemofiltration, but not during acetate or bicarbonate hemodialysis. Plasma noradrenaline levels (Fig. 3 e, f) increased considerably during ultrafiltration and hemofiltration, but not significantly during acetate hemodialysis and bicarbonate hemodialysis.

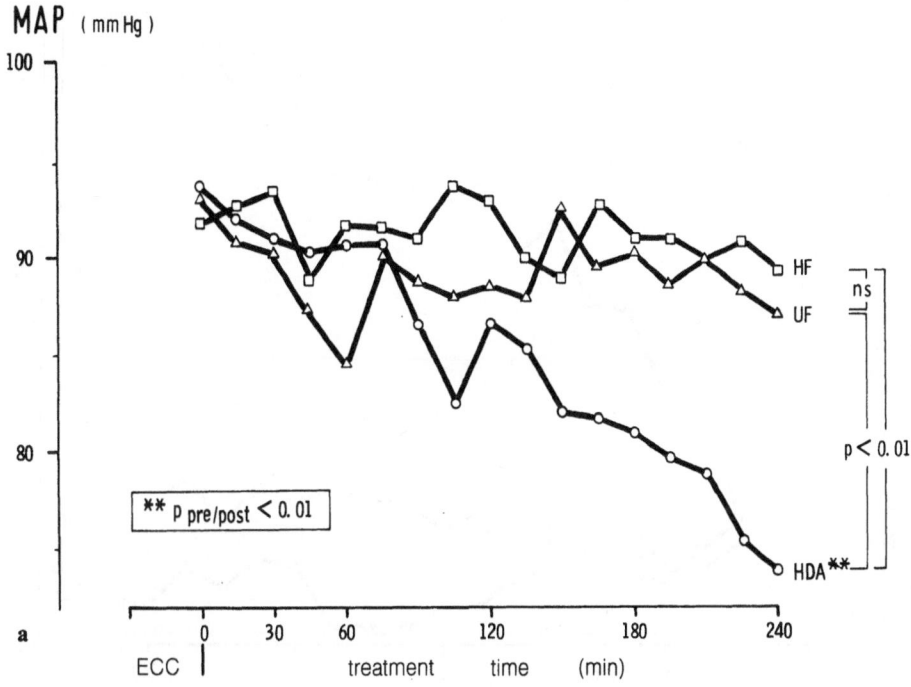

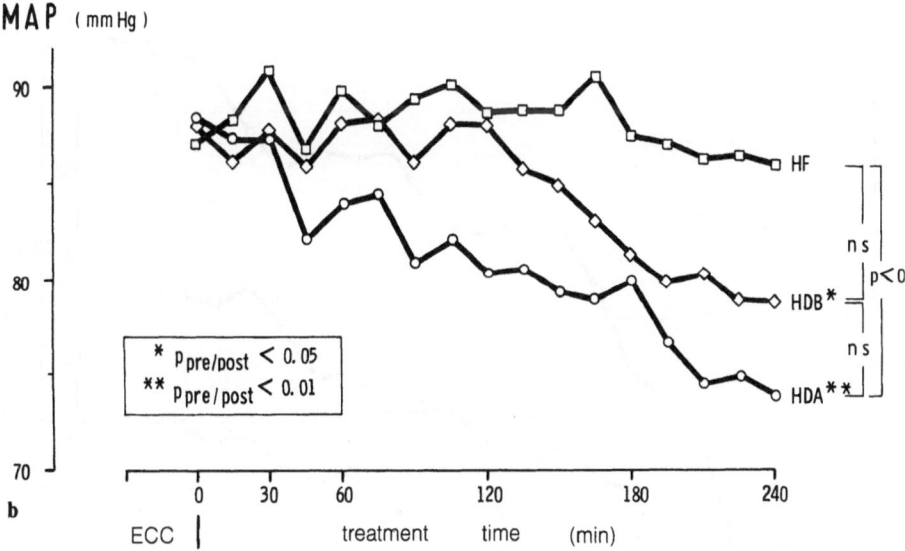

Fig. 2a–d. Mean arterial blood pressure *(MAP)* and heart rate *(HR)* after 30 min extracorporeal circulation without solute and volume flux *(ECC)* and during ultrafiltration *(UF)*, hemofiltration *(HF)*, acetate hemodialysis *(HDA)*, and bicarbonate hemodialysis *(HDB)*. (Redrawn from [22]). **a, b.** Mean arterial blood pressure

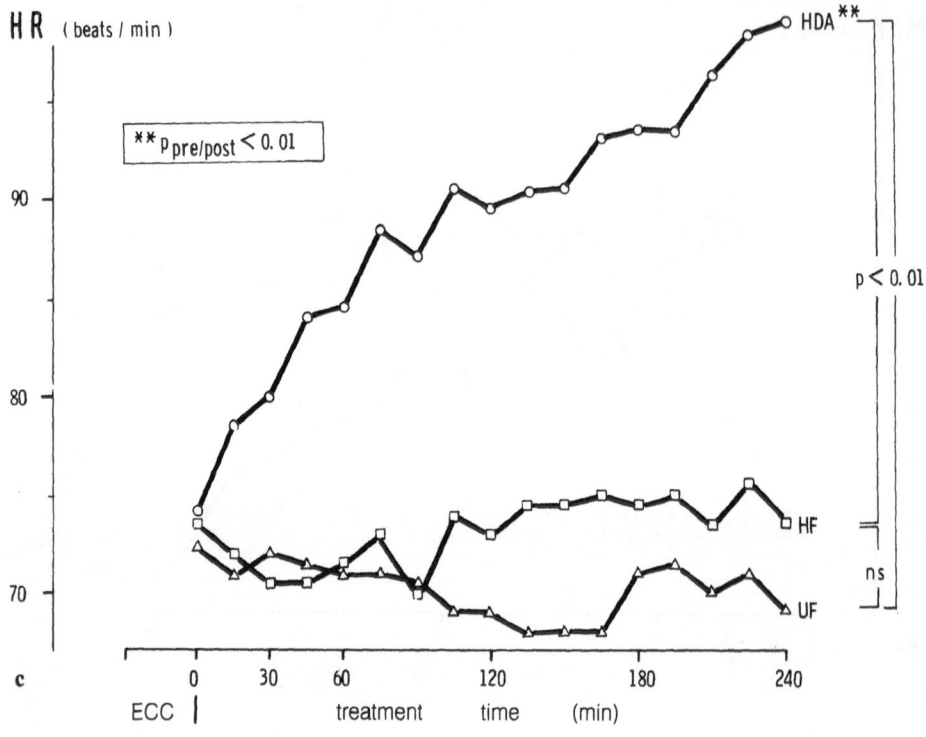

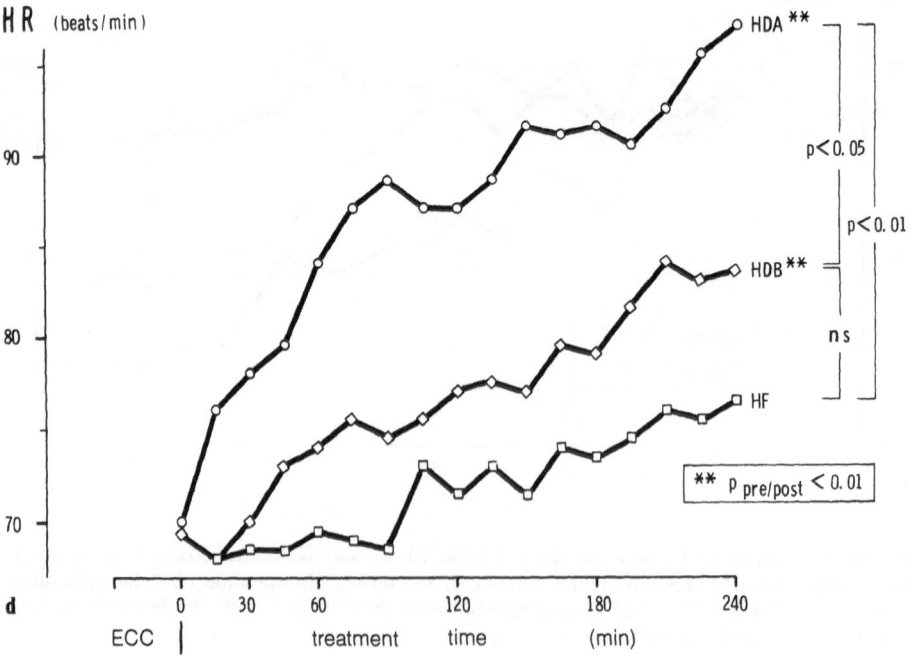

Fig. 2 c, d. Heart rate

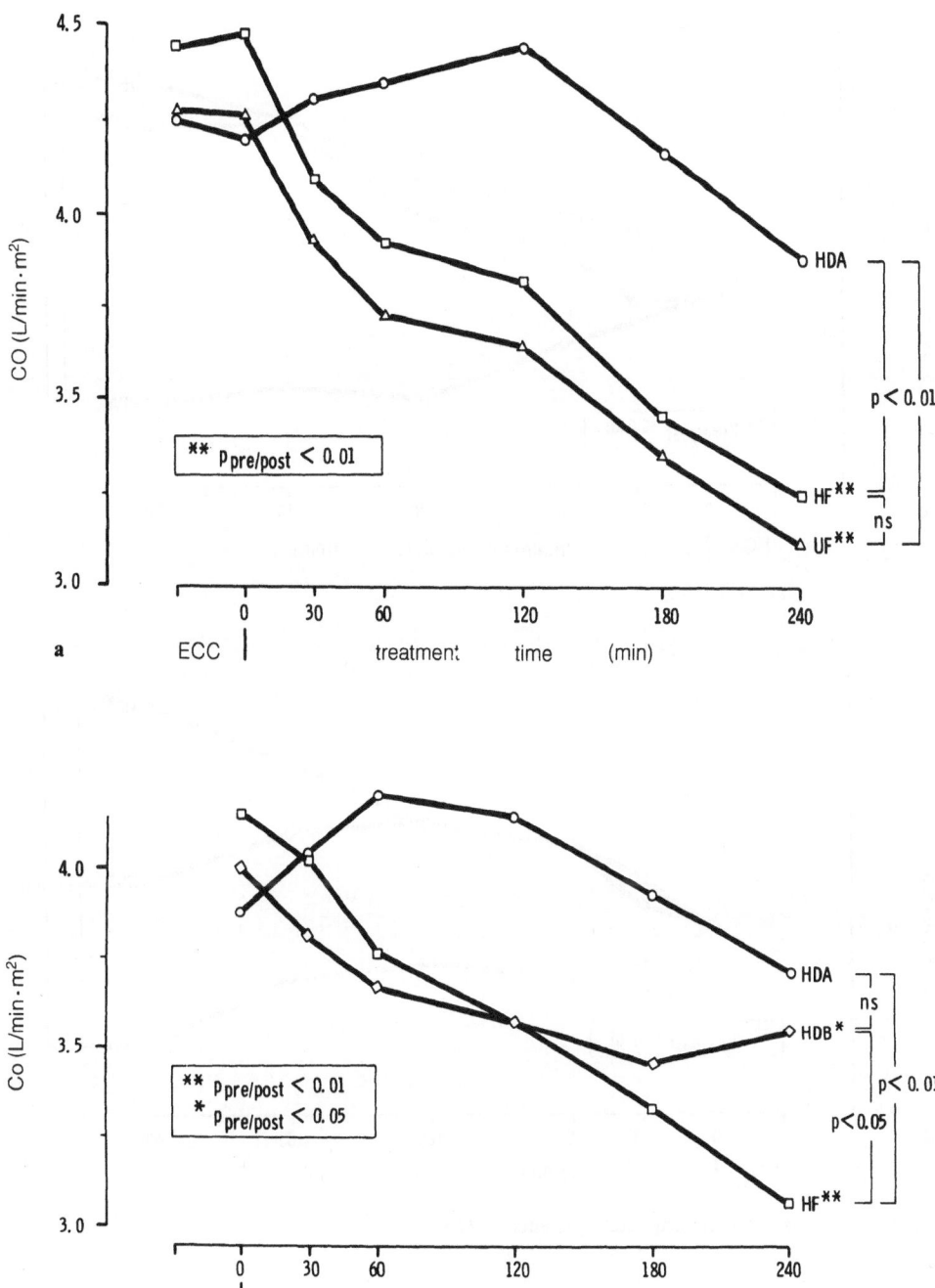

Fig. 3a–f. Cardiac output *(CO)*, change in total peripheral vascular resistance *(ΔTPR)*, and change in plasma noradrenaline concentrations *(PNA)* after 30 min extracorporeal circulation without solute and volume flux *(ECC)* and during ultrafiltration *(UF)*, hemofiltration *(HF)*, acetate hemodialysis *(HDA)*, and bicarbonate hemodialysis *(HDB)*. (Redrawn from [22]). **a, b.** Cardiac output (CO)

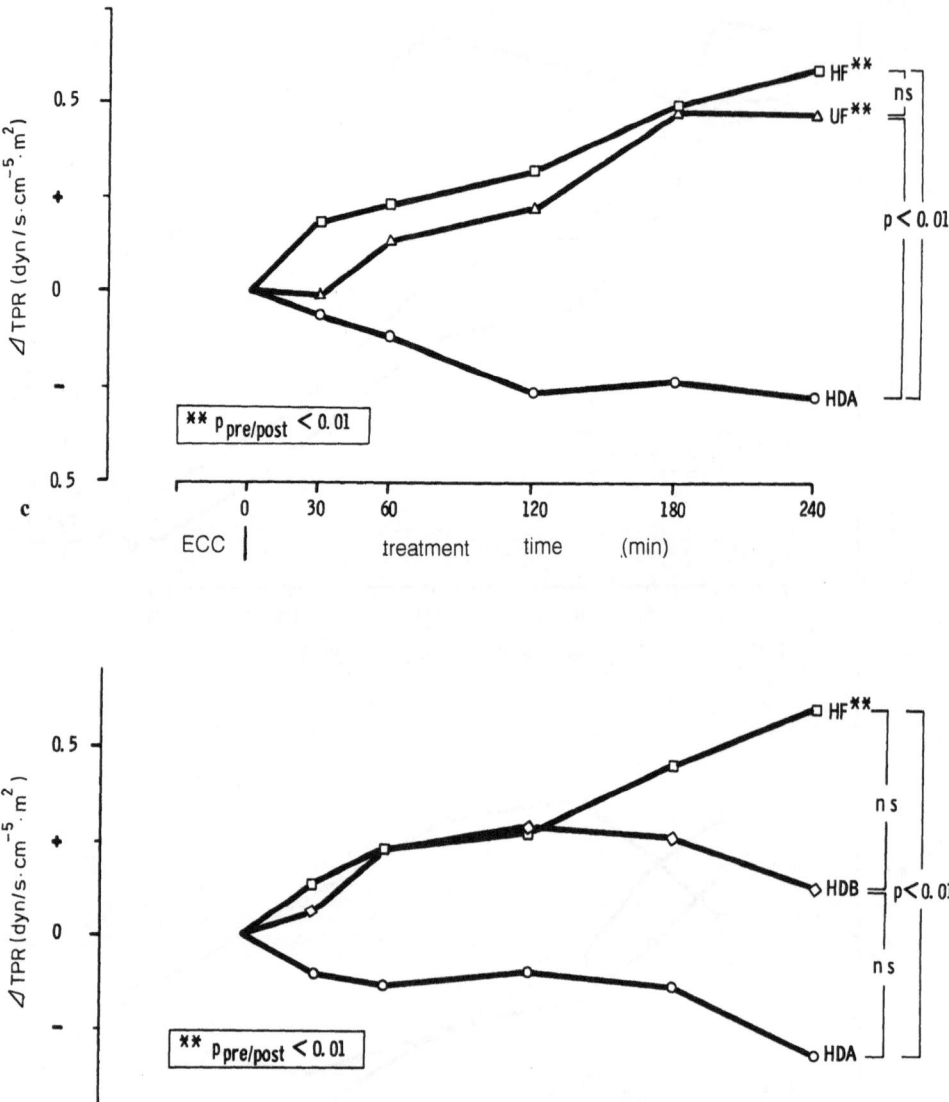

Fig. 3c, d. Change of total peripheral resistance (ΔTPR)

Table 1 gives a brief review of hemodynamic data reported in the literature, the vast majority of which support the described pattern shown in Figs. 2 and 3.

Ultrafiltration and hemofiltration are not the only treatment modalities with reported vascular stability. Improved hemodynamic stability has also been reported for hemodiafiltration [47, 48], and more recently for hemodialysis using dialysis membranes with high hydraulic permeability [45, 49].

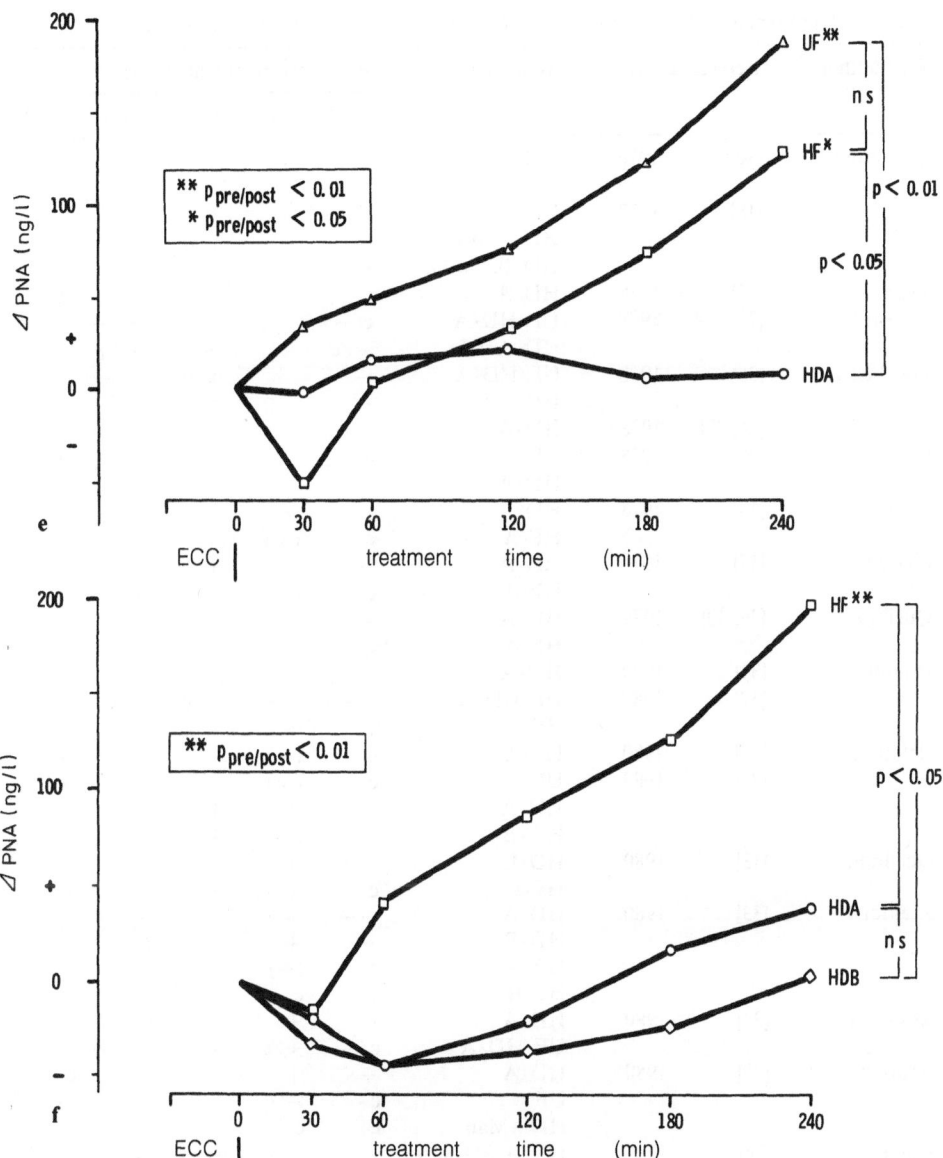

Fig. 3e, f. Change of plasma noradrenaline concentration (ΔPNA)

Summary

As is evident from Table 1, the majority of reports clearly show that the uremic patient on regular hemodialysis treatment is able to react physiologically, at least quantitatively, to volume removal. During hemofiltration this physiologic response is maintained. In contrast, during hemodialysis the same patient fails to react adequately to fluid withdrawal with an increased vascular resistance. There is some evidence that this coincides with a blunted increase in sympathetic tone. The actual cause of the different hemodynamics, however, remains unknown. The proposed factors (Table 2) will be discussed in detail.

Table 1. Hemodynamic changes during various extracorporeal treatments for uremia

First author	Reference	Year	Treatment	Pre-/post-treatment change				
				BP	HR	CO	TPR	PNA
Bergström	[10]	1976	HD·A	−	+			
			UF	c	c			
Graefe	[18]	1977	UF	c				
			HD·A, Na 133	−	−			
			HD·B, Na 133	−				
Brecht	[23]	1978	HD·A					c
Bergström	[20, 24]	1978	UF/HD·A	c/−		−/+	+/−	
			HD·A/UF	−/c		+/−	−/+	
Pogglitsch	[25]	1978	UF/HD·A	−/−		c/+	+/−	
			HD·A	−		c	−	
Zucchelli	[26, 27]	1978	HD·A			c		
Canella	[28]	1978	UF	c				+
			HD·A	−				c
Baldamus	[14]	1978	HD·A	−	+			
			HF·A	c	(+)			
Shaldon	[17]	1979	HD·A	−	+	+	c	
			HF·A	c	c	−	+	
Quellhorst	[29, 30]	1979	HD·A	−				
			HF·A	c				
Hampl	[31]	1979	HD·A	−	+	(−)	c	
	[32]	1980	UF/HD·A	c/−	c/+	−/c	+/c	
			HF·L	c	c	−	+	
Baldamus	[12]	1980	HF·A	c	(+)	−	+	+
	[22]	1982	UF	c	(+)	−	+	+
			HD·A	−	+	+	−	c
			HD·B	−	(+)	+	c	c
Quellhorst	[13]	1980	HD·L	−	+	+	c	c
			HF·L	c	+	−	+	+
Shaldon	[33]	1980	HD·A	− −	+		−	
			HD·B	−	+		c	
			HF·A	c	(+)		+	
			HF·B	c	c		+	
Keshaviah	[34]	1980	HD·A	−	+	−	c	
			UF/HD·A	c/−	+/c	−/c	+/−	
Henrich	[35]	1980	HD·A	−	+			c
			UF	c	−			+
			HD+Man	c	c			c
Wehle	[36]	1981	HD·A, Na140+U	−		+	−	
	[37]	1979	HD·B, Na140+U	−		+	−	
			HD·B, Na133+U	− −		c	−	
Aljama	[15]	1982	HD·A	−		c	−	
			HD·B	c		−	c	
			HF·A	c		−	+	
			UF	c		−	+	
Cini	[38]	1982	UF/HD·A	c/c	c/+	−/+	+/−	
			HD·A/UF	c/c	+/c	+/−	c/+	
Hampl	[39]	1982	HD·A	−	+	c	c	
			HD·B	c	c	−	+	
Kishimoto	[40]	1982	HD·A	−		c	−	
			UF	c		−	+	
Vincent	[41]	1982	HD·A	−	+	−	c	
			HD·B	c	c	−	(+)	

Table 1. continued

First author	Reference	Year	Treatment	Pre-/post-treatment change				
				BP	HR	CO	TPR	PNA
Schick	[42]	1983	HD·A	−	+	c	−	c
			HD·B	c	+	c	c	c
Frewin	[43]	1984	HD·A	−				−
Leenen	[44]	1984	HD·A	− .	+ +	+	−	
			HD·B	c	c	c	c	
Freyschuss	[46]	1984	UF	c	c	−	+	
			HD·A	c	+ +	(+)	−	
Zucchelli	[16]	1984	HD·A	−	+		c	c
			HF·A	c	c		+	+
Schneider	[45]	1985	HFD·A	−	+	−	c	+
			HFD·B	c	+	+	c	(−)
			HDF·A	c	+	−	+	+
			HDF·B	c	+	+	−	−
			HF·A	c	+	−	+	+
			HF·B	c	(+)	+	−	c

Treatments UF, ultrafiltration; HF, hemofiltration; HD, hemodialysis; UF/HD, HD/UF, sequential therapy, UF followed by HD or vice versa; HDF, hemodiafiltration; HFD, high-flux hemodialysis; ·A, acetate dialysate/replacement fluid; ·B, bicarbonate dialysate/replacement fluid; ·L, lactate dialysate/replacement fluid; Na 140, Na 133, sodium concentration in dialysate; +U, urea-containing dialysate; +Man, mannitol containing dialysate
Hemodynamic changes BP, blood pressure; HR, heart rate; CO, cardiac output; TPR, total peripheral vascular resistance; PNA, plasma noradrenaline concentration; c, pre- and post-treatment are comparable; −, decrease, (−) weak, − − strong; +, increase, (+) weak, + + strong

Mechanisms Involved

According to KJELLSTRAND [50], dialysis-induced hypotension is a multifactorial event. To understand the genesis of dialysis hypotension, the possible factors have to be classified as pathogenetic, mediating, pathophysiologic, and of underlying pathology. Pathogenetic factors are directly related to the treatment itself. Mediators are initiated by pathogenetic factors. Both pathogenetic mechanisms and/or mediators act on pathophysiologic pathways which might be altered by underlying pathological factors. The different hemodynamic factors which are believed to be involved in hemodialysis-associated hypotension are listed according to these distinctions in Table 2.

Hypovolemia

Hypotension during dialysis is primarily attributed to intravascular hypovolemia caused by ultrafiltration. Ultrafiltration leads to an increase in plasma protein concentration and in colloid osmotic pressure. This increases the volume shifted from the interstitial into the intravascular space (Fig. 4). Hypotension occurs only if ultrafiltration exceeds vascular refilling, and other mechanisms, such as increase in vas-

Table 2. Mechanisms which possibly interfere with blood pressure regulation during hemofiltration and hemodialysis

Pathogenetic factors	Mediators	Pathophysiologic factors	Underlying pathology
Ultrafiltration	Hypovolemia	Myocardial contractility	Heart disease
Solute removal	Electrolyte imbalance		Vascular disease
Solute uptake	Acid-base changes	Heart rate	Autonomic neuropathy
Membrane/blood interaction	Prostaglandins	Vascular volume	
	Complement activation	TPR	Medication
	White blood cell products		
	Platelet products		
	Antidiuretic hormone (ADH)		
	Atrial natriuretic factor		
	Interleukin-1		
	Catecholamines		

cular resistance or increase in heart rate, cannot compensate. Vascular refilling in dialysis patients exceeds that of normal patients after hemorrhage [51] and has been measured to be in the order of 300 ml/h [52, 53]. According to a study by KIM et al. [52], the critical point where systemic hypotension occurs is reached at a plasma volume of or below 50 ml/kg body weight.

The same group measured change in plasma volume during hemodialysis. Hemodynamic consequences of hypovolemia depend not only on the absolute blood volume but also on the mobility of blood from the venous capacitance vessels mainly in the lung [54]. CHAIGON et al. [53] concluded from their measurements of blood volume distribution and cardiac output in hemodialysis that the postdialysis reduction in cardiac output might be related more to the relocation of blood volume than to the absolute degree of blood volume reduction. Compliance of these venous capacitance vessels very much depends on sympathetic venous tone, and this might be impaired by autonomic neuropathy. Nothing is known about sympathetic regulation of the intrathoracic blood volume in response to ultrafiltration in uremic patients. Mobilization of venous blood from these capacitance vessels veils the strict relationship between decrease in central venous pressure and decrease in blood volume, devaluating the monitoring of central venous pressure as a control parameter for changes in blood volume. Hypovolemia leads to shock with all the deleterious consequences [7] at a point where the circulation no longer meets the needs of vital organ perfusion. This is not solely a function of circulatory volume, but also one of cardiac output and of TPR.

Summary
Intravascular hypovolemia occurs if ultrafiltration, an inevitable event of intermittent dialysis treatment, exceeds vascular refilling. It leads to intratreatment hypotension and shock if compensatory mechanisms such as mobilization of blood from venous capacitance vessels and increase in TPR, heart rate, and myocardial contractility are overstressed.

Osmotic Changes

Hypotension has frequently been associated with a fall in serum osmolality [10, 18, 35, 55–57] and has been linked to disequilibrium syndrome [35, 36]. The connection between changes in osmolality and symptoms of hypotension was further substantiated in 1976 by BERGSTRÖM et al. [10], who observed that in the same patients, fluid removal by ultrafiltration with no change in serum osmolality was well tolerated, but that the identical weight loss during conventional dialysis (acetate buffer) led to hypotension. SHALDON [58] then drew attention to the potential benefit of separating ultrafiltration from solute exchange by sequencing both treatment steps. Subsequently the improved tolerance of ultrafiltration, which was initially observed by KOBAYASHI et al. in 1972 [8], was confirmed by several investigators (Table 1).

BERGSTRÖM et al. suggested in their initial paper [10] that the change in serum osmolality might be a causative factor. They then conducted an experiment in which

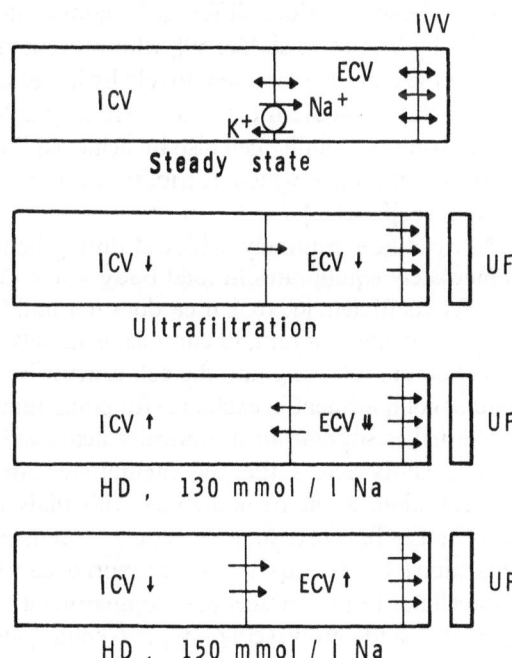

Fig. 4. Volume shifts during hemodialysis *(HD)*. In the steady-state body compartments are constant. Intravascular volume *(IVV)* is maintained mainly by the colloid oncotic pressure of proteins. Equilibrium of intracellular *(ICV)* and extracellular *(EVC)* volume is regulated mainly by the sodium-potassium pump, and by the passive permeability of the cell membrane. Ultrafiltration *(UF)* leads to a redistribution: ICV, ECV, and IVV decrease. During hemodialysis with low sodium concentration in the dialysate, the interstitial sodium concentration decreases. This leads to a volume flux from the ECV to the ICV and aggravates intravascular hypovolemia caused by UF. In contrast, during high-sodium dialysis, interstitial sodium concentration rises, which causes a volume flux from ICV to ECV and improves vascular refilling

they omitted or mitigated the drop in osmolality by increasing the sodium concentration of the dialysate [36, 37]. They, like others [18, 55], found an improved vascular stability with increasing dialysate sodium concentration and attributed this to less or no change in serum osmolality. In contrast to this interpretation, SHALDON et al. [21] compared hemodynamic stability in the same patient population at low- and high-efficiency treatment in a cross-over study. Patients had reached a metabolic steady state with increased serum urea concentrations during the low-efficiency treatment phase. Because of identical intratreatment removal of waste products – mainly urea – low- and high-efficiency treatments resulted in identical changes in serum osmolality, but symptomatology varied: hypotension occurred much more frequently during high- than during low-efficiency hemodialysis. Therefore, SHALDON et al. concluded that the absolute change in osmolality can not be the major contributing factor to hypotension during hemodialysis. The interpretation of BERGSTRÖM et al. must thus be reinterpreted.

The difference between the two studies is that the fall in serum osmolality is omitted in BERGSTRÖM's acute experiment by increasing the serum sodium concentration. In contrast, in SHALDON's steady-state study the change in serum osmolality was comparable, since he used identical dialysate sodium concentrations. Changes in body urea and sodium content, however, affect body compartments differently, and as a result produce different hemodynamic states. This view is supported by studies by WEHLE et al. [36, 59], who prevented a change in osmolality by adding urea to the dialysate, or alternatively by increasing dialysate sodium concentration. Only with high-sodium dialysate were they able to prevent hypotensive reactions. Hemodynamic stability can also be achieved if osmolality is maintained by solutes, such as mannitol, of which distribution volume is restricted to intravascular and/or interstitial space [35].

At clearances routinely achieved during hemodialysis and hemofiltration, urea immediately equilibrates in total body water. Owing to its high transcellular mass transfer coefficient [60–63], urea does not build up an intra-/extracellular concentration gradient. Sodium, in contrast, is mainly distributed in the extracellular volume. Sodium diffusing into the cell is actively transported outward into the extracellular compartment in exchange for potassium. This "restriction" to the interstitial space makes sodium an osmotically active substance, causing clinically relevant volume shifts across the cell membrane. An increase in extracellular sodium concentration, as in hemodialysis with dialysate of high sodium concentration (> 142 mEq/l), causes an extracellular volume shift. At low dialysate sodium concentration (< 138 mEq/l) fluid transport occurs in the opposite direction – from the extracellular to the intracellular compartment. The latter condition aggravates the interstitial and intravascular hypovolemia caused by ultrafiltration (Fig. 4). The dialysate sodium concentration of zero net diffusive sodium flux ($D_{Na=0}$) is dependent on the Donnan effect (α), which was found to be:

$$\alpha = 1 - 0.0073 \times C_{TPP}$$

for the operating conditions of hemodialysis [64]. It is further dependent on serum sodium concentration (C_{Na}):

$$D_{\mathrm{Na}=0} = \frac{C_{\mathrm{Na}}(1 - 0.0073 \times C_{\mathrm{TPP}})}{1 - 0.01 \times C_{\mathrm{TPP}}}$$

where C_{TPP} represents total plasma protein concentration in g%.

For clinical conditions this dialysate sodium concentration ($D_{\mathrm{Na}=0}$) is approximately 3 mEq/l higher than serum sodium concentration.

In view of these data, the hemodynamic differences described in the experiments of WEHLE et al. [36, 37] and SHALDON et al. [21] are easily understood. In SHALDON's study, ultrafiltration was not partially compensated for by an intra- to extracellular volume shift as was the case in WEHLE's study, where the intratreatment osmotic change was prevented by increasing dialysate sodium concentration. The magnitude of an intracellular fluid shift by low-sodium dialysate was measured to be of the order of 1–1.5 l, as demonstrated in early studies by OH et al. [65] and FALLS et al. [55] using dialysate sodium concentration of about 135 mEq/l. In thorough dog experiments KESHAVIAH et al. [66] separated the intercompartmental volume shifts during dialysis by sequencing ultrafiltration and diffusion. During ultrafiltration the change in interstitial space did not significantly differ from the ultrafiltered volume. During diffusion with a dialysate sodium concentration of 140 mEq/l and with zero net weight loss, they found a further decline of intravascular and interstitial volume. At the end of this sequential therapy, at a total ultrafiltrate of 700 ml, plasma volume had diminished by 340 ml and extracellular volume by 1170 ml. The extracellular volume shift (810 ml) was of about the same magnitude as the ultrafiltered volume. Conventional dialysis led to similar figures (820 ml).

VAN STONE et al. [67] studied the effect of dialysate sodium concentration on body fluid compartments in patients, and arrived at results similar to those of KESHAVIAH et al. [66] in dogs. At a total weight loss of 0 and of 2.0 kg they varied dialysate sodium concentration to 7% above and below pretreatment serum sodium

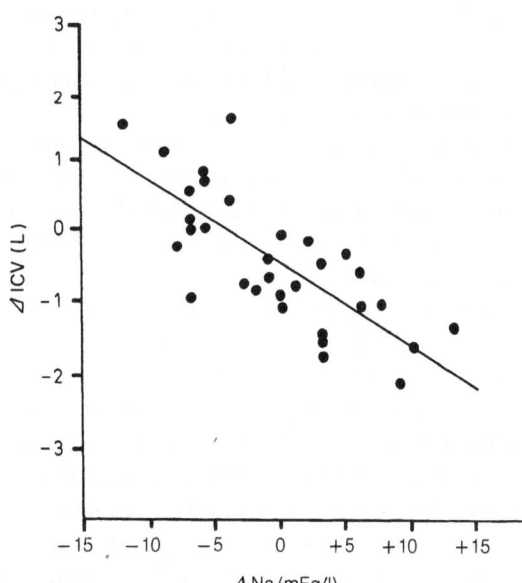

Fig. 5. Correlation between change in plasma sodium concentration and change in intracellular volume (ΔICV). (From [68])

concentration. Serum osmolality decreased in all groups and there was a significant inverse correlation between changes in intracellular volume and total serum osmolality. This correlation (Fig. 5) appeared to be entirely due to changes in serum sodium concentration, as there was no significant correlation between changes in intracellular volume and in serum urea concentration, the other major determinant of serum osmolality.

The discussion as to whether the hemodynamic benefits of hemofiltration were simply sodium related was initiated by GOTCH et al. [64, 69–71], who, on the basis of theoretical calculation, postulated that during hemofiltration protein concentration within the hemofilter increased owing to ultrafiltration along the device, and that therefore the Donnan factor would also increase. As a result of this, the sodium concentration of the ultrafiltrate would decrease with increasing plasma filtration fraction. This is in contrast to several reports which demonstrate that filtrate sodium concentration is independent of plasma protein concentration [72–74]. Additional data [75, 76] at single values of protein concentration show no net sodium holdback, i.e., filtrate and retentate sodium concentration are approximately equal. In an in vivo study LYSAGHT et al. [77] were able to demonstrate that the ratio of sodium concentration in the filtrate to that in the plasma (β_m) increases, results which LYSAGHT confirmed in a careful in vitro model study [75]. In an albumin sodium chloride solution, plasma water sodium sieving coefficient decreased with increasing protein concentration by only 1% (Fig. 6). This effect was counterbalanced by an increase in plasma water sodium concentration. The relative magnitude of these two oppositely directed effects differed from conditions in blood, so that the overall sieving coefficient changed slightly with plasma albumin level. Nevertheless, the same basic phenomenon was clearly operating in vitro as in vivo.

To further clarify this controversial issue, sodium balance was compared during hemodialysis and hemofiltration under defined and comparable experimental conditions [78]. Sodium balance was measured in hemofiltration, but could only be calculated according to the model of GOTCH and SARGENT [64]. The results showed essentially no difference in sodium flux between hemodialysis and hemofiltration using an identical sodium concentration of 140 mEq/l in dialysate and in hemofiltration replacement fluid. The hemodynamic benefit of hemofiltration became evident also from these experiments.

In order to compare the hemodynamic consequences of a changing sodium balance in hemodialysis and hemofiltration, BALDAMUS et al. [79, 80] measured the individual sodium loss (mEq/kg weight loss) and correlated it to the individual change in blood pressure and TPR (Fig. 7). Basic experimental conditions such as duration of treatment, small-solute clearances, weight loss (3 kg), and composition of dialysate and replacement fluid were the same for hemodialysis and hemofiltration. Whereas blood pressure remained stable over the entire scale of sodium removal in hemofiltration, it decreased during hemodialysis with increasing sodium loss. The corresponding TPR rose with increasing sodium loss only during hemofiltration, but decreased in hemodialysis with increasing sodium loss. Interpreting these data, hypovolemia, which is aggravated at high sodium loss by an intracellular volume shift, is hemodynamically compensated for by an increase in TPR during hemofiltration. This response is impaired, as was discussed before, during hemodialysis. The decreasing TPR with increasing sodium loss during hemodialysis may

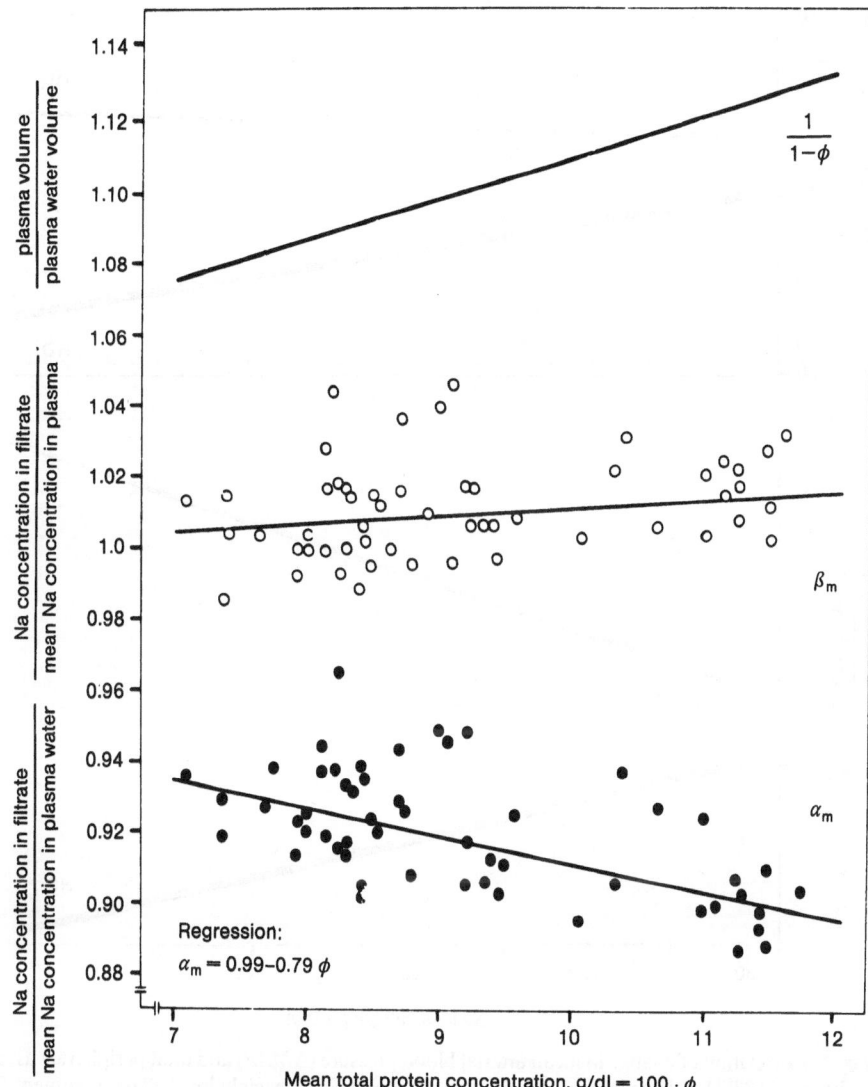

Fig. 6. In vivo sodium sieving coefficient, measured during hemofiltration [77]. Plasma volume relative to plasma water volume $\left(\dfrac{1}{1-\Phi}\right)$ increases with increasing plasma protein concentration. The ratio of sodium concentration in filtrate to mean sodium concentration in plasma water (α_m) decreases with increasing protein concentration. As a result of this, the ratio of sodium concentration in filtrate to mean sodium concentration in plasma (β_m) is practically uninfluenced by mean total protein concentration

be due to a stimulated production of prostaglandin E (see "Hormonal Changes", p. 182) as was found by SCHULTZE et al. in hemodialysis with low dialysate sodium concentration [81]. Decreased antidiuretic hormone (ADH) secretion could be another explanation (see "Hormonal Changes", p. 181).

The extreme experimental difficulty of measuring an exact sodium balance during hemodialysis results from multiplication of two high-number measures (vol-

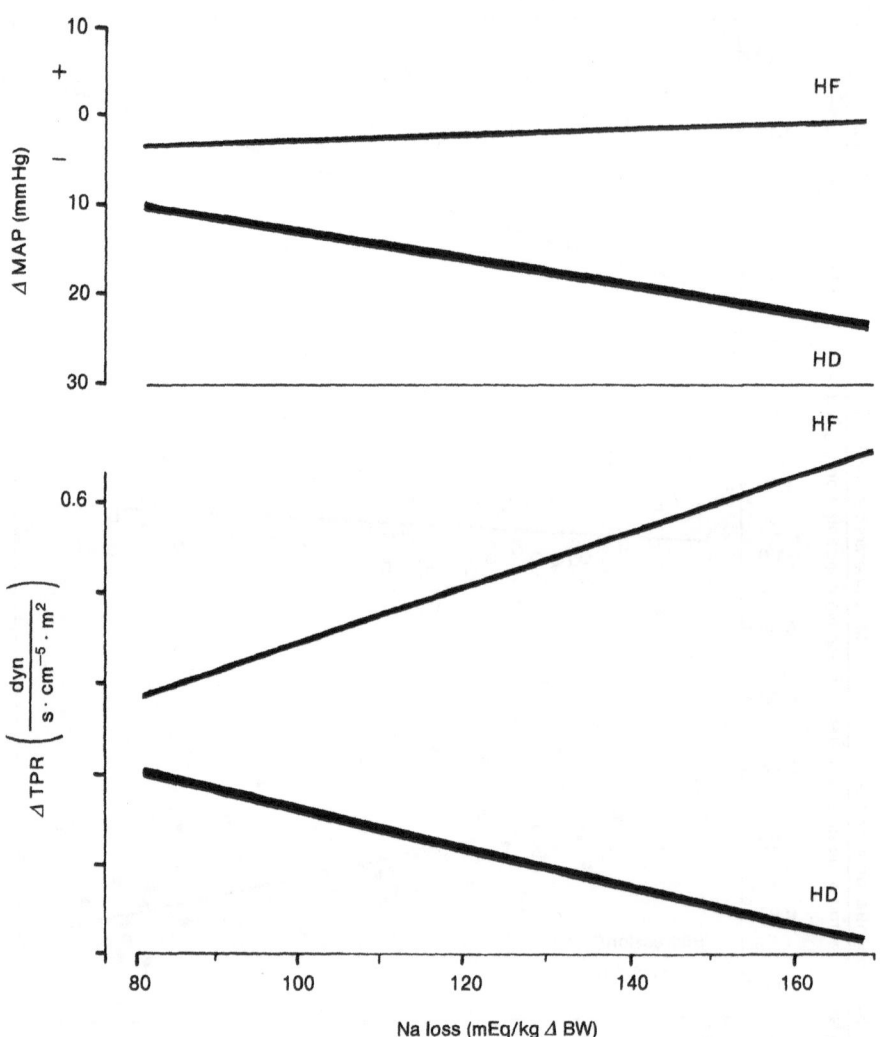

Fig. 7. Correlation of change in mean arterial blood pressure (ΔMAP) and total peripheral vascular resistance (ΔTPR) with individual sodium loss, given as mEq/kg weight loss [80] per treatment. The same patients underwent hemodialysis *(HD)* and hemofiltration *(HF)* at standardized working conditions: 3 kg linear weight loss and identical small-solute clearances and treatment time. Even at high sodium loss, i.e., a decrease in interstitial sodium concentration, blood pressure is maintained in HF by an increased TPR. In contrast, in HD TPR even decreases with increasing sodium loss and as a result of this blood pressure falls

ume × sodium concentration) and from the imprecision of sodium determination (± 2-3 mEq/l). Therefore, it is difficult to prove or disprove the hypothesis of GOTCH and SARGENT. The strongest argument against the hypothesis that hemodynamic stability during hemofiltration simply reflects a treatment with positive sodium balance is provided by the experimental observations by HENDERSON et al. [82]. They were able to show in a predilution hemofiltration experiment that hemodynamic stability was still greater than in comparable hemodialysis. During predilution hemofiltration, according to GOTCH and SARGENT [64], blood plasma protein concentration decreases, and therefore the sodium sieving coefficient should increase, resulting in a balance more negative than that in hemodialysis.

The fact that TPR increased in hemofiltration, a situation where GOTCH and SARGENT postulate a more positive sodium balance, but not during hemodialysis, seems to be an unphysiologic response.

Summary
As long as changes in serum osmolality during hemodialysis and hemofiltration are due to removal of solutes which equilibrate in total body water and have a high transcellular mass transfer coefficient (urea), the effect of these changes on blood pressure remains negligible. However, if solutes are moved selectively from or to the intravascular or interstitial space, this causes a fluid shift from the extra- to the intracellular compartment or vice versa. This fluid shift then compensates for or aggravates the hypovolemia caused by the unavoidable ultrafiltration. These fluid shifts have a greater hemodynamic effect during hemodialysis, because here the physiologic regulation of TPR is impaired. In contrast, during hemofiltration it still functions physiologically.

Electrolyte Changes

Intermittent ESRD treatment inevitably results in fast electrolyte changes. In addition, treatment-related acid-base changes cause an electrolyte shift at the cellular level.

Potassium

Extracellular potassium is vigorously removed during treatment by the dialysis procedure and by an intracellular shift parallel with normalization of uremic metabolic acidosis. These fast potassium concentration changes have been discussed as one causative factor in the increased incidence of cardiac arrhythmia during treatment. QUELLHORST et al. [83] studied the effect of potassium on intra- and posttreatment cardiac arrhythmia. They investigated the same patients during hemodialysis, hemofiltration, and hemodiafiltration, and reported a higher incidence of arrhythmia Lown class IV and V in all treatment regimes when patients were exposed to a bath with low potassium concentration. This was independent of the buffer (acetate or bicarbonate). The incidence was low in hemofiltration, increased in hemodiafiltration, and became frequent in hemodialysis. In addition, hypotension appeared to be a predisposing factor. MORRISON et al. [84] also observed an increase in ventricular arrhythmia at low dialysate potassium concentration. Intratreatment arrhythmia occurred more frequently in patients with ventricular hypertrophy and in those on digitalis medication.

Potassium itself is a vasoactive substance [85, 86]. A decrease in extracellular potassium concentration causes vasoconstriction [87]. This vasoactivity appears to result from actions on the sarcolemmal (Na-K)-ATPase.

Sodium

Depending on weight loss, net sodium balance during the dialytic process is negative. According to the sodium concentration in the dialysate or in the hemofiltration replacement fluid, extracellular sodium concentration increases or decreases. Sodium, beyond being a potent osmotic agent and causing intra-/extracellular fluid shifts (see "Osmotic Changes", p. 167) is known to induce vascular smooth muscle contraction [88, 89].

An increase in extracellular sodium increases passive intracellular sodium flux and hence reduces membrane potential. This sodium influx, however, depends upon intracellular ionic calcium. Whether the small changes in extracellular sodium concentration during hemodialysis or hemofiltration have an effect on TPR is still an unsettled issue.

Interstitial sodium concentration influences vascular resistance indirectly by its influence on vasopressin secretion (see "Hormonal Changes", p. 181). Vasopressin secretion is enhanced during increased sodium concentration and by decreased extracellular volume [90]. There are still no measurements of changes in plasma vasopressin concentration during ESRD treatment.

Sodium also influences TPR indirectly by its effect on the renin/angiotensin system (see "Hormonal Changes"). Lowering serum sodium concentration in isovolemic dialysis increases renin release and leads to an increase in blood pressure [91].

Calcium

One object of intermittent dialysis treatment is a positive calcium balance. A rise in ionized calcium increases TPR [92, 93] and improves cardiac contractility [94, 95]. Acidosis blunts this response [96]. So far, the effect of calcium on TPR during ESRD treatment has not been studied. HENRICH et al. [97], however, recently reported that calcium improves left ventricular contractility. In isovolemic hemodialysis, left ventricular contractility increased if plasma ionized calcium concentration was raised 0.25 mmol/l. Similar results were obtained by CHAIGNON et al. [98], but their experimental conditions were not as strictly controlled as those by HENRICH et al.

The indirect effect which calcium produces via parathyroid hormone secretion [99] on cardiac performance need be mentioned only briefly. It is difficult to monitor calcium balance during different ESRD treatments [100]. Here again hemofiltration is superior to hemodialysis, because of the simplicity with which in- and output can be measured. There are no hemodynamic studies comparing hemodialysis and hemofiltration under controlled conditions of intratreatment calcium balance.

Magnesium

Magnesium overload is a consequence of chronic renal failure, but it can be rectified by renal replacement therapy. A decrease in plasma magnesium concentration increases vascular reactivity and, concomitantly, vascular resistance [101], but vascular response differs from organ to organ and is closely linked to other ions, – in particular, calcium. Competition between magnesium and calcium is reported for the vascular smooth muscle cells [101] and for the heart [102, 103]. There are no studies of the effect of magnesium on cardiocirculatory parameters during dialysis.

The above-mentioned effects of ions on hemodynamics are oversimplified. The individual regulatory events of single ions during dialysis treatment cannot be separated from their interaction [87]. Beyond that, the ionic composition of body fluids alters the effect of many vasoactive hormones and substances.

Summary
Electrolyte changes influence hemodynamics in many ways. They cause fluid shifts between intra- and extracellular compartments and, consequently, change blood volume (sodium). They act directly on the peripheral vasculature and cause changes in TPR (sodium, potassium, etc.). In addition, they modulate cardiac performance (calcium). Individual ionic events depend on simultaneous changes in other ions. The complexity of ionic action on the cardiovascular system is further increased by its interaction with various hormonal systems.

Comparative studies on the effect of single ions on hemodynamics in hemodialysis and hemofiltration have not yet been performed.

Buffer-Related Changes

One essential requirement of ESRD treatment is the removal of hydrogen ions, which cause the metabolic hypochloremic acidosis of chronic renal failure. These hydrogen ions are mainly generated from protein metabolism. At a standard daily protein intake of 1 g/kg body weight, 50–60 mEq hydrogen ions are formed per day [104, 105]. During each renal replacement therapy these hydrogen ions have to be removed or neutralized.

Acetate/Bicarbonate

Up to 1972, acid-base balance during hemodialysis was achieved with bicarbonate as the dialysate buffer. It was MION et al. [106] who replaced bicarbonate in dialysate with acetate. Only physicochemical considerations led to this change; bicarbonate concentrate was unstable, and calcium and magnesium formed insoluble salts, problems which were solved with acetate. Under normal conditions metabolism of acetate generates equimolar amounts of bicarbonate, and the dialysance at zero ultrafiltration is about equal for both buffers. Bicarbonate is removed, but replaced by acetate. Ultrafiltration, however, decreases acetate dialysance, and under these circumstances bicarbonate removal exceeds acetate gain [107]. Acetate was and is used with great success and without major complications as a dialysate buffer. In 1976 GRAEFE et al. [19, 108] drew attention to the fact that acetate may play a role in the etiology of dialysis-induced hypotension and intradialytic symptomatology. Since then a great number of investigations have focused on the metabolism of acetate and its cardiovascular effects.

As early as 1928, BAUER and RICHARDS [109] were able to demonstrate that acetate is a potent vasodilator. This effect was subsequently confirmed by others [110–112]. While the vasodilating effect of acetate, decreasing TPR, is undisputed, there is controversy over the effect of acetate on myocardial contractility. KIRKENDOL et al. [113] found in anesthetized dogs a dose-dependent decrease in myocardial contractility and a fall in mean arterial pressure following a bolus injection of acetate; they postulated that acetate was a myocardial depressant. This view was supported by data from AIZAWA et al. [114, 115], showing that the ratio of the pre-ejection period to left ventricular ejection time (PEP:LVET), calculated from an electrocardiogram, increased during acetate infusion and during dialysis, indicating myocardial depression. Criticism of these data derived from the methodology. On the basis of echocardiography, CHEN et al. [116] were able to demonstrate during dialysis that the PEP:LVET ratio is an unreliable parameter for myocardial function. Their data showed a reduction in preload as well as in afterload at an increased heart rate; they interpreted this as a sign for improved myocardial contractility. This was also found in a study by LIANG and LÖWENSTEIN [117], who infused acetate in an increasing dosage into anesthetized dogs. As a consequence of this acetate application, cardiac output increased owing to an increase in heart rate and in stroke volume, while TPR decreased. This positive inotropic effect of acetate was confirmed in a later investigation by KIRKENDOL et al. [118], when they infused acetate instead of giving it as a bolus. Only at a high dosage of 1 mmol/min/kg body weight did they register a fall in blood pressure in dogs.

Similar results were obtained by KESHAVIAH [119]. In anesthetized dogs, acetate infusion was immediately followed by a rise in cardiac output and a fall in TPR (Fig. 8). Mean arterial pressure fell and pulmonary artery pressure rose. On the basis of the effects of acetate, namely an increase in cardiac output and a decrease in TPR, it is easy to explain the great variance of reported data on hemodynamics during hemodialysis [5, 12, 18, 22, 33, 36, 37, 39, 42, 44, 45]. In regular uncomplicated patients, no hemodynamic complications are observed. The increase in cardiac output compensates for the fall in TPR. However, patients with impaired cardiac function are unable to further increase cardiac output, and hypotension is the result of peripheral vasodilatation.

Cardiac performance can also be negatively influenced by a high acetate load during dialysis if plasma acetate concentration increases to toxic levels. Therefore it is important to briefly discuss acetate metabolism.

Acetate plasma concentration depends on acetate load and on acetate metabolic rate. Acetate load during standard hemodialysis amounts to 1100–1200 mEq per treatment, which leads to an increased mean plasma acetate concentration of 5 mEq/l, ranging from 2.5 to 12 mEq/l. As plasma acetate concentration rises, acetate metabolism reaches a maximum. The kinetics best fit the MICHAELIS MENTON

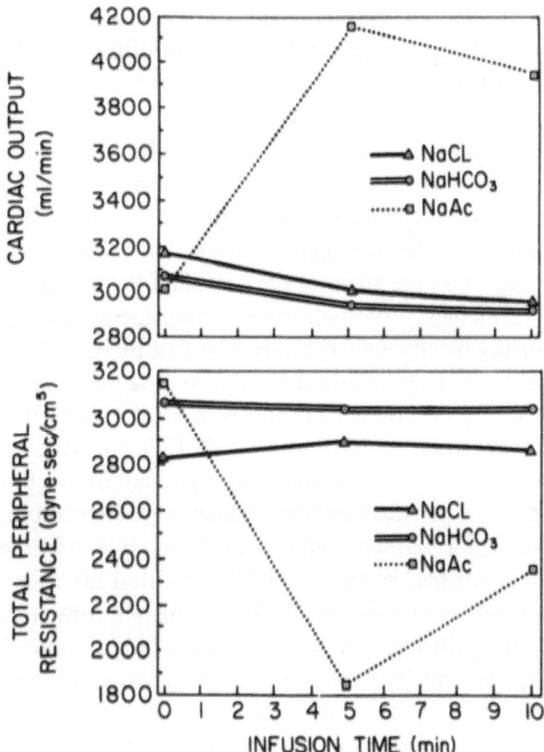

Fig.8. Changes in cardiac output and in TPR during infusion of sodium acetate, sodium chloride, or sodium bicarbonate (2.4 mmol/min) in anesthetized dogs. (From [119])

model, from which a maximal metabolic rate can be calculated ($V_{max} = 8.1$ mEq/min), as can the plasma concentration at which metabolic rate is half-maximal ($K_m = 8.6$ mEq/l) [105]. These are only mean figures with a great interindividual variance from acetate-intolerant patients, with V_{max} of only 5.6 mEq/min and a K_m of 2.3 mEq/l, to patients with high metabolic rates ($V_{max} = 50$ mEq/min; $K_m = 24$ mEq/l). From this great variability it can be concluded that there are a substantial number of patients who have only a limited capacity to metabolize acetate, who may suffer from the resultant but unwanted alteration of acid – base homeostasis, and who may also experience hemodynamic complications owing to the direct effects of acetate.

In view of data on acetate kinetics [120–122], it is hard to accept that at identical small-solute removal rates the acetate load would be higher in hemodialysis than in hemofiltration. SHALDON et al. [17] were the only investigators who measured plasma acetate concentrations during acetate hemodialysis and acetate hemofiltration under matched operating conditions. They did not observe any difference in plasma acetate concentrations. At a dialysance of more than 2 ml/min/kg body weight, bicarbonate loss (about equal to acetate gain) exceeds the metabolic production of bicarbonate. This is an important point, since modern dialysis equipment allows high acetate dialysance of far beyond this critical figure [123]. Here, acetate must be replaced by bicarbonate as the dialysis buffer.

There exists some experimental evidence that acetate metabolism differs between hemodialysis and hemofiltration. KISHIMOTO et al. [124] were able to show an improved acetate metabolism in hemofiltration. They attribute this to the improved hepatic blood flow in hemofiltration compared with that in hemodialysis [124, 219].

Beside the fact that acetate is a potent vasodilator, it is important to note that acetate might induce hypotension by a further mechanism. At a blood acetate concentration of 10 mEq/l and more [104] during hemodialysis, acetate stimulates interleukin-I (IL-1) production from monocytes [125]. The role of IL-1 in the pathogenesis of complications in hemodialysis will be discussed in a specific section (p. 183).

Several investigators have studied the incidence of hypotension and other intra-treatment symptomatology during acetate hemodialysis and compared it to that during bicarbonate dialysis. The first investigators to observe fewer hypotensive episodes during bicarbonate dialysis than during acetate dialysis were GRAEFE et al. [108, 19], and these findings were supported by a number of authors [22, 42, 44, 126]. Others found no differences [68, 127], and AIZAWA et al. even noticed a significant decrease in blood pressure during bicarbonate, but not during acetate, dialysis [115]. In a few publications differences were detectable only in specific situations and in particular patients [39]. A detailed analysis might help to understand the underlying mechanisms. WEHLE et al. [59] reported no differences at a dialysate sodium concentration of 140 mEq/l. At 133 mEq/l, however, hypotension occurred more frequently during acetate than during bicarbonate dialysis. In an additional series of experiments [68], they performed isovolemic dialysis at different dialysate sodium concentrations and with acetate and bicarbonate as buffers. They counterbalanced the change in osmolality with urea. TPR decreased significantly in acetate dialysis, and to a minor degree in bicarbonate dialysis. Neither urea nor sodium had an effect on TPR, but sodium still had an effect on blood pressure, most probably by its effect on the extracellular volume shift (see "Osmotic Changes", p. 167). Similar data were reported by RAIA et al. [128].

These reports indicate that acetate decreases vascular resistance, which is then counterbalanced by an increased cardiac output. Only if critical volume loss, caused either by ultrafiltration or by an intracellular volume shift (low-sodium dialysate), stresses the compensatory mechanisms to a maximum do clinical differences between acetate and bicarbonate dialysis become detectable. Comparing the hemodynamic data of acetate and bicarbonate hemodialysis with those of hemofiltration, the majority of authors report a decrease in vascular resistance during acetate dialysis and no increase during bicarbonate dialysis [12, 13, 22, 29, 33, 44]. In contrast, TPR increases in a physiological way during hemofiltration [12, 13, 33]. Only one report shows an increase in vascular resistance in acetate hemodialysis and hemofiltration but an unchanged or even decreased vascular resistance in bicarbonate dialysis [45].

Hypoxemia/Hypocapnia

Acetate may have an additional indirect effect on hemodynamics via hypoxemia, which occurs immediately after the start of hemodialysis; when acetate dialysate is used it persists throughout. According to a literature review [129, 130], pO_2 drops for a mean of 14.5 mmHg. Several mechanisms have been discussed:

1) Increased oxygen consumption, which is due either to acetate metabolism [131] or to the stress situation of a treatment with increased caloric turnover [132].
2) Decreased oxygen delivery, which is due to the Bohr effect, the acid – base-dependent change in oxygen affinity of the hemoglobin molecules [133]. The other possibility is related to membrane bioincompatibility (see below) of cellulosic membranes with complement activation and leukocyte sequestration in pulmonary capillaries [134, 135].
3) Depressed ventilatory drive, which is due to the CO_2 loss across the dialyzer [136, 137] or to acetate metabolism [130, 135, 137–139].

Beside its effect in hypoxemia, acetate may negatively influence cardiac performance in another way. HAMPL et al. [39] have demonstrated clinical evidence that in patients prone to hypotension the low pCO_2 (30.4 mmHg) during acetate dialysis when compared in the same patients to bicarbonate dialysis (pCO_2 38.2 mmHg) was associated with significant EEG changes and with an increased incidence of hypotension. It has been suggested that the EEG disturbances are a result of decreased cerebral blood flow, which is strongly regulated by pCO_2 [140, 141]. Hypocapnia leads to a decrease, whereas hypercapnia results in an increase in cerebral blood flow.

Differences in pCO_2 were reported for acetate hemodialysis and hemofiltration [142]. A low pCO_2 could be explained by generation and immediate loss of CO_2 within the dialyzer [143, 144], which, however, is not fully accepted [145]. A reduced pCO_2 decreases cerebral blood flow, which leads to a reduction in sympathetic activity [28, 146–148] and, consequently, to an impaired increase in TPR during acetate hemodialysis. But this does not explain why during bicarbonate dialysis TPR and plasma noradrenaline concentrations do not increase. KESHAVIAH [119] speculates, on the basis of a report by LIANG and LÖWENSTEIN [117], that byproducts of acetate metabolism, such as adenine nucleotides of adenosine, were inadequately removed during acetate hemodialysis, and that this may play a role in the etiology of dialysis-induced hypotension. Here again, the failure of TPR to increase during bicarbonate hemodialysis remains unexplained.

Summary
The use of acetate as a dialysate buffer is associated with vasodilatation, with increased cardiac output, with hypoxemia, and with hypocapnia. Only at a very high acetate load, which can be achieved with some forms of modern dialysis treatment [123], is maximal metabolic rate exceeded, leading to negative inotropic effects. In regular stable hemodialysis patients, the vasodilating action of acetate is compensated for by an increase in cardiac output. Only in patients with impaired cardiac and circulatory function does acetate lead to hemodynamic instability. Studies of acetate metabolism and its effect on the cardiovascular system explain why TPR decreases during acetate hemodialysis. However, is remains unclear why resistance in-

creases during hemofiltration in spite of the fact that the acetate load is comparable. Furthermore, there is still no explanation for the failure of TPR to increase during bicarbonate hemodialysis.

Hormonal Changes

Differences in removal of vasoactive substances have been suggested as the reason for the hemodynamic differences observed between hemodialysis and hemofiltration [22, 28]. Generation of one or more substances interfering with sympathetic activity during dialysis treatment, which are removed during hemofiltration but not during hemodialysis, or which are formed only during hemodialysis but not during hemofiltration, could explain all established findings: increase in sympathetic activity and TPR during ultrafiltration and hemofiltration, but no response during hemodialysis.

Catecholamines

Catecholamines are the most-discussed vasoactive substances. The finding that plasma noradrenaline concentration [23, 26] failed to increase during hemodialysis was ascribed to removal of this substance by the dialysis procedure. The difference from hemofiltration, where an increase was observed [13, 27], was explained by a higher removal rate during hemodialysis. This argument was invalidated when catecholamine dialysance was measured during hemodialysis and hemofiltration [22].

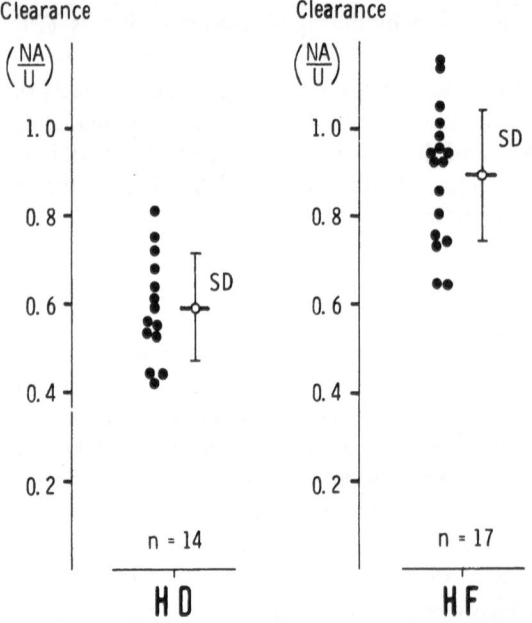

Fig. 9. Transmembranous noradrenaline *(NA)* transport relative to that of urea *(U)*, expressed as fractional clearance during hemodialysis *(HD)*, and hemofiltration *(HF)*. Mean values of HD and HF are significantly different

The ratio of noradrenaline to urea clearance was found to be 0.6 in hemodialysis 0.9 in hemofiltration (Fig. 9). Therefore at matched small-solute removal rates the observed increase in plasma noradrenaline during hemofiltration but not during hemodialysis can not be explained by an increased removal in hemodialysis. Just the opposite is the case [22]. As discussed in the section on autonomic neuropathy (see p. 186), the increase in sympathetic tone during hemofiltration and ultrafiltration but not during hemodialysis remains unexplained.

Vasopressin

Vasopressin was discussed by GOTCH and SARGENT [64] as a possible contributing factor to vascular stability, since it is a strong vasoconstrictor. Secretion is stimulated by even small changes in osmolality, sensed in the hypothalamus by osmoreceptors. Actually, it is not the change in osmolality of extracellular fluid which activates secretion, but rather the change in osmoreceptor cell size of the change in the intracellular concentration of a regulatory substance. When plasma osmolality is increased by urea, a solute rapidly equilibrating between intra- and extracellular fluid, ADH release is not enhanced. If, however, sodium or mannitol, solutes which remain in the extracellular space, are infused, ADH is released (Fig. 10) [149]. Therefore, ADH secretion has to be discussed in connection with intra-/extracellular volume shifts (see "Osmotic Changes," p. 167). In view of the observed hemodynamic changes during different treatment modalities, ADH secretion might help to ex-

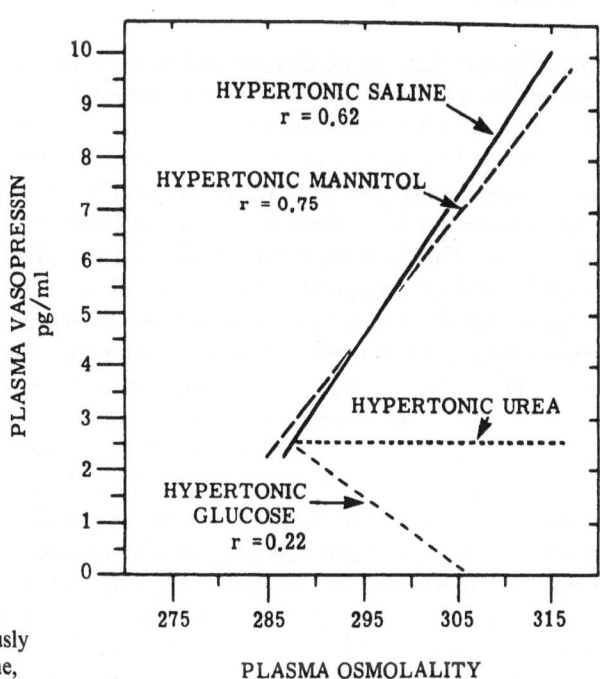

Fig. 10. Relationship of plasma vasopressin to osmolality [149] in healthy adults infused intravenously with hypertonic solutions of saline, mannitol, glucose, and urea

plain why during hemodialysis at high sodium loss, i.e., decrease in interstitial sodium concentration, TPR decreases (Fig. 7). The question, however, remains to be answered: Why at identically high sodium loss in both treatment modalities are the same patients able to increase TPR during hemofiltration but not during hemodialysis?

There are no comparative studies on ADH secretion during hemodialysis and hemofiltration.

Atrial Natriuretic Factor

Atrial natriuretic factor is a potent vasodilating hormone, which is secreted following atrial dilatation [150] and which is stimulated by volume loading [151]. As a polypeptide containing 28 amino acids, its molecular size was calculated to be about 3000 daltons [152]. Molecules of this size are removed effectively during hemofiltration, but not during hemodialysis. It is reasonable to assume increased secretion during the interdialytic period as a result of intertreatment fluid intake. During hemofiltration this vasodilator is removed, but not during hemodialysis, where it remains at high plasma concentrations if the endogenous half-life of this polypeptide is sufficiently long or prolonged in uremia. Increased susceptibility to hypotension in patients with cardiac impairment would also fit this hypothesis.

There are as yet no studies on atrial natriuretic factor in uremic patients.

Prostaglandins

Prostaglandins have to be divided into those with vasodilating and those with vasoconstricting potency. In addition, they may act differently on the peripheral systemic and pulmonary vasculature. To date there are only a few references which relate to hemodialysis, and none so far which focus on hemofiltration. Preliminary data suggest an increase in plasma prostaglandin (PGE_2) levels when using cellulosic membranes for hemodialysis; this is not observed with polyacrylonitrile membranes [153]. This increase is correlated with complement activation by cellulosic material and the consequent formation of leukocytic lung aggregates. BORGES et al. [154] speculated about a connection between increased incidence of intratreatment symptomatology and increased PGE_2 production. The only direct evidence that plasma PGE_2 rises during hemodialysis derives from data by SCHULTZE et al. [81], who were able to demonstrate an increase only if dialysis was performed at dialysate sodium concentrations of 125 mEq/l. Concomitantly with the rise of PGE_2, plasma renin activity (PRA) increased. An interaction PGE_2 synthesis and renin secretion is also known from other disease states [155-157]. A ratio of PGE:PRA correlated well with a decrease in systemic blood pressure. A principal argument against the direct influence of PGE_2 on peripheral vascular tone, which these authors discussed [156], is the high pulmonary clearance rate for PGE_2. Pulmonary clearance, however, might be severely altered as a result of sequestration of leukocytes. This would be an early event, but hypotension occurs late during dialysis.

Prostacyclin, a second vasodilating prostaglandin, is released during hemodialysis [158]. Using a cellulosic membrane an early rise is seen, which coincides with the peak of hypoxemia and occurrence of platelet aggregates, etc.

Thromboxane, a potent vasoconstrictor, also rises during the early phase of dialysis [159, 218, 219]. This can be shown in sheep to be induced by complement activation and pulmonary leukostasis [160].

So far these data do not contribute to the explanation of the difference in hemodynamics between hemodialysis and hemofiltration. Local secretion of prostaglandins may, however, play a role in the context of the IL-I hypothesis [161] (see "Blood/Device Interaction," p 184).

Summary

PGE_2, a potent vasodilator, is secreted early during hemodialysis with cellulosic membranes as a direct and/or indirect result of complement activation and pulmonary leukostasis. Prostacyclin and thromboxane are also stimulated. This does not occur if dialysis is performed with synthetic, "biocompatible" membranes. If the IL-I hypothesis proves to be true, late and local PGE_2 stimulation might help to explain dialysis hypotension.

So far, there are no reliable data which support the theory that prostaglandins play a contributory role in the hemodynamic differences between hemodialysis and hemofiltration.

Extracorporeal Temperature

MAGGIORE et al. [162] found that hemodynamic stability seen during ultrafiltration disappeared when returning extracorporeal blood was rewarmed to core body temperature. On the other hand, they were able to improve vascular stability during hemodialysis by decreasing the temperature of returning extracorporeal blood. They discussed the possibility that intratreatment vascular stability was at least partly a temperature-related phenomenon. Their finding was confirmed by several authors [163–167]. In an extended study, MAGGIORE et al. investigated hemodialysis and hemofiltration. They and others found that hemodynamic differences between cold hemodialysis and cold hemofiltration were partly diminished [168–170]. However, the maximal drop in blood pressure during warm hemofiltration was less than that during warm hemodialysis. In similar experiments, SCHÄFER et al. [171] and others [172] compared two situations in hemofiltration with replacement fluid at 35 °C and 40 °C and found no significant difference in hemodynamic stability. It appears that hemodialysis is more sensitive than hemofiltration to temperature changes. This might be related to temperature-dependent reactions within the dialyzer, the point of greatest heat exchange [173]. A report by ENIA et al. [174] is very interesting in this regard: membrane-related complement activation is prevented by decreasing dialysate temperature. The fact that hemodynamics are especially temperature-dependent during hemodialysis in contrast to hemofiltration would fit the IL-I hypothesis (see below): Complement activation and macrophage IL-I production are tempera-ture-sensitive [175].

Summary
Hemodynamic stability during dialysis and hemofiltration can be diminished by in-creasing the core body temperature. This lowers TPR. Temperature sensitivity seems to be higher during hemodialysis than during hemofiltration. This is in agree-ment with the IL-I hypothesis, since complement activation and macrophage IL-I production are both temperature-sensitive.

Blood/Device Interaction

In every extracorporeal treatment, blood comes into contact with the foreign mate-rial of dialyzer or filter, of blood lines, of connections, etc., and not only with the material of these devices, but also with substances diffusing from this material in minute concentration. These are substances of the manufacturing or sterilizing pro-cess of the dialysis equipment. Blood with its lipophilic properties bleaches out a number of substances which can not be rinsed out with saline.

Complement Activation

One of the most thoroughly investigated phenomena of blood/device interaction is the complement activation of cellulosic membranes, which occurs immediately af-ter blood/membrane contact [134, 176]. The sequence of events is a membrane-initi-ated complement activation, via the alternative pathway, with generation of com-plement products, one of which is C5a [177]. As a result of complement activation the peripheral leukocyte count drops and pulmonary leukostasis occurs, impairing circulation and function [178]. Leukostasis with increased formation of platelet aggregates initiates prostaglandin release [176]. The entire sequence of events fol-lowing complement activation by cellulosic membranes is reviewed in detail else-where [179]. It should be mentioned that complement activation in hemodialysis [174] seems to be temperature-sensitive (see "Extracorporeal Temperature"). In re-lation to dialysis-associated hypotension it is important to note that complement is activated immediately following the first blood/membrane contact. In contrast, however, hypotension occurs late during treatment.

Interleukin-I

HENDERSON et al. [161] offered a very interesting hypothesis. On the basis of several clinical observations in chronic dialysis patients, such as temperature increment during treatment, low plasma zinc levels [180], increased plasma levels of acute-

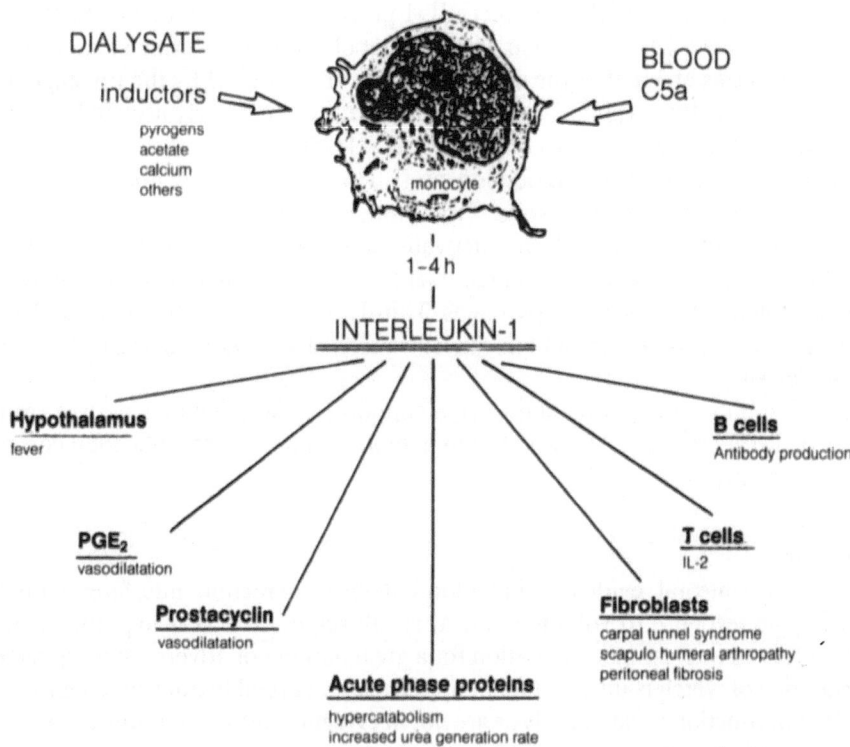

Fig. 11. Possible consequences of dialysis-associated IL-I production by activated monocytes

phase response proteins, etc., they postulated that IL-I is activated during dialysis. One pathway by which it can be activated is complement factor C 5 a. This complement component binds to macrophages and induces IL-I production [181, 182]. Once monocytes become activated they release IL-I after 3-4 h [183], a time lag which coincides with the peak incidence of hypotensive episodes during hemodialysis. A second pathway of IL-I activation can derive from dialysate containing endotoxin [188]. These exogenous pyrogens, which are extensively adsorbed to dialysis membranes, either penetrate the membrane and gain access to the blood stream or remain bound to the membrane while stimulating adherent monocytes to produce IL-I.

Beside its other effects (Fig. 11), IL-I induces PGE_2 release, which then leads to hypotension by its vasodilating potency. Another vasodilating effect is to be expected from IL-I-induced prostacyclin release [184].

Meanwhile, first experimental data seem to support the IL-I hypothesis [185]: Hemodialysis generates C 5 a [186,187] at correct concentrations for IL-I induction in vivo [179]. In view of the temperature dependence of complement activation [174], the improved vascular stability in cold hemodialysis reported by Maggiore et al. [162, 168] and others [209, 213, 215, 216] can be interpreted as an indirect support for the IL-I hypothesis.

In an ex vivo extracorporeal hemodialysis circuit, LONNEMANN et al. [188] were able to demonstrate monocyte IL-I production if the dialysate was contaminated with endotoxin. Hemodialysis induces IL-I production in the blood of ESRD patients during dialysis [183]. Muscle protein catabolism occurs during sham hemodialysis and peaks at 3 h after the start of dialysis. It is blocked by the prostaglandin inhibitor indomethacin [186]. Acetate in concentrations routinely used in hemodialysis induces monocytes in vitro to produce IL-I [125].

There is speculation that induction of IL-I production does not occur during hemofiltration for several reasons. First, noncellulosic synthetic membranes are used in hemofiltration, and do not activate the complement system. Secondly, replacement fluid is pyrogen-free in contrast to dialysate, which is often extensively contaminated with exogenous pyrogens. Thirdly, monocytes adherent to the membrane are not exposed to such high concentrations of IL-I inductors as is the case in hemodialysis.

The first indirect experimental in vivo support for these theories derives from a study by MINETTI et al. [189], who found hemofiltration less catabolic than comparable hemodialysis.

Summary
Direct experimental evidence that blood/device interaction interferes with the physiologic response to volume removal is still scarce. The IL-I hypothesis, however, offers an interesting explanation for a great number of adverse dialysis-related effects, one of which is intratreatment hypotension. Several factors which may initiate IL-I production in hemodialysis are not in evidence during hemofiltration. Time will show whether the IL-I hypothesis is correct.

Underlying Pathology

Autonomic Neuropathy

Hypohidrosis, impotence, loss of heart rate beat-to-beat variation, and severe hypotension during hemodialysis treatment indicate an impaired autonomic system [190–194] in many dialysis patients. With regard to hypotension during hemodialysis, the baroreflex, with its baroreceptors, the afferent limb, the central intersection, the vagal and sympathetic efferent limb, and the end organ response, is the critical determinant of acute blood pressure regulation. LILLEY et al. [193] investigated a group of hemodialysis patients with frequent hypotensive episodes and compared this group to one without hypotensive complications. They studied the entire baroreflex by analyzing the baroreflex sensitivity on the basis of beat-to-beat changes in pulse interval and in arterial pressure following an amyl nitrite inhalation. Plasma dopamine-β-hydroxylase activity and a cold pressor test served as indicators for the efferent sympathetic nervous system. The results obtained by Lilley et al. suggested that hypotension may result from a lesion in the baroreceptors, cardiopulmonary receptors, or visceral afferent nerves. NIES et al. [195] and others [191, 196, 198] confirmed that the lesions of the baroreflex were located at the baroreceptor site or in the afferent limb. They found a close correlation between this autonomic nervous lesion and the incidence of intertreatment hypotension. The blunted response of heart rate to a hypotensive stimulus and, more specifically, the pathologic diving test, [27] were interpreted as indicators of an efferent vagal lesion.

Uremic disturbance of end organ responsiveness is the subject of controversy. KERSH et al. [197] and NIES et al. [195] noted an adequate increase in blood pressure following a noradrenaline infusion, whereas ROMOFF et al. [199] interpreted the normal increase in plasma noradrenaline concentration after orthostasis, in combination with an inadequate rise in blood pressure, as an indicator of diminished end organ responsiveness. This view is supported by RASCHER et al. [198], who demonstrated a diminished increase in hind leg TPR following peripheral noradrenaline application in uremic rats.

In addition to an impaired baroreflex, uremia-related abnormalities in catecholamine metabolism, such as altered biosynthesis [200], reuptake [201], and density of sympathetic innervation [202], have been described, and are possibly responsible for the now well-established finding of increased basal plasma noradrenaline levels in uremic patients [27, 199, 203–205].

Although autonomic neuropathy is a common finding in uremia, and although severe lesions seem to provoke hypotension during treatment, the hemodynamic differences between hemodialysis and hemofiltration, as described above, cannot be explained by alterations in the autonomic nervous system. In controlled studies the hemodynamic behaviour of the same patients was different during hemodialysis and hemofiltration [12, 13, 15–17, 22, 40]. Only an acute impairment of the baroreflex during hemodialysis can explain the loss of the capacity to increase vascular resistance, which remains intact, at least qualitatively, during ultrafiltration and hemofiltration. Early studies of baroreflex sensitivity by PICKERING et al. [192] and more recent studies of the different segments of the baroreflex arc by BALDAMUS et al. [206] during hemodialysis and hemofiltration did not identify any acute changes during hemodialysis. Baroreflex sensitivity was the only parameter which improved during hemofiltration. These data are supported by ZUCCHELLI et al. [16], who also found an increase in Valsalva ratio during hemodialysis and hemofiltration, but the increase was significantly more pronounced in hemofiltration. So far, end organ responsiveness has not been tested comparatively during hemodialysis and hemofiltration, but even if it deteriorates during hemodialysis, this should enhance sympathetic tone, resulting in high plasma noradrenaline levels. This, however, was not found to be the case in hemodialysis [13, 22].

Summary
Autonomic neuropathy frequently exists in uremic patients [190–194, 207, 208] and predisposes to intratreatment hypotension [191, 193, 195–197]. Hemodynamic differences between hemodialysis and hemofiltration cannot be explained by autonomic insufficiency, because the same patients react differently during hemodialysis and hemofiltration. Acute treatment-induced impairment of the baroreflex, however, cannot be demonstrated [206]. Differences in end organ responsiveness, not yet tested, seem unlikely to explain the hemodynamic differences.

Cardiovascular Disorders

The heart very seldom escapes damage in chronic renal failure patients maintained on renal replacement therapy, and the term uremic cardiomyopathy [209-215] reflects myocardial dysfunction which becomes evident during the course of the renal failure and which is multifactorial in its pathogenesis. Among the etiologic factors, hypertension, atherosclerosis, anemia, and hypovolemia are the most important. Abnormal acid-base status and electrolyte metabolism, hyperparathyroidism, diabetes mellitus, and nutritional deficiency also contribute. Uremic toxins are usually listed, but not specifically identified. Regardless of etiology, patients suffering clinically from cardiomyopathy run a high risk of intratreatment hypotension. This can easily be explained by their very limited capacity to compensate for an acute additional workload.

In this critical situation the treatment modality with the least detrimental effect should be applied. HAMPL et al. [32] and others [12] clearly showed that especially cardiomyopathic patients benefit from hemofiltration. Comparative hemodynamic studies in these patients might help to amplify the effect of variants, which are completely compensated for in uncomplicated patients.

According to HUNG et al. [209], patients with impaired cardiac function benefit from hemodialysis with lower preload as well as afterload. This effect is not restricted to volume overload, but was also validated for patients with impaired left ventricular function. In patients with normal cardiac function ejection fraction did not increase. NIXON et al. [216] tried to separate the effect of volume removal from that of removal of uremic toxins. Ultrafiltration produced a pure Starling effect. In contrast, hemodialysis with and without volume loss produced a shift in the ventricular function curve to the left, which indicates an increase in left ventricular contractility. In a subsequent study the same group [97] was able to demonstrate that the increase in left ventricular contractility was due to an increase in ionized calcium. There are still no comparable detailed investigations of the cardiac state during hemofiltration.

Differences in patients' cardiac status might explain the different hemodynamic results reported by different authors [12, 22, 32], and clearly show, moreover, that studies comparing two treatment regimes should always be performed in the same patients.

Summary
Patients with "uremic cardiomyopathy" or any other form of cardiac impairment are especially sensitive to volume removal; intratreatment hypotension is the most frequent result. Hemofiltration is of particular benefit for these patients. Because of their high sensitivity, future studies in these patients might help to clarify specific pathogenetic aspects of hemodialysis-associated hypotension.

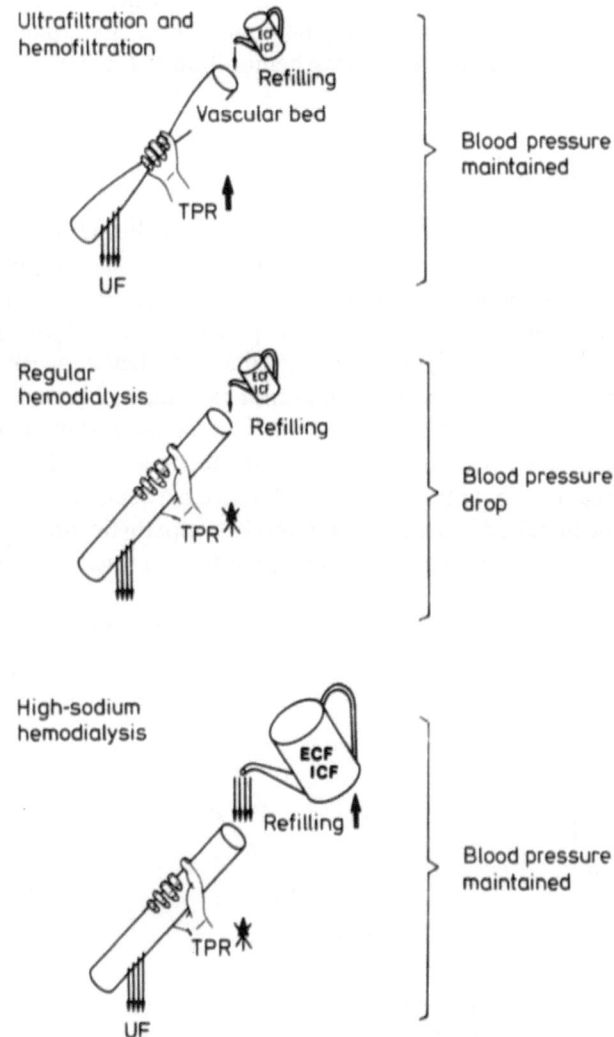

Fig. 12. Hemodynamic response to weight removal [78]. In ultrafiltration and hemofiltration blood pressure is maintained by an increase in total peripheral vascular resistance *(TPR)*. If weight removal rate *(UF)* exceeds vascular refilling from extra- *(ECF)* and intracellular *(ICF)* compartments, blood pressure drops during hemodialysis because here the same patient is unable to increase TPR. Only if vascular refilling rate increases, as in high-sodium hemodialysis, and counterbalances ultrafiltration, does blood pressure remain stable

Medication

Patients on regular renal replacement therapy very often receive medication affecting the cardiocirculatory system: antihypertensives, glycosides, antiarrhythmics, and bronchodilators. In addition, analgesics, narcotics, and psychotherapeutic drugs may interfere with hemodynamic compensatory mechanisms. Very little is known so far about pharmacokinetics and pharmacodynamics during hemofiltration. Differences are expected for drugs which are water soluble and too large for efficient elimination during hemodialysis (> 500 mol. wt.), but still small enough to be filtered effectively during hemofiltration (< 15000 mol. wt.).

Conclusion

Hemodynamic response to fluid removal during hemofiltration is physiologically adequate, at least qualitatively (Fig. 12): cardiac output decreases, TPR increases, most probably because of increased sympathetic tone, and blood pressure is maintained at a stable level. The same pattern is found during pure ultrafiltration, but not during hemodialysis. Here, regardless of whether acetate or bicarbonate is used as the dialysis buffer, cardiac output remains stable or is increased; TPR decreases (acetate) or remains unchanged (bicarbonate); sympathetic activity is unchanged; and blood pressure becomes labile, leading to the known high incidence of intra-treatment hypotension. The difference between hemodialysis and hemofiltration is the impaired increase in TPR and in sympathetic tone (Fig. 13) during hemodialysis, the causative mechanisms of which remain unclear. Since intratreatment hypoten-

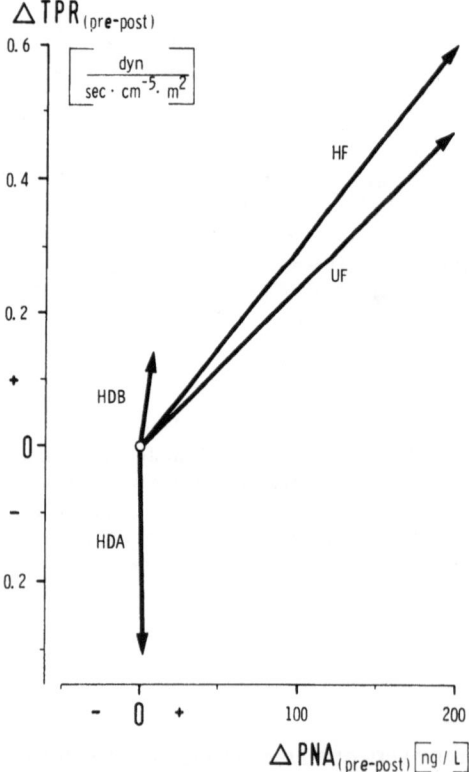

Fig. 13. Relation between intratreatment change in total peripheral vascular resistance (ΔTPR) and change in plasma noradrenaline concentration (ΔPNA) during ultrafiltration *(UF)*, hemofiltration *(HF)*, and acetate *(HDA)* and bicarbonate *(HDB)* hemodialysis. Pre- to posttreatment changes are drawn as vectors [78]

sion is a multifactorial phenomenon, several factors have been accused of causing the impairment in physiologic response to volume removal [217]. Important factors like intercompartmental fluid shifts, acetate, removal or induction of vasoactive hormones, and bioincompatibility have been discussed as playing a role in hemodialysis hypotension. But none of these factors has been proved to be the explanation for the principal hemodynamic difference between hemodialysis and hemofiltration.

The thought processe involved has delivered a very attractive and stimulating hypothesis, which might explain the hemodynamic differences and, beyond that, might help to understand late-occurring new diseases in long-term hemodialysis patients. This is the IL-I hypothesis [125, 168]. Its validity will be challenged in the near future.

It is desirable, and from a practical standpoint extremely important, to improve vascular stability during hemodialysis. This is done by varying factors which have been discussed as contributing to intratreatment vascular instability but which do not explain the hemodynamic difference between hemodialysis and hemofiltration. Hemodynamic stability during hemodialysis can be improved mainly by increasing dialysate sodium concentration, replacing acetate by bicarbonate as the dialysate buffer, using cold dialysate, and eventually by eliminating "bioincompatibility."

References

1. Degoulet P, Réach I, Rozenbaum W, Aime F, Devriés C, Berger C, Rojas P, Jacobs C, Legrain M (1979) Programme dialyse-informatique. VI Survie et facteurs de risque. J Urol Nephrol 85: 909–962
2. Degoulet P, Proulx J, Aime F, Berger C, Bloch P, Goupy F, Legrain M (1976) Programme dialyse - informatique. III - Données épidémiologiques. Stratégies de dialyse et résultats biologiques. J Urol Nephrol 82: 1001
3. Degoulet P, Réach I, Di Giulio S, Devriés C, Rouby JJ, Aimé F, Vonlanthen M (1981) Epidemiology of dialysis-induced hypotension. Proc Eur Dial Transplant Assoc 18: 133
4. Brynger H, Brunner FP, Chantler C, Donckerwolcke RA, Jacobs C, Kramer P, Selwood NH, Wing AJ (1979) Combined report on regular dialysis and transplantation in Europe. Proc Eur Dial Transplant Assoc 17: 4
5. Brunner FP, Giesecke B, Gurland HJ, Jacobs C, Parsons FM, Schärer K, Seyffart G, Spies G, Wing AJ (1974) Combined report on regular dialysis and transplantation in Europe. Prov Eur Dial Transplant Assoc 12: 3
6. Guyton AC, Coleman TG, Granger HJ (1972) Circulation: overall regulation. Annu Rev Physiol 34: 13
7. Guyton AC (1980) Circulatory physiology III: arterial pressure and hypertension. Saunders, Philadelphia
8. Kobayashi K, Shibata M, Kato K, Suo K (1972) Studies on the development of a new method of controlling the amount and contents of body fluids (extracorporeal ultrafiltration method, ECUM) and the application of this method for patients receiving long term hemodialysis. Jap J Nephrol 14: 1
9. Ing T, Ashbach DL, Kanter A, McIntosh J, Peter G (1975) Fluid removal and negative-pressure hydrostatic ultrafiltration using a partial vacuum. Nephron (BASEL) 14: 451
10. Bergström J, Asaba H, Fürst P, Oulés R (1976) Dialysis, ultrafiltration and blood pressure. Proc Eur Dial Transplant Assoc 13: 293
11. Quellhorst E, Rieger J, Doht B, Beckmann H, Jacob I, Kraft B, Mietzsch G, Scheler F (1976) Treatment of chronic uremia by an ultrafiltration kidney - first clinical experience. Proc Eur Dial Transplant Assoc 13: 314

12. Baldamus CA, Ernst W, Fassbinder W, Koch KM (1980) Differing haemodynamic stability due to differing sympathetic response: comparison of ultrafiltration, haemodialysis and haemofiltration. Proc Eur Dial Transplant Assoc 17: 205
13. Quellhorst E, Schuenemann B, Hildebrand U, Falda Z (1980) Response of the vascular system to different modifications of haemofiltration and haemodialysis. Proc Eur Dial Transplant Assoc 17: 197
14. Baldamus CA, Schoeppe W, Koch KM (1978) Comparison of haemodialysis and post-dilution haemofiltration on an unselected dialysis population. Proc Eur Dial Transplant Assoc 15: 228
15. Aljama P, Martin-Malo A, Sanz R, Pasalodos J, Sancho M, Moreno E, Gómez J, Pérez R, Burdiel LG, Andrés E (1982) Left ventricular function during haemofiltration and haemodialysis: a comparative study. Proc Eur Dial Transplant Assoc 19: 281
16. Zucchelli P, Santoro A, Sturani A, Degli Esposti E, Chiarini C, Zuccalà A (1984) Effects of hemodialysis and hemofiltration on the autonomic control of circulation. Trans Am Soc Artif Intern Organs 30: 163
17. Shaldon S, Deschodt G, Beau MC, Claret G, Mion H, Mion C (1979) Vascular stability during high flux haemofiltration. Proc Eur Dial Transplant Assoc 16: 695
18. Graefe U, Milutinovich J, Follette WC, Babb AL, Scribner BH (1977) Improved tolerance to rapid ultrafiltration with the use of bicarbonate in dialysate. Proc Eur Dial Transplant Assoc 14: 153
19. Graefe U, Milutinovich J, Follette WC, Vizzo JE, Babb AL, Scribner BH (1978) Less dialysis-induced morbidity and vascular instability with bicarbonate in dialysate. Ann Intern Med 88: 332
20. Bergström J (1978) Ultrafiltration without simultaneous dialysis for removal of excess fluid. Proc Eur Dial Transplant Assoc 15: 260
21. Shaldon S, Deschodt G, Beau MC, Ramperez P, Mion C (1978) The importance of serum osmotic changes in symptomatic hypotension during short hemodialysis. Proc Dial Transplant Forum 8: 184
22. Baldamus CA, Ernst W, Frei U, Koch KM (1982) Sympathetic and hemodynamic response to volume removal during different forms of renal replacment therapy. Nephron (BASEL) 31: 324
23. Brecht HM, Schoeppe W, Scheuermann E, Nassauer A, Baldamus C, Koch KM (1978) Factors involved in hemodialysis hypotension (Abstract). 7th Congress Int Soc Nephrol, Montreal
24. Wehle B, Asaba H, Castenfors J, Fürst P, Gunnarsson B, Shaldon S, Bergström J (1979) Hemodynamic changes during sequential ultrafiltration and dialysis. Kidney Int 15: 411
25. Pogglitsch H, Holzer H, Waller J, Pristautz H, Leopold H, Katschnigg H (1978) The cause of inadequate haemodynamic reactions during ultradiffusion. Proc Eur Dial Transplant Assoc 15: 245
26. Zucchelli P, Catizone L, Esposti ED, Fusaroli M, Ligabue A, Zuccala A (1978) Influence of ultrafiltration on plasma renin activity and adrenergic system. Nephron (BASEL) 21: 317
27. Zuccala A, Degli Esposti E, Sturani A, Chiarini C, Santoro A, Catizone L, Zucchelli P (1978) Autonomic function in hemodialyzed patients. Int J Artif Organs 1: 76
28. Cannella G, Picotti GB, Mioni G, Cristinelli L, Maiorca R (1978) Blood pressure behaviours during dialysis and ultrafiltration. A pathogenic hypothesis on hemodialysis-induced hypotension. Int J Artif Organs 1: 69
29. Quellhorst E (1979) Hämofiltration – Differentialindikation zur Hämodialyse unter Berücksichtigung hämodynamischer und metabolischer Aspekte. Klin Wochenschr 57: 1061
30. Quellhorst E, Schuenemann B (1979) Postdilution hemofiltration is rational and preferable. Proc Dial Transplant Forum 9: 54
31. Hampl H, Paeprer H, Unger V, Kessel MW (1979) Hemodynamics during hemodialysis, sequential ultrafiltration and hemofiltration. J Dialysis 3: 51
32. Hampl H, Paeprer H, Unger V, Fischer C, Resa I, Kessel M (1980) Hemodynamic changes during hemodialysis, sequential ultrafiltration, and hemofiltration. Kidney Int 18: S-83
33. Shaldon S, Beau MC, Deschodt G, Ramperez P, Mion C (1980) Vascular stability during hemofiltration. Trans Am Soc Artif Intern Organs 26: 391
34. Keshaviah P, Illstrup K, Constantini E, Berkseth R, Shapiro F (1980) The influence of ultrafiltration and diffusion on cardiovascular parameters. Trans Am Soc Artif Intern Organs 26: 328
35. Henrich WL, Woodard TD, Blachley JD, Gomez-Sanchez C, Pettinger W, Cronin RE (1980)

Role of osmolality in blood pressure stability after dialysis and ultrafiltration. Kidney Int 18: 480

36. Wehle B, Asaba H, Castenfors J, Gunnarsson B, Bergström J (1981) Influence of dialysate composition on cardiovascular function in isovolaemic haemodialysis. Proc Eur Dial Transplant Assoc 18: 153

37. Wehle B, Asaba H, Castenfors J, Fürst P, Gunnarsson B, Bergström J (1979) Hämodynamische Veränderungen während Ultrafiltration and Hämodialyse bei Urämikern. Z Urol Nephrol 72: 3

38. Cini G, Camici M, Pentimone F, Palla R (1982) Echocardiographic hemodynamic study during ultrafiltration sequential dialysis. Nephron (BASEL) 30: 124

39. Hampl H, Klopp H, Wolfgruber M, Pustelnik A, Schiller R, Hanefeld F, Kessel M (1982) Advantages of bicarbonate hemodialysis. Artif Organs 6: 410

40. Kishimoto T, Sugimura K, Nakatani T, Yamagami S, Ezaki K, Okazaki S, Maekawa M (1982) The effects of diffusion and ultrafiltration on cardiac output and organ blood flows. Proc Eur Dial Transplant Assoc 19: 275

41. Vincent JL, Vanherweghem JL, Degaute JP, Berré J, Dufaye P, Kahn RJ (1982) Acetate-induced myocardial depression during hemodialysis for acute renal failure. Kidney Int 22: 653

42. Schick EC Jr, Idelson BA, Liang C, Redline RC, Bernard DB (1983) Comparison of the hemodynamic response to hemodialysis with acetate or bicarbonate. Trans Am Soc Artif Intern Organs 29: 25

43. Frewin DB, Bartholomeusz FDL, Cummings MF, Clarkson AR, Barry LA, Furber B, De Lorenzo C, Jonsson JR, Taylor WB (1984) Changes in plasma catecholamine levels during hemodialysis. Aust NZ J Med 14: 31

44. Leenen FHH, Buda AJ, Smith DL, Farrel S, Levine DZ, Uldall PR (1984) Hemodynamic changes during acetate and bicarbonate hemodialysis. Artif Organs 8: 411

45. Schneider H, Liomin E, Streicher E (1985) Hemodynamic studies of diffusive and convective procedures using a polysulfone membrane. Contrib Nephrol 46: 134

46. Freyschuss U, Asaba H, Danielsson A, Bergström J (1984) Cardiovascular adaptation to dialysis in healthy man. Contrib Nephrol 41: 376–379

47. Wizemann V, Sychla M, Leber HW (1980) Simultaneous hemofiltration/hemodialysis versus hemofiltration and hemodialysis: hemodynamic parameters. Proc Eur Soc Artif Organs 7: 143

48. Wizemann V, Kramer W, Knopp G, Sychla M, Schmidt H, Rawer P, Schütterle G (1982) Cardiovascular function during hemodialysis, hemofiltration and hemodiafiltration. In: Schütterle G, Wizemann V, Seyffart G (eds) Hemodiafiltration. Hygieneplan, Oberursel, p 89

49. Schmidt M, Schoeppe W, Baldamus CA (1985) Hemodynamics during hemodialysis with dialyzers of high hydraulic permeability. Contrib Nephrol 46: 127

50. Kjellstrand CM (1980) Can hypotension during dialysis be avoided? In: Schreiner GE (ed) Controversies in nephrology. Georgetown University, Washington, p 12

51. Skillman JJ, Awwad HK, Moore FD (1967) Plasma protein kinetics of the early transcapillary refill after hemorrhage in man. Surg Gynecol Obstet 125: 983

52. Kim KE, Neff M, Cohen B et al (1970) Blood volume changes and hypotension during hemodialysis. Trans Am Soc Artif Int Organs 16: 508

53. Chaignon M, Chen WT, Tarazi RC, Bravo EL, Nakamoto S (1981) Effect of hemodialysis on blood volume distribution and cardiac output. Hypertension 3: 327

54. Ashkar E, Hamilton WF (1963) Cardiovascular response to graded exercise in the sympathectomized-vagotomized dog. Am J Physiol 204: 291

55. Falls WF Jr, Stacy WK, Bear ES et al (1972) Dialysis-induced change of extracellular fluid volume in man. Proc Dial Transplant Forum 2: 155

56. Rodrigo R, Shideman J, McHigh R, Buselmeier T, Kjellstrand C (1977) Osmolality changes during hemodialysis. Ann Intern Med 86: 554

57. Port FK, Johnson WJ, Klass DW (1973) Prevention of dialysis disequilibrium syndrome by use of high sodium concentration in the dialysate. Kidney Int 3: 327

58. Shaldon S (1976) Sequential ultrafiltration and dialysis. Proc Eur Dial Transplant Assoc 13: 300

59. Wehle B, Asaba H, Castenfors J et al (1978) The influence of dialysis fluid composition on the blood pressure response during dialysis. Clin Nephrol 10: 62

60. Bell RL, Curtis FK, Babb AL (1965) Analog simulation of the patient-artificial kidney system. Trans Am Soc Artif Intern Organs 11: 183
61. Rastogi RP, Frost T, Anderson J, Schroft R, Kerr DNS (1968) The significance of disequilibrium between body compartments in the treatment of chronic renal failure by hemodialysis. Proc Eur Dial Transplant Assoc 5: 102
62. Frost TH, Kerr DNS (1977) Kinetics of hemodialysis: theoretical study of the removal of solutes in chronic renal failure compared to normal health. Kidney Int 12: 41
63. Borah MF, Schoenfeld PY, Gotch FA, Sargent JA, Wolfson M, Humphreys MH (1978) Nitrogen balance during intermittent dialysis therapy of uremia. Kidney Int 14: 491
64. Gotch FA, Sargent JA (1983) Hemofiltration: an unnecessarily complex method to achieve hypotonic sodium removal and controlled ultrafiltration. Blood Purif 1: 9
65. Oh MS, Levison SP, Carroll HJ (1975) Content and distribution of water and electrolytes in maintenance hemodialysis. Nephron (BASEL) 14: 421
66. Keshaviah P, Berkseth RO, Shapiro FL et al (1978) Mechanisms and control of fluid removal by ultrafiltration. Proceedings of the 11th annual contractor's conference, artificial kidney program. National Institutes of Arthritis, Metabolism, and Digestive Diseases
67. Van Stone JC, Bauer J, Carey J (1980) The effect of dialysate sodium concentration on body fluid distribution during hemodialysis. Trans Am Soc Artif Intern Organs 26: 383
68. Van Stone JC, Cook J (1978) The effect of replacing acetate with bicarbonate in the dialysate of stable chronic hemodialysis patients. Proc Clin Dial Transplant Forum 9: 103
69. Gotch FA, Lam MA, Prowitt M, Keen M (1980) Preliminary clinical results with sodium-volume modeling of hemodialysis therapy. Proc Dial Transplant Forum 10: 12
70. Gotch FA (1981) Net sodium flux in postdilution hemofiltration. Kidney Int 19: A 146
71. Gotch FA, Sargent JA (1982) Hemofiltration: an unnecessarily complex method to achieve hypotonic sodium removal and controlled ultrafiltration. Contrib Nephrol 4: 279
72. Shaldon S, Baldamus CA, Koch KM, Mion CA, Lysaght MJ (1982) Is better sodium balance responsible for maintenance of blood pressure with hemofiltration? Or the logical fallacy of the undistributed middle. Controversies in Nephrology 4: 267
73. Ramenofsky JA, Prestidge H, Ford C, Sanfelippo ML, Henderson LW (1982) Novel applications for hemofiltration membranes. Trans Am Soc Artif Intern Organs 27: 613
74. Bosch JP, Lauer AP, Belledone M, Constantiner A, Glabman S (1982) Effect of protein concentration on the ultrafiltrate (Qf) electrolyte composition. Am Soc Artif Intern Organs 11: 42
75. Lysaght MJ (1983) An experimental model for the ultrafiltration of sodium ion from blood or plasma. Blood Purif 1: 25
76. Shaldon S, Baldamus CA, Beau MC, Koch MK, Mion CM, Lysaght MJ (1983) Acute and chronic studies of the relationship between sodium flux in hemodialysis and hemofiltration. Trans Am Soc Artif Intern Organs 29: 641
77. Lysaght MJ, Baldamus CA, Koch KM, Mion CA, Pusch W, Shaldon S (1982) Relevance of sodium flux to vascular stability in postdilution hemofiltration. Kidney Int 21: A172
78. Shaldon S, Baldamus CA, Koch KM, Lysaght MJ (1983) Of sodium, symptomatology and syllogism. Blood Purif I: 16
79. Baldamus CA, Ernst W, Lysaght MJ, Shaldon S, Koch KM (1983) Hemodynamics in hemofiltration. Int J Artif Organs 6: 27
80. Baldamus CA (1983) Hemofiltration. In: D'Amico G, Colasanti G (eds) Nephrology '83. Wichtig, Milan, p 163
81. Schultze G, Maiga M, Neumayer H-H, Wagner K, Keller F, Molzahn M, Nigam S (1984) Prostaglandin E_2 promotes hypotension in low-sodium hemodialysis. Nephron (BASEL) 37: 250
82. Henderson LW, Sanfelippo ML, Stone RA (1979) Comparison of hemodialysis and hemofiltration. Proceedings 12th annual contractor's conference. Artificial kidney-chronic uremia program. NIAMDD (National Institutes of Health), Bethesda
83. Quellhorst E (1984) Herzrhythmusstörungen während und nach Hämodialyse, Hämofiltration und Hämodiafiltration bei Patienten mit chronischer Niereninsuffizienz - vergleichende Langzeit-EKG-Untersuchungen. In: Braun J (ed) Die Behandlung von Herzrhythmusstörungen bei Nierenkranken. Karger, Basel, p 23
84. Morrison G, Michelson EL, Brown S, Morganroth J (1980) Mechanism and prevention of cardiac arrhythmias in chronic hemodialysis patients. Kidney Int 17: 811

85. Haddy FJ (1983) The role of potassium ions in regulating vascular resistance. In: Altura BM (ed) Advances in microcirculation vol II. Karger, Basel, p 43
86. Fukuchi S, Hanata M, Takahashi H, Demura H, Goto K (1965) The relationship between vascular reactivity and extracellular potassium. Tohoku J Exp Med 85: 181
87. Haddy FJ, Scott JB, Emerson TE Jr, Overbeck HW, Daugherty RM (1969) Effects of generalized changes in plasma electrolyte concentration and osmolarity on blood pressure in the anesthetized dog. Circ Res (Suppl 1) 24: 59
88. Friedman SM (1983) Sodium ions and regulation of vascular tone. In: Altura BM (ed) Advances in microcirculation vol II. Karger, Basel, p 20
89. Lang S, Blaustein MP (1980) The role of the sodium pump in the control of vascular tone in the rat. Circ Res 46: 463
90. Dunn FL, Brennan TJ, Neson AE, Robertson GL (1973) The role of blood osmolality and volume in regulating vasopressin secretion in the rat. J Clin Invest 52: 3212
91. Brecht HM (1980) Wirkung der Hyponatriämie und der Hypovolämie auf die Sympathikus- und Reninaktivität bei der terminalen Niereninsuffizienz. In: Rosenthal J, Knauf H (eds) Diuretika, Edition Medizin, Weinheim, p 219
92. Altura BT (1983) Influence of calcium ions on microvascular permeability, contractility and reactivity. In: Altura BM (ed) Advances in microcirculation vol II. Karger, Basel, p 62
93. Overbeck HW, Molnar JI, Haddy FJ (1961) Resistance to blood flow through the vascular bed of the dog forelimb. Local effects of sodium, potassium, calcium, magnesium, acetate, hypertonicity and hypotonicity. Am J Cardiol 8: 533
94. Bristow MR, Schwartz HD, Binetti G, Harrison DC, Daniels JR (1977) Ionized calcium and the heart: elucidation of in vivo concentration-response relationships in the open-chest dog. Circ Res 41: 565
95. Connor TB, Rosen BL, Blaustein MP, Applefeld MM, Doyle LA (1982) Hypocalcemia precipitating congestive heart failure. N Engl J Med 307: 869
96. Wei EP, Thames MD, Kontos HA, Patterson JL Jr (1974) Inhibition of the vasodilator effect of hypercapnic acidosis by hypercalcemia in dogs and rats. Circ Res 35: 890
97. Henrich WI, Hund JM, Nixon JV (1984) Increased ionized calcium and left ventricular contractility during hemodialysis. N Engl J Med 310: 19
98. Chaignon M, Chen WT, Tarazi RC, Nakamoto S, Salcedo E (1982) Acute effects of hemodialysis on echographic-determined cardiac performance: improved contractility resulting from serum increased calcium with reduced potassium despite hypovolemic-reduced cardiac output. Am Heart J 103: 374
99. Drüecke T, Fauchet M, Fleury J et al (1980) Effect of parathyroidectomy on left-ventricular function in haemodialysis patients. Lancet I: 112
100. Schneider H (1982) Die Kinetic des Kalziumtransports bei Dialyse und Filtration. In: Streicher E, Schoeppe W (eds) Die adäquate Dialyse. Springer, Berlin Heidelberg New York, p 119–132
101. Altura BM (1983) Magnesium and regulation of contractility of vascular smooth muscle. In: Advances in microcirculation Vol II. Karger, Basel, p 77
102. Langer GA, Serena SD, Nudd LM (1974) Cation exchange in heart cell culture: correlation with effects on contractile force. J Mol Cell Cardiol 6: 149
103. Shine II (1979) Myocardial effects of magnesium. Am J Physiol 237: H413
104. Weiner MW (1982) Acetate metabolism during hemodialysis. Artif Organs 6: 370
105. Vreman HJ, Assomull VM, Kaiser BA, Blaschke TF, Weiner MW (1980) Acetate metabolism and acid-base homeostasis during hemodialysis: influence of dialyzer efficiency and metabolic capacity for acetate metabolism. Kidney Int 18 (Suppl 10): S62
106. Mion CR, Hegstrom RM, Boen ST, Scribner BH (1964) Substitution of sodium acetate for sodium bicarbonate in the bath fluid for hemodialysis. Trans Am Soc Artif Intern Organs 10: 110
107. Kaiser BA, Assomull VM, Vreman HJ, Weiner MW (1979) Dialysance of acetate and bicarbonate: effect of ultrafiltration. Proc Clin Dial Transplant Forum 9: 104
108. Graefe U, Follette WC, Vizzo JE, Gutisman LD, Scribner BH (1976) Reduction in dialysis-induced morbidity and vascular instability with the use of bicarbonate in dialysate. Proc Clin Dial Transplant Forum 6: 203–206
109. Bauer W, Richards JW (1928) A vasodilator action of acetate. J Physiol (Lond) 66: 371
110. Olinger GN, Werner PH, Bonchek LI, Boerboom LE (1979) Vasodilator effects of the sodium acetate in pooled protein fraction. Ann Surg 190: 305

111. Frohlich ED (1965) Vascular effects of the Krebs intermediate metabolites. Am J Physiol 208: 149
112. Molnar JI, Scott JB, Frohlich ED, Haddy FJ (1962) Local effects of various anions and H^+ on dog limb and coronary vascular resistances. Am J Physiol 203: 125
113. Kirkendol PL, Devia CJ, Bower JD, Holbert RD (1977) A comparison of the cardiovascular effects of sodium acetate, sodium bicarbonate and other potential sources of fixed base in hemodialysate solution. Trans Am Soc Artif Intern Organs 23: 399–405
114. Aizawa Y, Shibata A (1978) Hemodynamic effects of acetate in man. J Dial 2: 235
115. Aizawa Y, Ohmori T, Imai K, Nara Y, Matsuoka M, Hirakawa Y (1977) Depressant action of acetate upon the human cardiovascular system. Clin Nephrol 8: 477
116. Chen TS, Friedman HS, Del Monte M, Smith AJ (1979) Hemodynamic changes during dialysis. Proc Clin Dial Transplant Forum 9: 66
117. Liang CS, Lowenstein JM (1978) Metabolic control of the circulation: effects of acetate and pyruvate. J Clin Invest 62: 1029
118. Kirkendol PL, Robie NW, Gonzalez FM, Devia CJ (1978) Cardiac and vascular effects of infused sodium acetate in dogs. Trans Am Soc Artif Intern Organs 24: 714
119. Keshaviah PR (1982) The role of acetate in the etiology of symptomatic hypotension. Artif Organs 6: 378
120. Sargent JA, Gotch FA (1978) Principles and biophysics of dialysis. In: Drukker, Parsons, Maker (eds) Replacement of renal function by dialysis. Nijhoff, Boston, pp 38–68
121. Gotch FA, Sargent JA, Keen ML, Lam M, Provitt MH (1978) Solute kinetics of intermittent dialysis therapy. Annual progress report. Artificial kidney – chronic uremia programm. NIAMDD (National Institute of Health), Bethesda
122. Gotch FA, Sargent JA, Keen ML (1982) Hydrogen ion balance in dialysis therapy. Artif Organs 6: 388
123. Albertini B von, Miller JH, Gardner PW, Shinaberger JH (1984) Performance characteristics of high flux haemodiafiltration. Proc Eur Dial Transplant Assoc 21: 447
124. Kishimoto T, Yamamoto K, Yamamoto T, Mizutani Y, Horiuchi N, Hirata S, Yamagami S, Yamakawa M, Maekawa M (1983) Acetate intolerance in hemodialysis. Trans Am Soc Artif Intern Organs 29: 402
125. Shaldon S, Deschodt G, Branger B, Oulés R, Granolleras C, Baldamus CA, Koch KM, Lysaght MJ, Dinarello CA (1985) Haemodialysis hypotension: the interleukin hypothesis restated. Proc Eur Dial Transplant Assoc 22 (in press)
126. Iseki K, Onoyama K, Maeda T, Shimamatsu K, Harada A, Fijimí F, Omae T (1980) Comparison of hemodynamics induced by conventional acetate hemodialysis, bicarbonate hemodialysis and ultrafiltration. Clin Nephrol 14: 294
127. Weitzman RE, Gorbaty I, Davidson WD (1978) The effect of bath composition on blood pressure and vasoactive hormone levels during hemodialysis. Kidney Int 14: 690A
128. Raja R, Kramer M, Rosenbaum JL (1980) Prevention of hypotension during iso-osmolar hemodialysis with bicarbonate dialysate. Trans Am Soc Artif Intern Organs 26: 375
129. Nissenson AR, Kraut JA, Shinaberger JH (1984) Dialysis-associated hypoxemia: pathogenesis and prevention. asaio Journal 7: 1
130. Davidson WD, Dolan MJ, Whipp BJ, Weitzman RE, Wasserman K (1982) Pathogenesis of dialysis-induced hypoxemia. Artif Organs 6: 406
131. Ward RA, Wathen RL (1982) Utilization of bicarbonate for base repletion in hemodialysis. Artif Organs 6: 396
132. Wathen RL, Ward RA, Harding GB, Myer LC (1982) Acid-base and metabolic responses to anion infusion in the anesthetized dog. Kidney Int 21: 592
133. Wathen RL (1977) The impact of acetate and bicarbonate containing dialysate on hydrogen ion balance. Proc Renal Physicians Assoc 1: 19
134. Craddock PR, Fehr J, Brigham KL, Kronenberg RS, Jacob HS (1977) Complement and leukocyte-mediated pulmonary dysfunction in hemodialysis. N Engl J Med 296: 769
135. Bischel MD, Scoles BG, Mohler TG (1975) Evidence for pulmonary microembolization during hemodialysis. Chest 67: 335
136. Sherlock J, Ledwith J, Letteri J (1977) Hypoventilation and hypoxemia during hemodialysis: reflex response to removal of CO_2 across dialyzer. Trans Am Soc Artif Intern Organs 23: 406

137. Aurigemma NM, Feldman NT, Gottlieb M, Ling G, Sutter LS (1977) Arterial oxygenation during hemodialysis. N Engl J Med 297: 871
138. Oh MS, Uribarri JV, Del Monte ML, Friedman EA, Carrol HJ (1979) Consumption of CO_2 in metabolism of acetate as an explanation for hypoventilation and hypoxemia during hemodialysis. Proc Clin Dial Transplant Forum 9: 226
139. Romaldini H, Rodriguez-Roisin R, Lopez FA, Ziegler TW, Bencowitz HZ, Wagner PD (1984) The mechanisms of arterial hypoxemia during hemodialysis. Am Rev Respir Dis 129: 780
140. Wasserman AJ, Patterson JL (1961) The cerebral vascular response to reduction in arterial carbon dioxide tension. J Clin Invest 40: 1297
141. Finnerty FA Jr, Witkin L, Fazekas JF (1954) Cerebral hemodynamics during cerebral ischemia induced by acute hypotension. J Clin Invest 33: 1227
142. Hampl H, Fischer Ch, Resa I, Paeprer H, Kessel M (1979) Recirculation dialysis (RD) (20 to 40 liters of dialysate) with venous bicarbonate buffering – an alternative procedure to hemofiltration (HF). Int J Artif Organs 2: 235
143. Bosch JP, Glabman S, Moutoussis G, Belledonne M, Albertini B von, Kahn T (1984) Carbon dioxide removal in acetate hemodialysis: effects on acid base balance. Kidney Int 25: 830
144. Bosch J, Constantiner A, Belledonne M, MacMoune F, Glabman S, von Albertini B (1981) Bicarbonate generation and red blood cell hypocapnia during acetate hemodialysis. Trans Am Soc Artif Intern Organs 27: 172
145. Bosch JP, Gotch FA, Kjellstrand CM, Scribner BH (1981) Acetate versus bicarbonate in dialysis. Trans Am Soc Artif Intern Organs 27: 655
146. Gregory GA, Egerli EI, Smith NT, Cullen BF (1974) The cardiovascular effects of carbon dioxide in man awake and during diethyl ether anesthesia. Anesthesiology 40: 301
147. Burnum JF, Hickam JB, McIntosh HD (1954) The effect of hypocapnia on arterial blood pressure. Circulation 9: 89
148. Suutarinen T (1966) Cardiovascular response to changes in arterial carbon dioxide tension. Acta Physiol Scand 67 (Suppl 266): 1
149. Robertson GL, Athar S, Shelton RL (1977) Disturbances in body fluid osmolality. Am Physiol Soc Bethesda, Maryland, p 133
150. Maack T, Marion DN, Camargo MJF, Kleinert HD, Laragh JH, Vaughan ED Jr, Atlas SA (1984) Effects of auriculin (atrial natriuretic factor) on blood pressure, renal function, and the renin-aldosterone system in dogs. Am J Med 77: 1069
151. Lang RE, Thoelken H, Ganten D, Luft FC, Ruskoaho H, Unger T (1985) Atrial natriuretic factor is a circulating hormone stimulated by volume loading. Nature 314: 6008
152. Kangawa J, Matsuo H (1984) Purification and complete amino acid sequence of alpha-human atrial natriuretic polypeptide (alpha-hANP). Biochem Biophys Res Commun 118: 131
153. Schmitt G, Tobin M, Metheson J, Flamenbaum W (1981) Prostaglandin E (PGE) blood levels during hemodialysis comparison of cellulosic and polycralonitrile membranes. Kidney Int 19: A158
154. Borges H, Shideman J, Kjellstrand CM (1981) Hypotension during chronic hemodialysis: on the effects of prostaglandin inhibition. Proceedings 8th International Congress Nephrol, Athens 1981, p 433
155. Friedrich T, Lichey J, Nigam S, Heidrich E, Doye K, Schultze G, Wegscheider K, Priesnitz M (1982) Levels of prostaglandins and complement activity in plasma of patients with acute myocardial infarction. Proceedings 5th International Conference on Prostaglandins, Florence
156. Lichey J, Nigam S, Friedrich T, Maiga M, Schultze G, Heidrich E, Doye K, Wegscheider K, Priesnitz M (1982) Elevated levels of prostaglandins in arterial and venous blood of patients with pulmonary embolism. Proceedings 5th International Conference on Prostaglandins, Florence
157. Dzau VJ, Packer M, Lilly LS, Swartz SL, Hollenberg NK, Williams GH (1984) Prostaglandins in severe congestive heart failure. Relation to activation of the renin-angiotensin system and hyponatremia. N Engl J Med 310: 347
158. Leithner C, Sinzinger H, Silberbauer K, Stummvoll HK (1981) Platelet microaggregates and release of endogenous prostacyclin during the initial phase of hyemodialysis. Proc Eur Dial Transplant Assoc 18: 122
159. Branger B, Oulés R, Bonardet A, Deschodt G, Rey R, Treissede D, Granolleras C, Balducchi

JP, Shaldon S, Mion H, Fourcade J (1984) Hemodynamic and prostaglandin level changes during acetate hemodialysis versus bicarbonate hemodialysis. Contrib Nephrol 41: 388

160. McDonald JW, Ali M, Morgan E, Townsend ER, Cooper JD (1983) Thromboxane synthesis by sources other than platelets in association with complement-induced pulmonary leukostasis and pulmonary hypertension in sheep. Circ Res 52: 1

161. Henderson LW, Koch KM, Dinarello CA, Shaldon S (1983) Hemodialysis hypotension: the interleukin hypothesis. Blood Purif 1: 3

162. Maggiore Q, Pizzarelli F, Zoccali C, Sisca S, Nicolò F, Parlongo S (1981) Effect of extracorporeal blood cooling on dialytic arterial hypotension. Proc Eur Dial Transplant Assoc 18: 597

163. Sherman RA, Faustino EF, Bernholc AS, Eisinger RP (1984) Effect of variations in dialysate temperature on blood pressure during hemodialysis. Am J Kidney Dis 4: 66

164. Coli U, Landini S, Lucatello S, Fracasso A, Morachiello P, Righetto F, Scanferla F, Onesti G, Bazzato G (1983) Cold as cardiovascular stabilizing factor in hemodialysis: hemodynamic evaluation. Trans Am Soc Artif Intern Organs 29: 71

165. Mahida BH, Dumler F, Zasuwa G, Fleig G, Levin NW (1983) Effect of cooled dialysate on serum catecholamines and blood pressure stability. Trans Am Soc Artif Intern Organs 29: 384

166. Lindholm T, Thysell H, Yamamoto Y, Forsberg B, Gullberg CA (1985) Temperature and vascular stability in hemodialysis. Nephron (BASEL) 39: 130

167. Sherman RA, Rubin MP, Cody RP, Eisinger RP (1985) Amelioration of hemodialysis-associated hypotension by the use of cool dialysate. Am J Kidney Dis 5: 124

168. Maggiore Q, Pizzarelli F, Sisca S, Catalano C, Delfino D (1984) Vascular stability and heat in dialysis patients. Contrib Nephrol 41: 398

169. Maggiore Q, Pizzarelli F, Sisca S, Zoccali C, Parlongo S, Nicolò F, Creazzo G (1982) Blood temperature and vascular stability during hemodialysis and hemofiltration. Proc Trans Am Soc Artif Intern Organs 28: 523

170. Absolom DR, Policova Z, Neumann AW, Zingg W (1983) The effect of temperature on the extent of platelet adhesion to foreign surfaces. Trans Am Soc Artif Intern Organs 29: 425

171. Schaefer K, von Herrath D, Hüfler M (1983) Failure to show a temperature-dependent vascular stability during hemofiltration. Int J Artif Organs 6: 75–76

172. Vanholder R, Piron M, Ringoir S (1984) Absence of a beneficial haemodynamic effect of bicarbonate versus acetate haemodialysis. Proc Eur Dial Transplant Assoc 21: 195

173. Pizzarelli F, Sisca S, Zoccali C, Parlongo S, Nicolò F, Greazzo G, Delfino D, Maggiore Q (1983) Blood temperature and cardiovascular stability in hemofiltration. Int J Artif Organs 6: 37

174. Enia G, Catalano C, Pizzarelli F, Greazzo G, Zaccuri F, Mundo A, Iellamo D, Maggiore Q (1984) The effect of dialysate temperature on haemodialysis leucopenia. Proc Eur Dial Transplant Assoc 21: 167

175. Dinarello CA (1984) Interleukin-1. Rev Infect Dis 6: 51

176. Craddock PR, Fehr J, Dalmasso AP, Brigham KI, Jacob HS (1977) Hemodialysis leukopenia: pulmonary vascular leukostasis resulting from complement activation by dialyzer cellophane membranes. J Clin Invest 59: 879.

177. Craddock PR, Hammershmidt DE, White JG, Dalmasso AP, Jacob HS (1977) Complement (C5a)-induced granulocyte aggregation in vitro: a possible mechanism for complement-mediated leukostasis and leukopenia. J Clin Invest 60: 260

178. Walker JF, Lindsey M, Sibbald WJ, et al (1984) Cuprophane hypersensitivity. The cardiopulmonary phenomenon and its modification in an animal model. Trans Am Soc Artif Intern Organs 30: 168

179. Arnaout MA, Hakim RM, Todd RF, Dana N, Colten HR (1985) Increased expression of an adhesion-promoting surface glycoprotein in the granulocytopenia of hemodialysis. N Engl J Med 312: 457

180. Condon CJ, Freeman RM (1970) Zinc metabolism in renal failure. Ann Intern Med 73: 531

181. Chenoweth DE, Goodman MG, Wiegle WO (1982) Demonstration of a specific receptor for human C5a anaphylatoxin on murine macrophages. J Exp Med 156: 68

182. Goodman MG, Chenoweth DE, Wiegle WO (1982) Induction of interleukin-1 secretion and enhancement of humoral immunity by binding of human C5a to macrophage surface C5a receptors. J Exp Med 156: 912

183. Dinarello CA, Wolff SM (1982) Molecular basis of fever in humans. Am J Med 72: 799

184. Rossi V, Rivario F, Ghezzi P, Mantovani L (1985) Interleukin-I induces prostacyclin synthesis in vascular cells. Science (in press)
185. Port FK, Weingast JA, van de Kerkhove K, Eiger SM, Kluger MJ (1985) Release of pyrogens during clinical hemodialysis. Trans Am Soc Artif Intern Organs 31 (in press)
186. Gutierrez A, Alvestrand A, Wahren J, Bergström J (1985) Blood-membrane interaction without dialysis induces increased protein catabolism in normal man. 22nd Congress of the European Dialysis and Transplant Association, Brussels 1985, p 107
186. Hakim RM, Lowrie EG (1982) Hemodialysis-associated neutropenia and hypoxemia: the effect of dialyzer membrane materials. Nephron (BASEL) 32: 12
187. Hakim RM, Fearon DT, Lazarus JM (1984) Biocompatibility of dialysis membranes: effects of chronic complement activation. Kidney Int 26: 194
188. Lonneman G, Bingel M, Koch KM, Shaldon S, Dinarello CA (1985) Interleukin-I induction during in vitro dialysis. Blood Purification 2: 198 A
189. Minetti L, Civati G, Guastoni C, Teatini U, Perego A, Perrino ML, Brunati C (1985) Evaluation of physiology and efficacy of hemofiltration without substitution fluid after 2000 sessions. Blood Purification 2: 226 A
190. Röckel A, Hennemann H, Sternagel-Haase A, Heidland A (1979) Uraemic sympathetic neuropathy after haemodialysis and transplantation. Eur J Clin Invest 9: 23
191. Lazarus JM, Hampers CL, Lowrie EG, Merrill JP (1973) Baroreceptor activity in normotensive and hypertensive uremic patients. Circulation 47: 1015
192. Pickering TG, Gribbin B, Oliver DO (1972) Baroreflex sensitivity in patients on long-term haemodialysis. Clin Sci 43: 645
193. Lilley JJ, Golden J, Stone RA (1976) Adrenergic regulation of blood pressure in chronic renal failure. J Clin Invest 57: 1190
194. Koch KM, Baldamus CA, Ernst W, Fassbinder W, Georges J, Brecht HM (1980) Autonome Kreislaufregulation in der Urämie. Klin Wochenschr 58: 1037
195. Nies AS, Robertson D, Stone WJ (1979) Hemodialysis hypotension is not the result of uremic peripheral autonomic neuropathy. J Lab Clin Med 94: 395
196. Cohn JN, Gombos FA, Tristani FF (1966) Disturbed baroreceptor and peripheral vascular control in chronic uremia. Clin Res 14: 374
197. Kersh ES, Kronfield SJ, Unger A, Popper RW, Cantor S, Cohn K (1974) Autonomic insufficiency in uremia as a cause of hemodialysis-induced hypotension. N Engl J Med 290: 650
198. Rascher W, Schömig A, Kreye VA, Ritz E (1982) Diminished vascular response to noradrenaline in experimental chronic uremia. Kidney Int 21: 20
199. Romoff MS, Campese VM, Lane K, Massry SG (1978) Mechanism of autonomic dysfunction in uremia: evidence for reduced end organ response to norepinephrine. Kidney Int 14: A 731
200. Horler E, Hennemann H, Heidland A (1974) Intraneuronaler Stoffwechsel von Noradrenalin bei experimenteller Urämie und Hypertonie. Verh Dtsch Ges Inn Med 80: 237
201. Hennemann H, Horler E (1976) Sympathicopathy in uremia. In: Heidland A (ed) Renal insufficiency. Thieme, Stuttgart, p 41
202. Winckler J, Hennemann H, Heidland A, Wiegand ME (1976) Katecholamingehalt adrenerger Nerven in Speicheldrüsen mit gestörter Elektrolytausscheidung bei Urämie. Klin Wochenschr 51: 479
203. Brecht HM, Ernst W, Koch KM (1976) Plasma noradrenaline levels in regular haemodialysis patients. Proc Eur Dial Transplant Assoc 12: 281
204. Ksiazek A (1979) Dopamine-beta-hydroxylase activity and catecholamine levels in the plasma of patients with renal failure. Nephron (BASEL) 24: 170
205. McGrath BP, Ledingham JGG, Benedict CR (1978) Catecholamines in peripheral venous plasma in patients on chronic haemodialysis. Clin Sci Mol Med 55: 89
206. Baldamus CA, Mantz P, Kachel HG, Koch KM, Schoeppe W (1984) Baroreflex in patients undergoing hemodialysis and hemofiltration. Contrib Nephrol 41: 409
207. Tomiyama O, Shiigai T, Ideura T, Tomita K, Mito Y, Shinohara S, Tekeuchi J (1980) Baroreflex sensitivity in renal failure. Clin Sci 58: 21
208. Ewing DJ, Winney R (1975) Autonomic function in patients with chronic renal failure on intermittent haemodialysis. Nephron (BASEL) 15: 424
209. Hung J, Harris PJ, Uren RF, Tiller DJ, Kelly DT (1980) Uremic cardiomyopathy - effect of hemodialysis on left ventricular function in end-stage renal failure. N Engl J Med 302: 547

210. Prosser D, Parsons V (1975) The case for a specific uraemic myocardiopathy. Nephron (BASEL) 15: 4
211. Raab W (1944) Cardiotoxic substances in the blood and heart muscle in uremia (their nature and action). J Lab Clin Med 29: 715
212. Bailey GL, Hampers CL, Merrill JP (1967) Reversible cardiomyopathy in uremia. Trans Am Soc Artif Intern Organs 13: 263
213. Ianhez LE, Lowen J, Sabbage E (1975) Uremic myocardiopathy. Nephron (BASEL) 15: 17
214. Drueke L, Pailleur AJ, Mailhac B et al (1977) Congestive cardiomyopathy in uraemic patients on long term hemodialysis. Br Med J 1: 350
215. Gueron M, Berlyne GM, Nord E, Ben Ari J (1975) The case against the existence of a specific uremic myocardiopathy. Nephron (BASEL) 15: 2
216. Nixon JV, Mitchell JH, McPaul JJ Jr, Henrich WL (1983) Effect of hemodialysis on left ventricular function. J Clin Invest 71: 377
217. Keshaviah P, Shapiro FL (1982) A critical examination of dialysis-induced hypotension. Am J Kidney Dis II: 290
218. Ylikorkala O, Huttunen K, Järvi J, Viinikka L (1982) Prostacyclin and thromboxane in chronic uremia: the effect of hemodialysis. Clin Nephrol 18: 83
219. Kishimoto T, Yamamoto T, Yamamoto K, Yamagami S, Nishitani H, Mizutani Y, Yamakawa M, Maekawa M (1984) Acetate kinetics during hemodialysis and hemofiltration. Blood Purif 2: 81

Blood Pressure Control

E. A. QUELLHORST

Table of Contents

Mechanisms responsible for the maintenance of high blood pressure have been investigated extensively in essential as well as in renovascular hypertension. The pathogenesis of hypertension in end-stage renal failure (ESRF), however, has evidently evoked little interest despite the fact that, due to a diminishing interference of the natural kidneys and an increasing potential allowing a modulation of several factors by the application of an artificial kidney, observations made in patients with advanced renal insufficiency would have been of great value for the elucidation of essential hypertension. Whereas the fractional sodium excretion is increased in mild or moderate renal insufficiency, this compensatory mechanism of the natural kidney is abolished in severe renal failure. Thus, hypertension in patients with renal insufficiency requiring artificial kidney treatment in most cases is a consequence of fluid and sodium overload. In a minor proportion of patients (about 10% of the dialysis population) hypertension may be volume independent, e.g., hypertension continues to exist in spite of adequate fluid removal. Whereas, an inverse relation exists between renin secretion and exchangeable sodium under physiological conditions [1], this individually determined equilibrium may be disturbed in those patients demonstrating an increased renin activity in spite of an augmentation of their exchangeable sodium (Fig. 1). Disorders of the autonomic nervous system or catecholamine metabolism seem to be of minor importance, at least as factors for the maintenance of severe hypertension in advanced renal insufficiency.

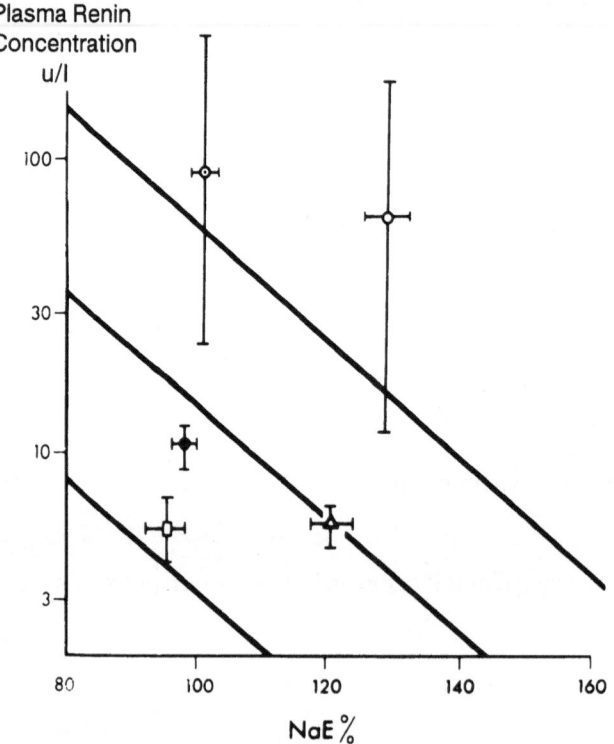

Plasma Renin
Concentration
    u/l

Fig. 1. Relation between total body exchangeable sodium (NaE) and plasma renin concentration in normal individuals and patients with various renal or renovascular disorders [1]. ☉, renal artery stenosis; ○, chronic renal failure; ●, essential hypertension, normal renin; □, low-renin hypertension; △, primary adolsteronism

Mechanisms by which Hemofiltration Influences Hypertension in Chronic Renal Insufficiency

Volume Dependent Hypertension

Fluid and sodium overload can be identified as the main cause of hypertension in the majority of patients depending on artificial kidney therapy. As an adequate blood pressure can be achieved even when dialysis fluids with iso- or hypertonic sodium concentrations are applied, fluid removal seems to be of greater importance for the maintenance of normal blood pressure than is total body sodium. Fluid removal can be assessed more precisely by hemofiltration (HF) than by conventional dialysis therapy. Moreover, a linear reduction of body weight during the whole procedure is an important measure for prevention of sudden blood pressure depression or collapse reaction, inducing saline infusion for its control, while at the same time compromising an adequate fluid removal. Generally, a higher fluid removal is tolerated with HF than with HD, during which the adjustment of the transmembrane pressure (TMP) allows only an approximation of the dehydration per treatment procedure (Fig. 2). It is, thus, easy to understand that volume-dependent hy-

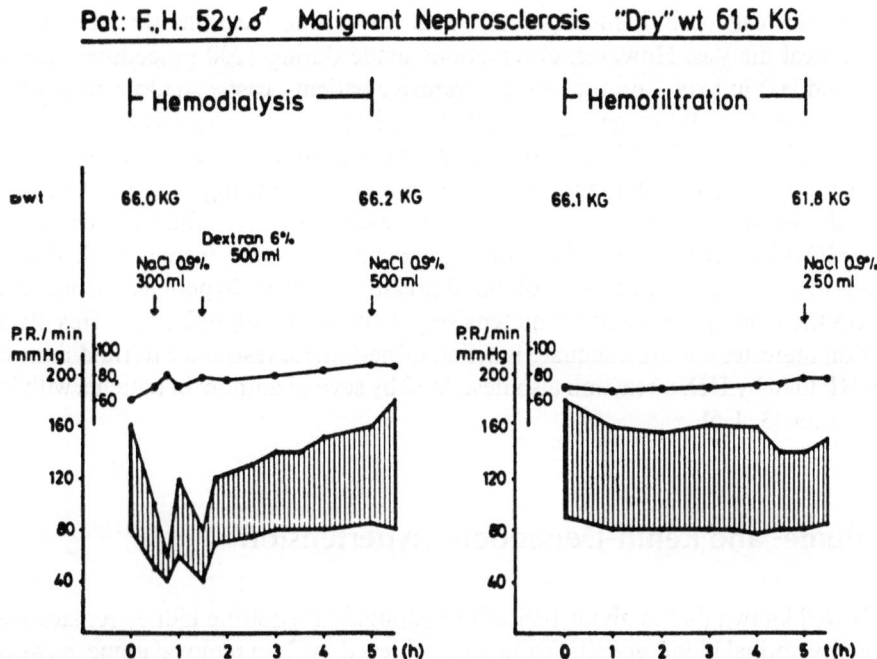

Fig. 2. Reaction of arterial blood pressure and pulse rate on fluid removal by hemodialysis and postdilution hemofiltration

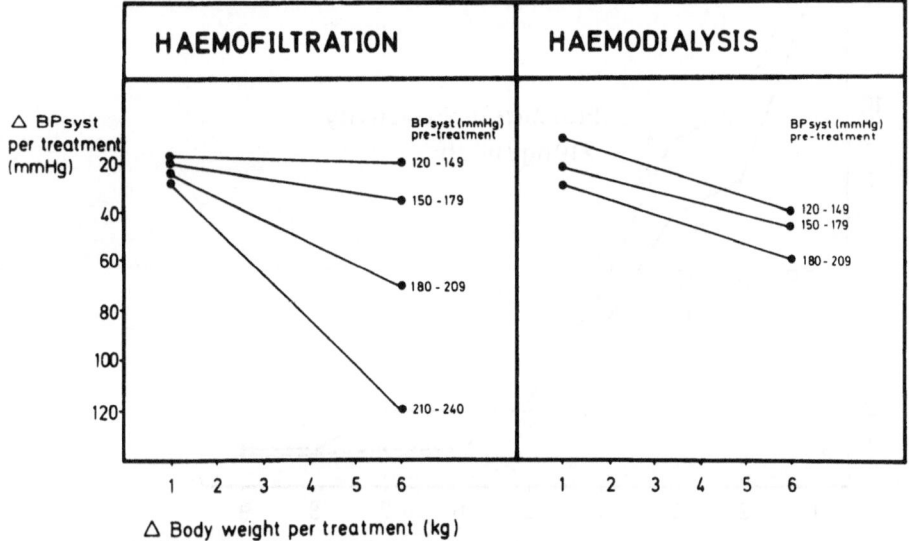

Fig. 3. Reaction of systolic blood pressure (BP syst) per treatment on fluid removal (Δ body weight) related to the pretreatment blood pressure in 1000 procedures each of hemofiltration and hemodialysis

pertension can be influenced by HF with fewer side reactions than by HD or peritoneal dialysis. However, observations made during 1000 procedures each of HF and HD in hypo-, normo-, or hypertensive patients, cast a shadow on this harmonious picture. When trying to correlate body weight loss per treatment and the decrease in systolic blood pressure with the systolic blood pressure at the start of the procedure, it could be demonstrated, at least in HF, that the higher the pretreatment blood pressure was, the more it could be influenced by a given fluid withdrawal [2]. For HD this correlation was not as obvious (Fig. 3). The same degree of dehydration leads to a considerable decrease of blood pressure in severe hypertension, but influences the blood pressure in normotensive patients only insignificantly. This observation indicates a more adequate reaction of peripheral resistance to fluid removal by HF than by HD, a reaction also described by several authors in patients with hypotension [3, 4, 5].

Volume- and Renin-Dependent Hypertension

It is well known that in about 10% of the population requiring kidney replacement therapy normal blood pressure cannot be achieved by fluid removal alone, however distinct it might be. In those patients demonstrating an unusually high plasma renin

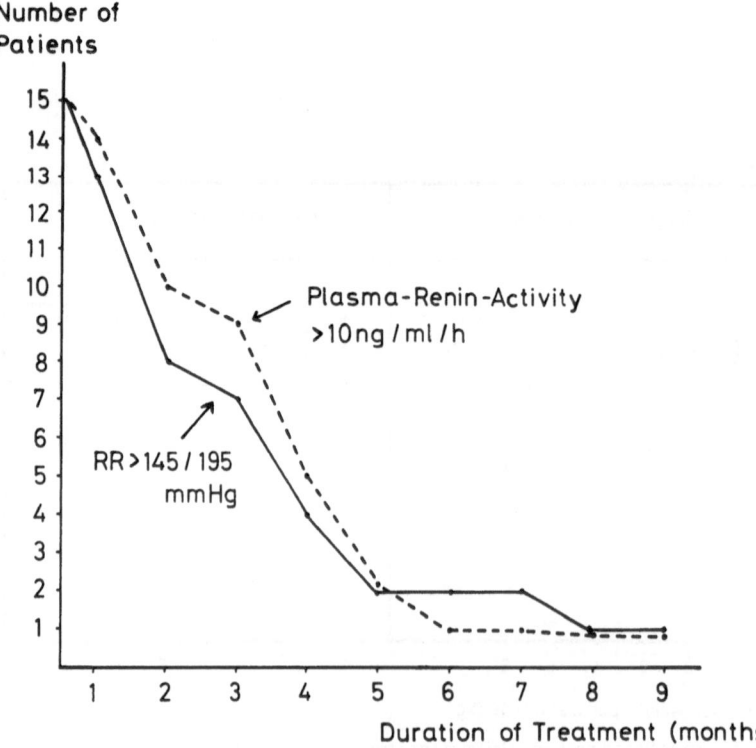

Fig. 4. Normalization of blood pressure and plasma renin activity in 14 patients with dialysis and drug-resistant hypertension during regular hemofiltration

activity, bilateral nephrectomy had to be performed to normalize the blood pressure; this surgical procedure may soon be replaced by the administration of converting enzyme blockers (e. g., captopril). It has been shown that even in those patients a normalization of blood pressure in tandem with a decline of plasma renin activity can be expected with HF, but not with HD (Fig. 4). The favorable effects of HF may be explained by the absence of collapse reactions during treatment, thereby eliminating the repetitive stimulus for the renin-angiotensin system [6]. Thus, one important mechanism responsible for the maintenance of hypertension in chronic renal failure (CRF), an inadequately high plasma renin activity related to total exchangeable sodium [1], may be eliminated by HF.

Clinical Observations

Soon after the development of HF as a method of treatment in patients with chronic renal insufficiency, HENDERSON et al. [7] published preliminary observations on blood pressure response to regular HF. In two patients with severe hypertension, blood pressure was normalized after transfer from intermittent HD to HF, the effect being reversable after reinitiation of HD. As one of these patients has been bilaterally nephrectomized before starting therapy, the authors concluded that the renin-angiotensin system could not have had an influence on the blood pressure regulation. It has to be stressed that normal blood pressure was obtained no earlier than about 2 months after transfer to the test treatment. The authors discussed a more adequate removal of sodium and water by HF, or equally possible, the withdrawal of some intermediate molecular weight substances, with a pressor function, as mediators of blood pressure normalization.

In a further study, HENDERSON et al. [8], investigated six patients with severe hypertension due to chronic renal insufficiency who underwent a cross-over protocol (3 months on HD, 3 months on predilution HF, and again 3 months on HD). Three patients, responding to HF with blood pressure normalization, in contrast to the remaining three, showed a decrease of plasma dopamine-β-hydroxylase activity, but no changes in plasma renin activity, blood volume, or body weight (Fig. 5). The authors conclude that a defective baroreceptor reflex, present in patients with chronic renal insufficiency and hypertension, might be improved by HF rather than by HD. According to their view, a normalization of blood pressure in all patients could have been achieved if the patients had been treated by HF for longer than 3 months. The role of dopamine-β-hydroxylase as a method of predicting the influence of HF on blood pressure behavior in hypertension was queried by SPOHR et al. [9], who detected a uniform increase of dopamine-β-hydroxylase activity in both HF and HD, depending on the amount of fluid being removed by ultrafiltration.

QUELLHORST et al. [6, 10] observed a normalization of blood pressure even in patients with dialysis and drug-resistant hyperreninemic hypertension during a HF phase of up to 9 months: eight of nine patients with hyperreninemic and 12 of 13 patients with normoreninemic hypertension responded to postdilution HF, the effect being reversible on returning to HD (Fig. 6). In the hyperreninemic group, a considerable number of collapse reactions during HD induced not only stimulation

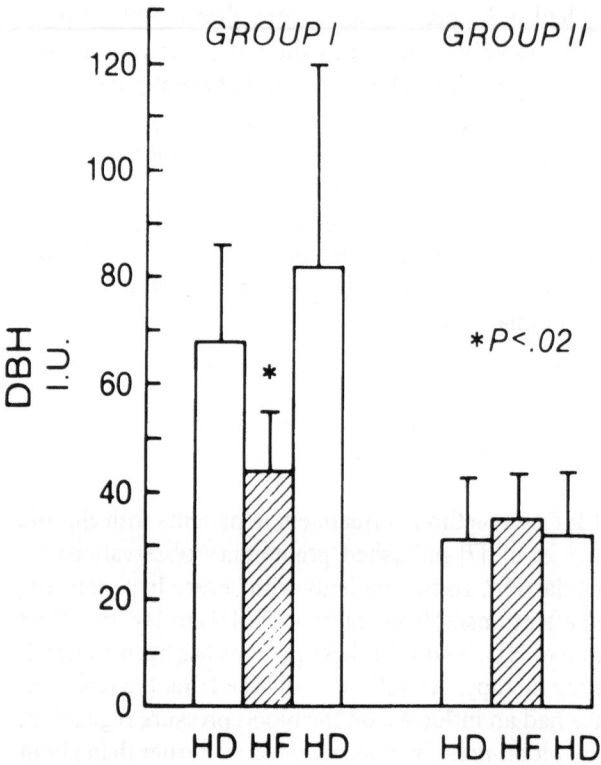

Fig. 5. Behavior of plasma dopamine-β-hydroxylase (DBH) in the course of a 3-month hemodialysis (HD) or hemofiltration (HF) period in responders (group I) and nonresponders (group II) concerning blood pressure normalization by hemofiltration [8]

of the renin-angiotensin system, but also an increased number of saline infusions to overcome the depression of blood pressure obstructing its normalization during this phase of treatment. On the other hand, these interventions proved unnecessary during HF therapy.

The favorable results of HF on blood pressure normalization in renal hypertension are not without contradiction. SCHNEIDER et al. [11] reported on nine patients who had been subjected to intermittent HF because of dialysis-resistant hypertension. Besides three nonresponders, there were six patients in whom antihypertensive drug therapy could be reduced significantly. The behavior of plasma dopamine-β-hydroxylase levels did not differ between responders and nonresponders. The authors concluded that changes in dopamine-β-hydroxylase activity, inso far as it reflects sympathetic activity, "are not essential for an improvement in dialysis-resistant hypertension."

NAKAGAWA [12] investigated several hemodynamic and metabolic parameters in nine patients having been transferred to regular postdilution HF treatment after a HD period of 17.8 months on average. Although the frequency of hypotensive reactions could be reduced from 8% to 2% by HF, hypertension persisted in two of six patients even after adequate fluid removal by HF. In these patients, however, the dosage of antihypertensive drugs could be reduced after 5 months of HF treatment.

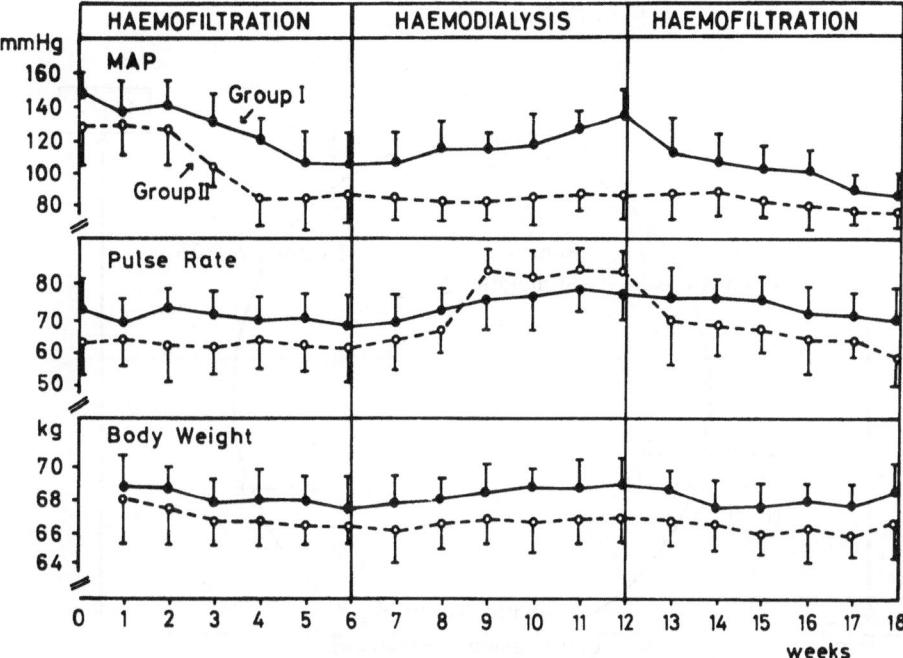

Fig. 6. Mean arterial pressure (MAP), pulse rate, and body weight in nine patients with hyperreninemic (group I) and 13 patients with normoreninemic hypertension (group II). The steep increase in pulse rate during hemodialysis in group II patients deserves special attention [6]

BALDAMUS et al. [13], performing an ABA study (A, hemodialysis; B, hemofiltration), did not observe significant blood pressure response in three hypertensive patients in the course of a 4-month HF period. However, the body weight was kept constant during the whole HF phase. It may be speculated that a more vigorous dehydration would have influenced blood pressure favorably.

Potential Mechanisms Normalizing Blood Pressure in Hyper- as in Hypotension

In an attempt to explain the obviously controversial reactions of the vascular system to HF, namely, the prevention of collapse reactions with hypotension and the normalization of blood pressure [6], the following concept may be proposed (Fig. 7): The stability of the vascular system during and after HF is maintained by a more rapid refilling of the extracellular space during ultrafiltration and by an increase in total peripheral vascular resistance which occurs even with severe hypertension in HF but not in HD [3, 4]. During a controlled ultrafiltration period lasting between 30 and 90 min ROUBY et al. [14] observed a plasma refilling rate of 65% of the ultrafiltration; whereas, this parameter was as low as 40% in HD. SCHUENEMANN et al. [15], assessing the behavior of the extracellular space in HD in comparison with HF by the application of a modified inulin method, observed a marked reduction of the

HAEMOFILTRATION

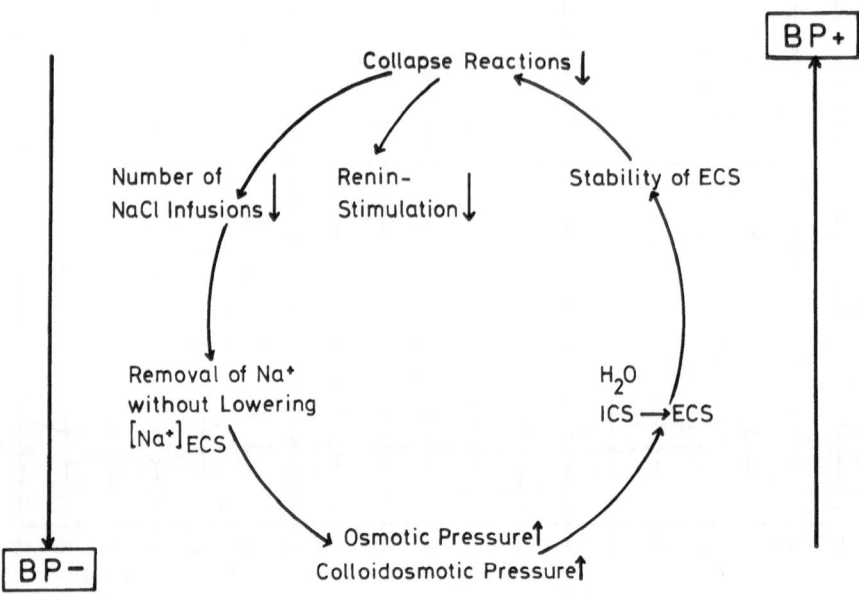

Fig. 7. Hypothetical concept of blood pressure regulation by hemofiltration (BP, blood pressure; ICS, intracellular space; ECS, extracellular space)

inulin space in HD but not in HF. The authors interpret their observation as indication for a more rapid refilling of the extracellular space in HF. Vascular stability enables fluid removal without collapse reaction which generally involves less saline infusions. A depression of the renin-angiotensin system and an adequate dehydration without deterioration of the vascular stability induce a normalization of blood pressure even with hyperreninemic hypertension.

References

1. Brown JJ, Fraser R, Lever AF, Morton JJ, Robertson JIS, Schalekamp MADH (1977) Mechanisms in hypertension: A personal view. In: Genest J, Koiw E, Kuchel O (eds) Hypertension. McGraw-Hill, New York, pp 529–548
2. Quellhorst E, Schuenemann B, Doht B (1977) Treatment of severe hypertension in chronic renal failure by haemofiltration. Proc Eur Dial Transplant Assoc 14: 129–135
3. Baldamus CA, Ernst W, Fassbinder W, Koch KM (1980) Differing haemodynamic stability due to differing sympathetic response: Comparison of ultrafiltration, haemodialysis and haemofiltration. Proc Eur Dial Transplant Assoc 17: 205–212
4. Quellhorst E, Schuenemann B, Hildebrand U, Falda Z (1980) Response of the vascular system to different modifications of haemofiltration and haemodialysis. Proc Eur Dial Transplant Assoc 17: 197–203
5. Quellhorst E, Schuenemann B, Hildebrand U (1981) How to prevent vascular instability: Haemofiltration. Proc Eur Dial Transplant Assoc 18: 243–249

6. Quellhorst E, Schuenemann B, Hildebrand U, Neumann W (1982) Hypertension and hemofiltration. Contrib Nephrol 32: 46-55
7. Henderson LW, Ford CA, Lysaght MJ, Grossman RA, Silverstein ME (1975) Preliminary observations on blood pressure response with maintenance diafiltration. Kidney Int 7: S-413-417
8. Henderson LW, Sanfelippo ML, Stone RA (1980) Hemofiltration for long-term maintenance of patients with end stage renal disease: Impact on hypertension. Adv Nephrol 9: 21-32
9. Spohr U, Ritz E, Kaden F (1977) Plasma dopamin-β-hydroxylase-activity in dialysed patients. Klin Wochenschr 55: 1089-1093
10. Quellhorst E (1979) Hämofiltration - Differentialindikation zur Hämodialyse unter Berücksichtigung hämodynamischer und metabolischer Aspekte. Klin Wochenschr 57: 1061-1068
11. Schneider H, Streicher E, Hövelborn U, Müller HAG, Spohr U, Schmidt-Gayk H (1979) Haemofiltration - critical evaluation of clinical benefits. Proc Eur Dial Transplant Assoc 16: 218-223
12. Nakagawa S (1980) Multifactorial evaluation of hemofiltration therapy in comparison with conventional hemodialysis. Artif Organs 4: 94-102
13. Baldamus CA, Schoeppe W, Koch KM (1978) Comparison of haemodialysis (HD) and post dilution haemofiltration (HF) on an unselected dialysis population. Proc Eur Dial Transplant Assoc 15: 228-235
14. Rouby JJ, Rottembourg J, Durande JP, Basset JY, Legrain M (1978) Importance of the plasma refilling rate in the genesis of hypovolaemic hypotension during regular dialysis and controlled sequential ultrafiltration-hemodialysis. Proc Eur Dial Transplant Assoc 15: 239-244
15. Schuenemann B, Borghardt J, Falda Z, Jacob I, Kramer P, Kraft B, Quellhorst E (1978) Reactions of blood pressure and body spaces to hemofiltration treatment. Trans Am Soc Artif Intern Organs 24: 687-689

Impact of Hemofiltration on Various Metabolic and Endocrine Disturbances of Chronic Uremia

K. SCHAEFER and D. VON HERRATH

Table of Contents

The chronic uremic state is characterized by various organ complications which are in general not improved, or at least not healed, by even an intensive dialytic strategy.

Important disturbances regularly encountered in patients suffering from chronic uremia concern calcium and phosphorus metabolism, anemia, disorders of lipid metabolism, and disturbances of the nervous system.

Chronic hemodialysis does not permit the removal of medium-sized and larger molecules retained in the uremic organism, as the permeability of most of the dialysis membranes facilitates an efficient transport only of solutes with a molecular weight of below 1000.

It was anticipated in the past that hemofiltration might be an advantageous therapeutic method for some of the above-mentioned complications, as it was assumed that this method would allow the removal even of substances with a molecular weight of 15000 and more, which are considered by some workers to be of pathogenetic importance for uremic complications [9, 12].

There are many reports inplying that some of the uremic complications are at least partially caused by larger molecules. One of the most interesting substances in this context is parathyroid hormone. However, as chronic hemofiltration on a larger scale has only been available for a few years, knowledge about the impact of hemofiltration on certain uremic complications is limited. Therefore it is not possible at the present time to draw final conclusions as to whether or not this alternative blood

purification treatment is more capable of alleviating uremic complications than hemodialysis or peritoneal dialysis.

In the following paragraphs we will try to sumarize the effects of hemofiltration
on various uremic complications. As parathyroid hormone could, as already mentioned, be the culprit in many uremic complications, it is evident that this hormone
deserves a special place in the following discussion [5, 6].

Parathyroid Hormone Metabolism in Acute and Chronic Hemofiltration

There are various reports which indicate that acute hemofiltration induces a significant decrease in the serum concentration of parathyroid hormone. Figure 1 shows
that this decrease is related not only to changes in serum calcium concentration, but
is caused also by the removal of parathyroid hormone during a hemofiltration session [18, 19]. Futhermore, there is clear evidence that not only biologically inactive
fragments of parathyroid hormone, but also the intact hormone, are removed during one treatment session (Fig. 2). On the other hand, it is of note that the serum concentration of parathyroid hormone returns to normal a few hours after an acute
hemofiltration treatment [7]. Long-term observations collected in our department
and by others seem to indicate that chronic hemofiltration treatment could induce a
sustained reduction in the serum parathyroid hormone levels which, however, is
certainly mainly due to a decrease in the number of parathyroid hormone fragments
excreted by the diseased kidneys [7, 15-17].

To summarize the available data on parathyroid hormone metabolism, it appears
that chronic hemofiltration, in contrast to chronic hemodialysis, induces a decrease
in the serum parathyroid hormone concentration. Whether the change is of any
benefit for parathyroid hormone-associated disorders will be discussed later.

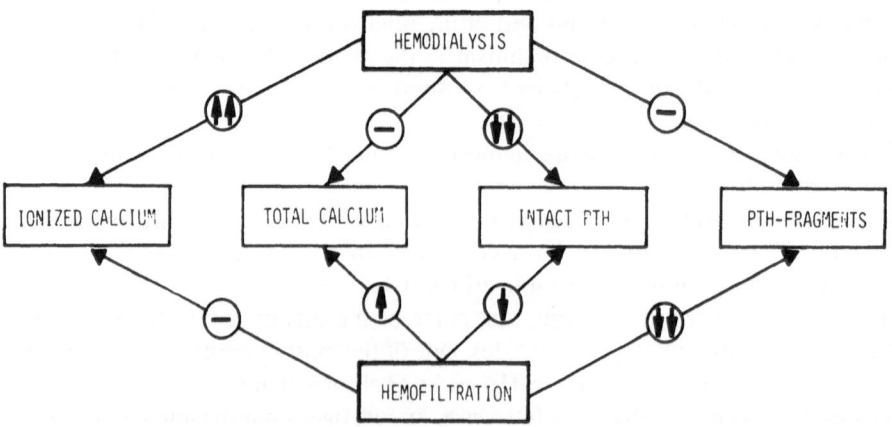

Fig. 1. Parathyroid hormone *(PTH)* metabolism in hemodialysis and hemofiltration. -, no influence; ↓, weak; ↓↓, strong

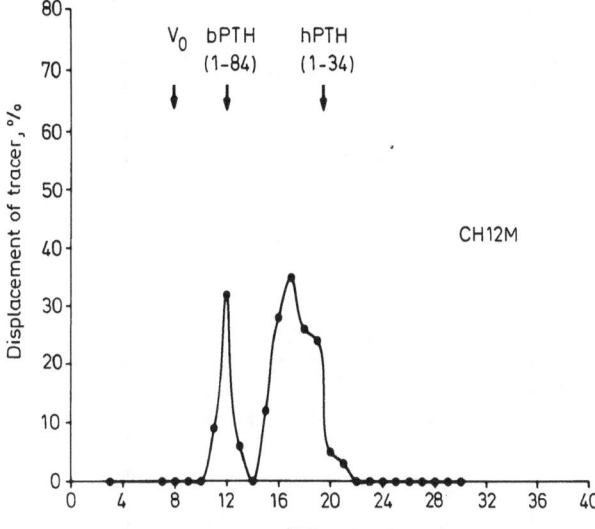

Fig. 2. Chromatography of parathyroid hormone *(PTH)* and fragments in hemofiltration. V_0, vehicle; b, bovine; h, human; CHI2M, chicken no. 12

Uremic Bone Disease

Secondary hyperparathyroidism is a universal finding in patients with renal insufficiency. Chief cell hyperplasia of the parathyroid glands and high levels of parathyroid hormone are among the earliest alterations in mineral metabolism in patients with chronic renal failure. The most important factor for the development of secondary hyperparathyroidism is the reduction in the serum level of ionized clacium. Although many factors are responsible for the regulation of the secretion of parathyroid hormone, the most important appear to be

a) a retention of phosphorus,
b) an altered vitamin D metabolism,
c) a skeletal resistance to the calcemic action of parathyroid hormone,
d) an altered point for calcium-regulated parathyroid hormone release, and
e) impaired degradation of parathyroid hormone [24].

It is evident that hemofiltration could interfere with some of the listed pathogenetic factors, as the removal of phosphate is satisfactorily achieved by chronic hemofiltration and, on the other hand, sufficient calcium could be administered to ensure a positive calcium balance [7, 21]. In addition, as mentioned earlier, parathyroid hormone is partially removed by hemofiltration [13].

The data reporting on the influence of hemofiltration on the underlying renal

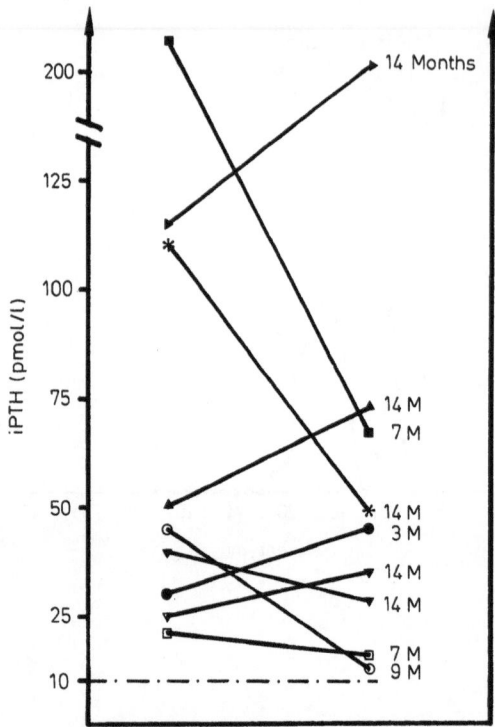

Fig. 3. Parathyroid hormone *(PTH)* levels in hemofiltration patients before hemofiltration and after various time periods. iPTH, immunoreactive parathyroid hormone

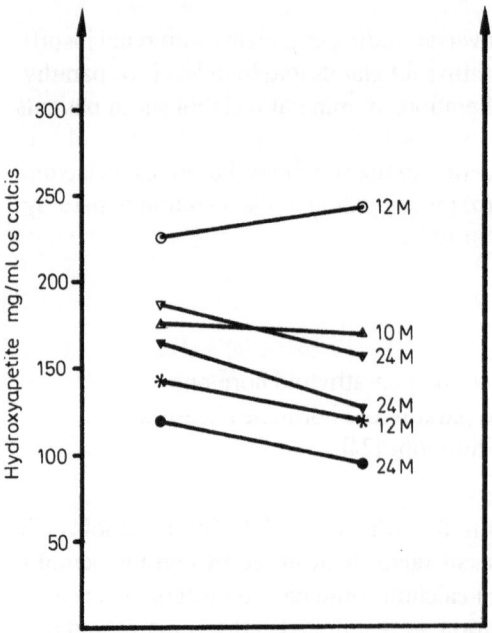

Fig. 4. Hydroxyapatite concentration in the os calcis at the beginning of hemofiltration and after various time periods. *M,* months

osteodystrophy are, however, conflicting. Our own data showed in some patients a certain decrease in serum parathyroid hormone concentration, whereas in others it remained stable [13, 15] (Fig. 3). Data about the hydroxyapatite concentration in the os calcis reveal no dramatic improvement after months of hemofiltration (Fig. 4). In addition, regularly performed x-ray investigations did not show a significant amelioration of the underlying bone disease. PIERIDES and coworkers reported on the elimination of parathyroid hormone and phosphorus during hemofiltration [7]. They observed a considerable decrease in serum parathyroid hormone and found that approximately 850 mg of phosphorus were removed during one treatment session. Long-term observation up to 30 months showed no progression of preexisting subperiosteal bone lesions, but on the other hand no changes in the underlying serum parathyroid hormone concentration. These authors conclude "that long term hemofiltration should allow an excellent control of calcium and phosphorus, parathyroid hormone and vitamin D metabolism, and that symptomatic bone disease should not be allowed to develop" [7].

SCHULZ and coworkers also observed lower parathyroid hormone values in hemofiltration patients than in hemodialysis patients, but no significant changes in the underlying bone disease [23]. SCHNEIDER and coworkers observed an elimination of phosphorus comparable to that observed by other workers during hemofiltration. However, in contrast to others, they reported an increase in the parathyroid hormone levels determined by a C-terminal radioimmunoassay in eight out of ten chronically treated patients, using mainly a replacement solution with 3.75 m val/l of calcium. Radiological assessment of the renal osteodystrophy revealed no significant changes in the Barnet-Nordin index over a longer time period [22]. In none of the patients did acro-osteolysis develop, or deteriorate when already present [22]. SCHNEIDER et al. concluded that calcium intake should be adequate with a calcium concentration of not lower than 4.0–4.25 m val/l in the replacement solution.

To summarize the available data, it seems evident that chronic hemofiltration does not generally promote a significant amelioration of an underlying uremic bone disease. It appears, however, that the removal of parathyroid hormone (active hormone and/or fragments), which does not occur during hemodialysis, could on a long-term basis be advantageous for the treatment of secondary hyperparathyroidism [15, 18]. Further observation is certainly necessary to establish the final role of hemofiltration for this uremic complication. As far as the aluminum-related bone disorders are concerned, it appears that hemofiltration could be the superior method, as it has been shown that during hemofiltration a larger amount of aluminum can be removed after desferrioxamine treatment than during hemodialysis [1].

Anemia

Patients with advanced chronic renal failure almost always have marked anemia. Decreased production and shortened survival of erythrocytes have been implicated as main causes of anemia in the uremic state. However, both clinical and experimental data point toward an important role for the excess blood levels of parathyroid hormone in the genesis of the anemia [6, 8]. Corresponding to the hopes which were expressed concerning a possible beneficial influence of hemofiltration on the development and course of uremic bone disease, it was also suggested and reported that hemofiltration might improve the underlying anemia to a greater extent than hemodialysis [10, 11]. It was suggested that this would be due not only to the removal of parathyroid hormone, but also to the eliminatation of currently unknown toxic compounds which are not normally removed by conventional hemodialysis [11]. In contrast to some earlier reports which were very optimistic, it appears, however, that chronic hemofiltration is not capable of improving uremic anemia, as long-term observations have not shown any significant rise in hemoglobin values.

Lipid Metabolism

Hyperlipidemia is usually present in patients with chronic uremia. An increase in the production of triglyceride-rich lipoproteins by the liver, a reduction in their removal by peripheral tissues, or a combination of both may be contributing factors. There are several studies indicating that besides these factors, parathyroid hormone might be involved in the genesis of the abnormal lipid metabolism. As mentioned

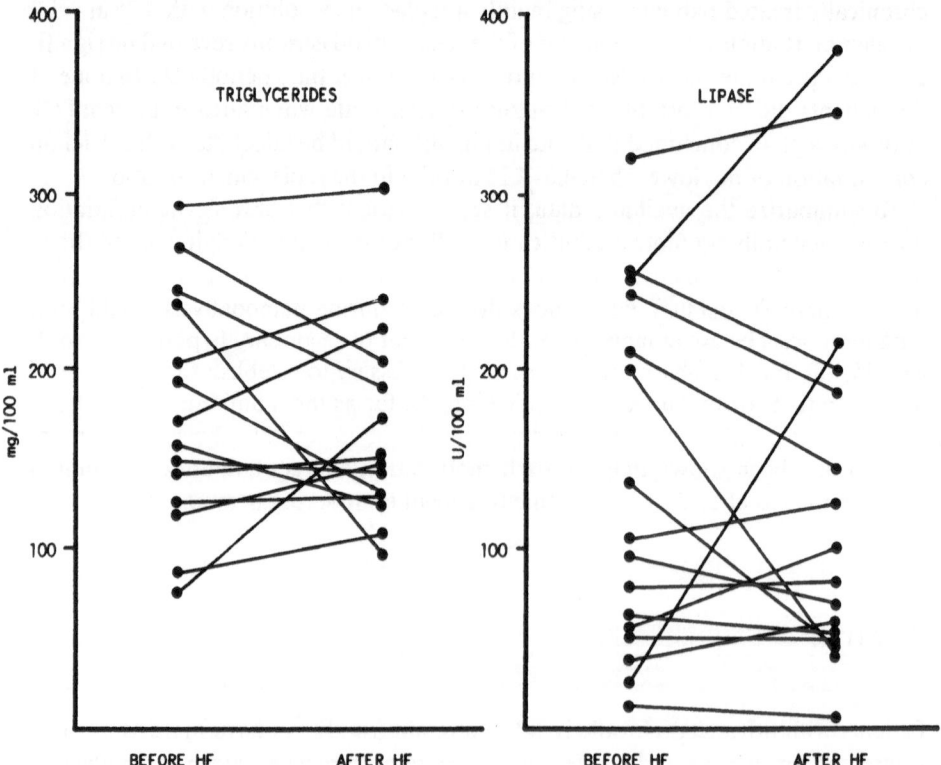

Fig. 5. Triglyceride concentration and lipoprotein lipase concentration before and after a hemofiltration session

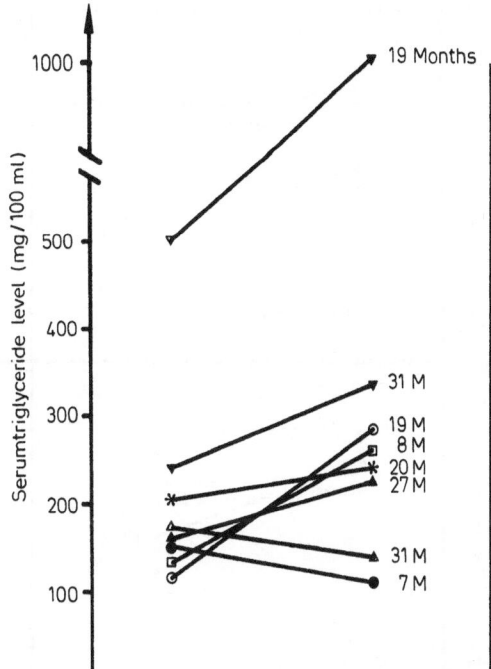

Fig. 6. Serum triglyceride levels at the beginning of hemofiltration and after various time periods. *M,* months

earlier, it has been suggested that hemofiltration could ameliorate lipid metabolism, especially as preliminary investigations showed an improvement in hypertriglyceridemia [3, 9]. Some authors considered the removal of uremic toxins responsible [9]; others favored the theory that the alkali equivalent used in the substitution fluid might be responsible for the observed effects. A summary of our own data is given in Figs. 5, 6. We observed no significant differences between the levels of serum triglyceride before and after a hemofiltration session in various uremic patients [4]. Our long-term observations lasting up to 31 months did not reveal any significant decrease in the serum triglyceride level [13, 15]. Fuchs et al. also observed no changes in different serum lipids and lipoproteins after a comparable time period [2]. Furthermore, these authors, comparing patients treated by hemofiltration, hemodialysis, or peritoneal dialysis, were unable to detect any improvement in lipid profiles of hemofiltration patients compared with patients being maintained by conventional hemodialysis [2]. To summarize the available evidence on the influence of hemofiltration on the various lipid disorders, it is thus currently impossible to state that hemofiltration offers any advantages in the treatment of this uremic complication.

Polyneuropathy

Patients with advanced renal failure display a variety of disturbances in the functioning of the nervous system. Of special interest here is the development of a pe-

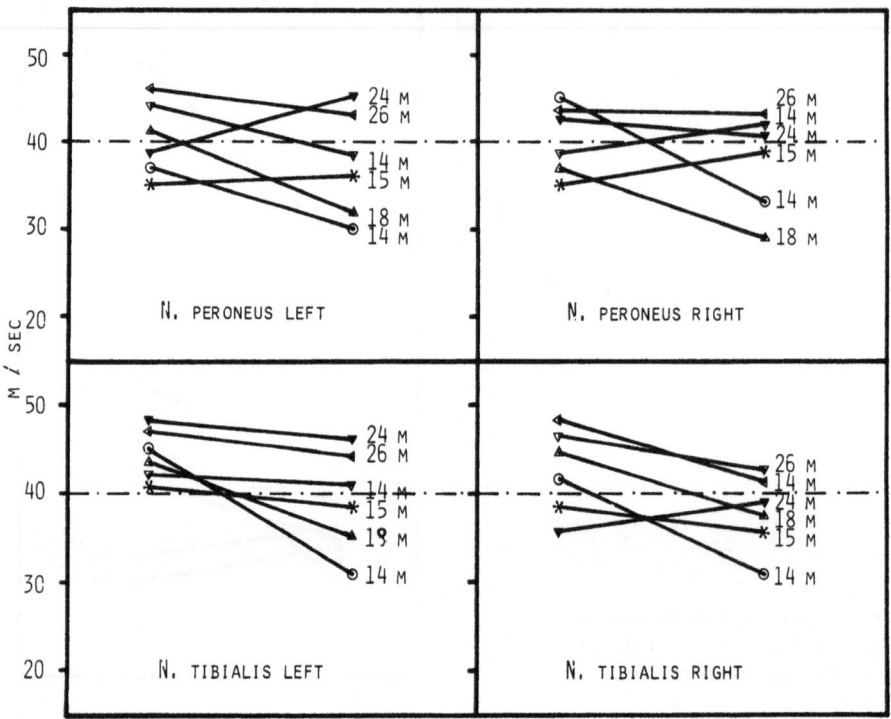

Fig. 7. Conduction velocities of the peroneal and tibial nerves at the beginning of hemofiltration and after various time periods. *M,* months

ripheral neuropathy. Considerable evidence based on studies in animals and in man suggests that parathyroid hormone is a very important agent also in this disorder [6]. However, data are also aviailable which indicate that dialysis patients with abnormal nerve conduction velocity values do not have higher parathyroid hormone levels than those with normal values [20]. Anyhow, in spite of the contradictory role of parathyroid hormone as a neurotoxin, there is evidence that hemofiltration patients have less severe neuropathy than patients treated by hemodialysis. Although the reports claiming a beneficial effect of hemofiltration have not tried to correlate the nerve conduction velocities with the prevailing parathyroid hormone concentration, it is tempting to speculate whether these changes could be the result of a decrease in the serum parathyroid hormone concentration. On the other hand, data are also available which fail to reveal any positive effect of hemofiltration on peripheral neuropathy [13]. Our own data did not show any positive influence of hemofiltration on nerve conduction velocity; however, it is important to note also that no deterioration could be detected after more than 2 years of hemofiltration (Fig. 7).

Summary

A critical evaluation of the available literature reveals that chronic hemofiltration is generally no more capable of ameliorating some of the typical uremic complications than hemodialysis [14, 20]. In the past it was erroneously assumed that hemofiltration might be superior to hemodialysis, as the membranes used in hemofiltration facilitate the removal of so-called middle and large molecules, which are sometimes considered more important uremic toxins than the so-called small molecules. One of the large molecules which has aroused great interest as a uremic toxin is parathyroid hormone, the serum concentration of which is frequently raised in chronic renal failure and which has been shown to be deleterious to many organs.

There is clear evidence that hemofiltration is capable of lowering the serum concentration of parathyroid hormone not only in acute treatment but presumably also during long-term treatment. Nevertheless, it is currently not possible to relate these findings to an improvement of certain uremic complications such as the lipid disorders, anemia, or neuropathy. Also, as far as renal osteodystrophy is concerned, no clear-cut positive effect could be demonstrated in patients treated by hemofiltration compared with those treated by hemodialysis. This failure does not necessary argue against parathyroid hormone as an important uremic toxin, but rather shows that 15 or 18 h of blood purification per week are not as efficient as the intact human kidney, which works for 24 h every day. Nevertheless, it has to be stated that no uremic complication has deteriorated in patients undergoing chronic hemofiltration treatment even for 5 and more years. This finding is very important for patients who are being transferred to hemofiltration for various other medical problems.

References

1. Baldamus CA, Schmidt H, Scheuermann EH, Werner E, Kaltwasser JP, Schoeppe W (1983) Iron (Fe) and aluminium (Al) removal in ESRD patients treated with deferrioxamine (DFO). Am J Kidney Dis (National Kidney Foundation) 2: (Abstract)
2. Fuchs C, Armstrong VW, Cremer P, Henning H, Wieland H, Quellhorst E, Seidel D (1982) An investigation of the lipoprotein profiles of patients on hemofiltration as compared to those on hemodialysis and intermittent peritoneal dialysis. Contrib Nephrol 32: 92–96
3. Henning HV, Balusek E (1977) Lipid metabolism in uremia: effect of regular hemofiltration and hemodialysis. J Dial 1: 595–605
4. von Herrath D, Asmus G, Hüfler M, Schaefer K (1978) Klinische Erfahrungen und Probleme bei chronischer Hämofiltration. Nieren Hochdruckkrankheiten 1: 16–20
5. Massry SG (1978) Is parathyroid hormone a uremic toxin? Nephron 19: 125–130
6. Massry SG (1983) The toxic effects of parathyroid hormone in uremia. Semin Nephrol 4: 306–328
7. Pierides AM, Giacherio D, Schniepp B, Burritt M (1982) Calcium, phosphorus and parathyroid hormone metabolism in chronic hemofiltration. Contrib Nephrol 32: 77–85
8. Potasman I, Better OS (1983) The role of secondary hyperparathyroidism in the anemia of chronic renal failure. Nephron 33: 229–231
9. Quellhorst E, Doht B, Schuenemann B (1977) Hemofiltration: treatment of renal failure by ultrafiltration and substitution. J Dial 1: 529–543
10. Quellhorst E, Rieger H, Doht B, Beckmann H, Jacob I, Kraft B, Mietzsch G, Scheler F (1976) Treatment of chronic uremia by an ultrafiltration kidney - first clinical experience. In: Robinson BHB, Vereerstraeter P, Hawkins JB (eds) Dialysis, transplantation, nephrology. Pitman Medical London, p 314
11. Quellhorst E, Schuenemann B (1978) Metabolic and hemodynamic aspects of hemofiltration. Dial Transplant 7: 369–372

12. Röckel A, Gilge U, Ohl B, Liewald A, Heidland A (1982) Elimination of low molecular weight proteins during hemofiltration. Contrib Nephrol 32: 40–45
13. Schaefer K, von Herrath D (1981) Einfluß der Hämofiltration auf Sekundärerkrankungen des Dialysepatienten. Medizintechnik 5: 129–132
14. Schaefer K, von Herrath D, Asmus G, Offermann G (1979) Is chronic hemofiltration better than chronic hemodialysis? Artif Organs 3 [Suppl]: 40–43
15. Schaefer K, von Herrath D, Gullberg CA, Asmus G, Hüfler M, Offermann G, Cremer H, Heuck CC, Ritz E (1978) Chronic hemofiltration. A critical evaluation of a new method for the treatment of blood. Artif Organs 2: 386–394
16. Schaefer K, von Herrath D, Hüfler M (1982) Hemofiltration 1982: a stocktaking. Contemp Dial 8: 14–18
17. Schaefer K, von Herrath D, Offermann G (1980) Long-term experiences with chronic hemofiltration. J Artif Organs 3: 219–220
18. Schaefer K, Offermann G, Asmus G, von Herrath D (1978) Das Verhalten von Calcium, Phosphat und Parathormon unter chronischer Haemofiltration. Nieren Hochdruckkrankheiten 1: 40–43
19. Schaefer K, Offermann G, von Herrath D, Asmus G, Hüfler M (1977) Parathyroid hormone, 25-OH-vitamin D, and digoxin levels in patients treated by chronic hemofiltration. J Dial 1: 619–630
20. Schaefer K, Offermann G, von Herrath D, Schröter R, Stölzel R, Arntz HR (1980) Failure to show a correlation between serum parathyroid hormone, nerve conduction velocity and serum lipids in hemodialysis patients. Clin Nephrol 2: 81–88
21. Schneider H, Streicher E (1978) Klinische Erfahrungen mit der intermittierenden Haemofiltrationsbehandlung. Nieren Hochdruckkrankheiten 2: 21
22. Schneider H, Streicher E, Schmidt-Gayk H, Bosnjakovic S (1979) Does long-term haemofiltration provoke hyperparathyroidism? Proc Eur Dial Transplant Assoc 15: 532–539
23. Schulz W, Baier E, Hümpfner A, Delling G (1982) Clinical problems of renal osteopathy in patients on hemofiltration. Contrib Nephrol 32: 86–91
24. Slatopolsky E, Lopez-Hilker S, Chan LY, Weaver M, Morrisey J, Martin K (1985) Parathyroid hormone secretion in renal failure. In: Norman AW, Schaefer K, Grigoleit HG, von Herrath D (eds) Vitamin D. A chemical, biochemical and clinical update. Walter de Gruyter, Berlin, p 844

Long-Term Survival

E. A. QUELLHORST

Table of Contents

After a long period of exclusive reliance on hemodialysis (HD) or peritoneal dialysis, the therapeutic options for patients with advanced renal insufficiency have expanded substantially since the beginning of the last decade. After a spell of enthusiasm and a phase of serious reservations regarding the contamination of commercially produced substitution fluid [1], hemofiltration (HF) has found – at least in Europe and Japan – its place among other methods of blood purification.

With hemodialysis serving as the standard reference procedure, other techniques will be accepted only if they offer advantages in terms of patient well-being and survival, or reduction of treatment costs. With an increasing scope of application (advances in the regeneration of substitution fluid [2] or its production from tap water and concentrate [3]), as well as the reuse of filters, HF will undoubtedly reduce the treatment costs. However, an extensive analysis of survival rates, morbidity, and medical and technical complications has not been made. Even though the number of patients is still small and the period of observation relatively short, these parameters can be compared with those which characterize HD, and intermittent or continuous ambulatory peritoneal dialysis (CAPD), employed in the same centers under identical conditions.

Methods

Since 1972 HF has been performed in the postdilution mode. A transmembranous pressure (TMP) of 300–400 mmHg produces 80–100 ml filtrate per minute on average [4]. Three treatment procedures are performed per week in patients with chronic renal failure (CRF). Whereas during the first 2 years 20 liters of fluid were exchanged per treatment procedure, later on the amount of dilution fluid was individualized. According to our experience the exchange of one third of the body weight per treatment leads to pretreatment BUN and serum creatinine levels similar to those of patients on intermittent HD. The dilution fluid had the following composition: Na^+ 142, Ca^{2+} 2.0, Mg^{2+} 0.75, Cl^- 103, and lactate 44.5 mmol/l.

Intermittent HD was performed three times weekly for 5–6 h, using capillary or plate Cuprophan dialyzers with an exchange area of 1.0–1.2 m^2.

Intermittent peritoneal dialysis (IPD) was done for 12 h three times weekly, with the fluid volume amounting to 80–100 liters per treatment. CAPD was practised as originally described by POPOVICH et al. [5] and OREOPOULOS et al. [6], exchanging 2 liters of dialysis fluid four times daily. Only those patients who were treated for at least 6 months with a particular modality were considered for statistical evaluation. Survival rates were calculated according to the recommendations of CUTLER and EDERER [7].

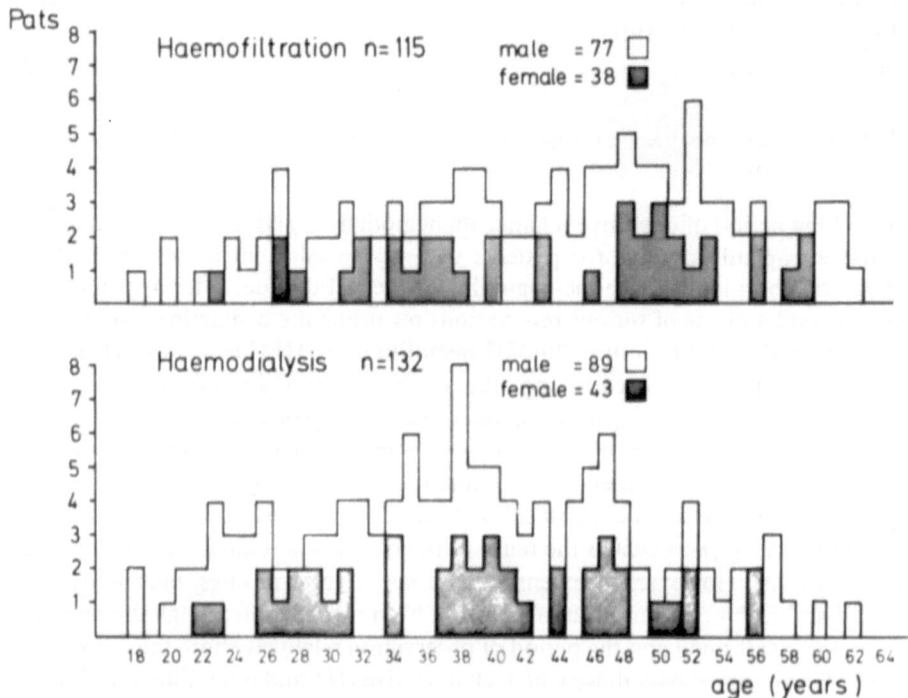

Fig. 1. Age and sex distribution of 247 patients with chronic renal insufficiency

Morbidity and Mortality in a "Standard" Population of Patients with Chronic Renal Insufficiency

Patients

A comparative study in which patients were randomly admitted to HD or HF was conducted [8] from 1974 to 1978. "Poor risk" patients with complications such as diabetes mellitus, malignant tumors, and systemic or severe cerebrovascular or cardiovascular diseases, as well as patients younger than 15 years and older than 60 years of age, were excluded. This group (Fig. 1) comprises 115 HF patients (mean age, 43 years) and 132 HD patients (mean age, 38.5 years). The diagnosis of the underlying renal disease is depicted in Table 1.

Results

The migration of patients between HD and HF is shown in Table 2. The main reasons for withdrawal from HF were renal transplantation and fistula complications; whereas, overhydration, hypotension, and hypertension were the main factors necessitating transfer to HF.

Table 3 lists the complications observed during 33 112 HF and 41 510 HD procedures. Whereas the incidence of hypertensive and febrile reactions did not differ significantly between the two modalities, hypotensive episodes occurred much more frequently in HD than in HF. Hypotensive episodes were defined as a drop in systolic blood pressure by more than 30 mmHg within 10 min, accompanied by clinical symptoms. Hypertensive episodes were defined as an increase in systolic blood pressure by more than 30 mmHg within 10 min, again accompanied by clinical symptoms. Febrile reactions were defined as an increase in body temperature by more than 1.5 °C in the course of treatment. In spite of a considerably more rapid

Table 1. Survey of patient number, mean age, and treatment duration in the different groups of "low risk" patients

	Group I		Group II	
Observation period	1974–1978		1978–1982	
Number of patients	247		125	
Treatment modality	HF	HD	HF	CAPD
No. of patients	115	132	57	68
Male	77	89	41	50
Female	38	43	16	18
Mean age (years)	43.0	38.5	49.5	41.5
Patient months	5196	6690	1428	1464

HF, hemofiltration; HD, hemodialysis; CAPD, continuous ambulatory peritoneal dialysis

Table 2. Causes of patient migration between hemofiltration and hemodialysis

	From HF to HD	From HD to HF
Transplantation	3	2
Fistula complications	3	–
Hyperkalemia	2	–
Overhydration	–	5
Hypotension	–	3
Hypertension	1	3
Uremia	1	–
Technical reasons	1	–
	11	13

Table 3. Intratreatment complications of hemofiltration and hemodialysis

	Hemofiltration		Hemodialysis	
No. of treatment procedures	33 112		41 510	
	Number	%	Number	%
Muscle cramps	1125	3.4	2360	5.7
Hypotensive reactions	1035	3.1	4152	10.0
Hypertensive reactions	950	2.9	1270	3.1
Fever reactions	84	0.3	112	0.3
Fluid removal (ml/h)	680 ± 210		395 ± 122	

fluid removal in HF than in HD, the incidence of muscle cramps was remarkably higher in HD than in HF.

An objective index of morbidity is provided by the number of days spent in hospital for each treatment group. Figure 2 outlines the impact of the most common complications, expressed in hospital days per month of treatment, excluding those hospital days due to fistula creation or transplantation. Infections were the main reasons for hospital admission in both subgroups. Hypotension, hypertension, and cerebrovascular disease prevailed in HD; whereas, fistula problems, cardiac infarction, and malignancies were more common in HF. On the average, HF patients spent 1.3 ± 1.2 and HD patients 1.8 ± 0.9 days per month in hospital, the difference being statistically significant. Death eliminated 18 patients from the HD and 16 patients from the HF subgroup. Myocardial infarction and septicemia were observed in both subgroups, but cardiac insufficiency, the cause of death in HD therapy occurred in HF only in one case (Table 4).

The overall survival rate was the same for both subgroups, amounting to about 90% after 3 years and about 80% after 6 years (Fig. 3). No statistically significant difference could be demonstrated between HD and HF patients except for year 8, in which the survival rate was significantly lower for HD than for HF. Survival rates of the French dialysis registry "Diaphane" [9] and the European Dialysis and Trans-

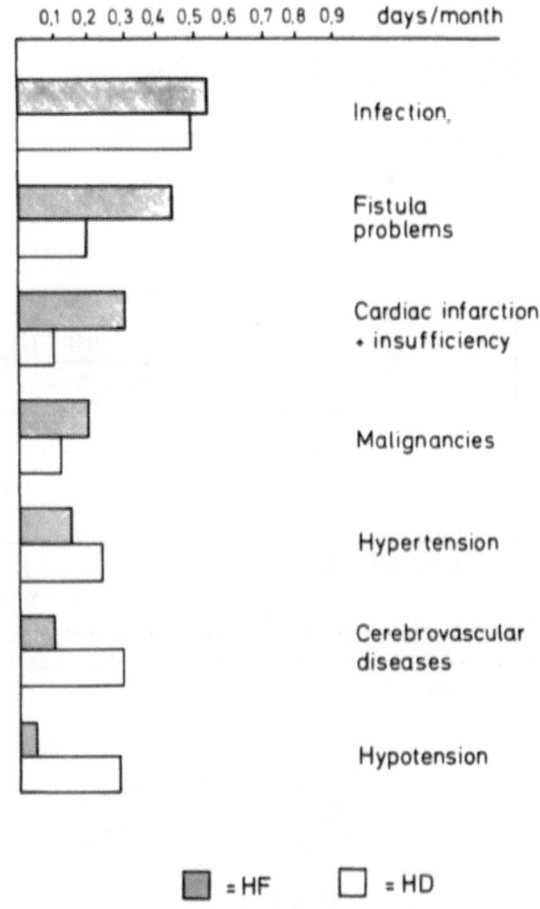

Fig. 2. Days of hospitalization per treatment month in patients with chronic renal insufficiency ("low risk group")

Table 4. Causes of death in 16 hemofiltration and 18 hemodialysis patients (8)

	Hemofiltration		Hemodialysis	
	Early	Late	Early	Late
Cerebrovascular	2	1	1	2
Myocardial infarction	2	1	2	1
Malignancy	2	–	1	1
Pneumonia	2	1	1	–
Cardiac insufficiency	1	–	1	4
Septicemia	1	–	2	–
Tuberculosis	1	–	1	–
Pancreatitis	1	1	1	–
	12	4	10	8

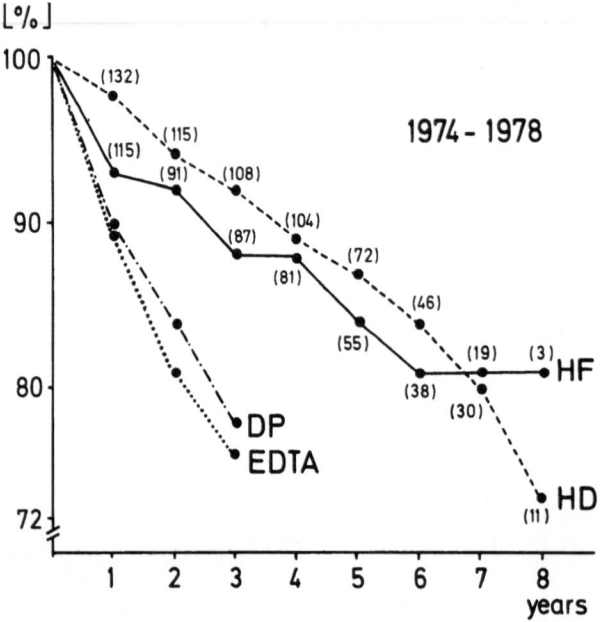

Fig. 3. Survival rates of patients starting regular hemofiltration or hemodialysis treatment between 1974 and 1978 ("standard dialysis population"); data of EDTA registry and Diaphane (DP) shown for comparison

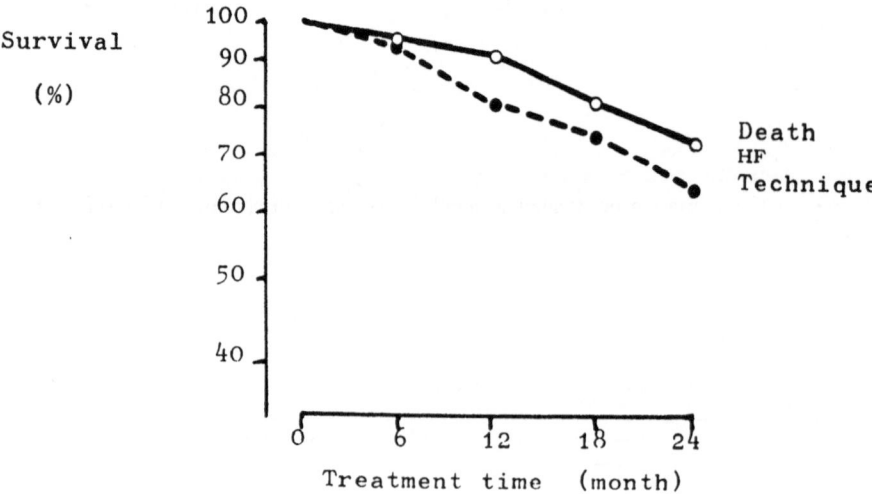

Fig. 4. Patients and techniques survival data, according to BALDAMUS [11]

plant Association (EDTA) registry for patients aged 40 to 45 years [10] are shown for comparison.

"Technique" survival data have been calculated by BALDAMUS [11] based on 56 patients with chronic renal insufficiency. "Technique survival" was defined as time on HF treatment, transplantation being excluded as reason for abandonment of HF (Fig. 4).

Morbidity and Mortality in "Poor Risk" Patients

Patients

Diabetic Nephropathy

Regular postdilution HF was performed in 178 patients with chronic renal insufficiency, 28 of whom were suffering from type I diabetic nephropathy. Data of these patients were compared with those of 168 patients on intermittent HD (32 diabetic nephropathy), 72 patients on CAPD (16 diabetic nephropathy), and 82 patients on IPD treatment (32 diabetic nephropathy). Details concerning mode of treatment, sex distribution, mean age, and duration of treatment in the diabetic group in relation to the whole group of patients on kidney replacement therapy are depicted in Table 5. Table 6 provides information about the development of diabetes mellitus. Mean age at diabetes onset was between 21 and 29 years; whereas, replacement therapy had to be started at a mean age of 31.4 to 38.5 years.

Table 5. Treatment modality, sex, and age distribution as well as duration of treatment in 99 patients with end-stage renal failure due to diabetic nephropathy and in 500 patients with end-stage renal failure of various origin

	All patients				Diabetics			
	HD	HF	CAPD	IPD	HD	HF	CAPD	IPD
No. of patients	168	178	72	82	32	28	16	23
Male	92	104	41	21	17	16	10	14
Female	76	74	31	61	15	12	6	9
Mean age (years)	39.2	43.5	42.4	55.6	41.4	32.5	34.6	38.6
Duration of treatment (Patient months)	4202	4628	1944	1804	752	652	421	572

Table 6. Mean age at diabetes onset and at the start of renal replacement therapy in 99 patients with end-stage renal failure due to diabetic nephropathy

	HD	HF	CAPD	IPD
No. of patients	32	28	16	23
Mean age at diabetes onset (years)	23 (17–26)	21 (12–34)	24 (14–36)	29 (12–48)
Mean age at start of replacement therapy (years)	38.5 (22–41)	31.4 (17–44)	32.5 (19–39)	36.1 (16–52)

Patients Older than 60 Years

Table 7 shows data characterizing mode of treatment, sex distribution, mean age at the start of treatment, and duration of treatment for patients older than 60 years of

Table 7. Treatment modality, sex, and age distribution as well as duration of treatment in 113 patients with end-stage renal failure, older than 60 years of age and in 500 patients with end-stage renal failure of various origin

	All patients				Patients > 60 years			
	HD	HF	CAPD	IPD	HD	HF	CAPD	IPD
No. of patients	168	178	72	82	32	41	18	22
Male	92	104	41	21	12	22	9	9
Female	76	74	31	61	20	19	9	13
Mean age (years)	39.2	43.5	42.4	55.6	64.1	66.4	63.5	66.2
Duration of treatment (Patient months)	4202	4628	1944	1804	742	1224	452	541

age in comparison with the whole group of dialysis patients. It has to be stressed that patients with the highest age are concentrated in the IPD group.

Results

Diabetic Nephropathy

The period of hospitalization per year of treatment, shown in Fig. 5 for diabetic patients treated by intermittent HD or HF, may serve as a rough parameter for the morbidity to these groups. Whereas infections, fistula problems, and gangrene gave reason for equally frequent hospitalization in both subgroups, malignancies, hypertension, hypotension, and myocardial insufficiency prevailed in the HD subgroup. On average, HD patients with diabetic nephropathy remained in hospital for 13.5 days and HF patients for 9.2 days per year, the difference being statistically significant at a level of $P < 0.005$.

Figure 6 shows the survival rates for the diabetic group in relation to the whole group of dialysis patients. In the diabetic patients, the 5-year survival rate amounts to 70% in the HF, 56% in the CAPD, but only 34% in the HD and 29% in the IPD subgroups. After 2 years of treatment during which the survival rates as related to the methods of treatment do not differ significantly, there is a steep decrease for IPD and HD. On the other hand, HF, HD, and CAPD show almost identical results in the whole group of dialysis patients, IPD being the least successful. Causes of death are listed in Table 8, demonstrating the presumed prevalence of cardiovascular complications.

Patients Older than 60 Years

For the group of patients above 60 years of age the rate of hospitalization, expressed in days per year of treatment, is shown in Fig. 7. Differences in favor of HF can only be detected for cerebrovascular diseases, myocardial infarction, and hypotension.

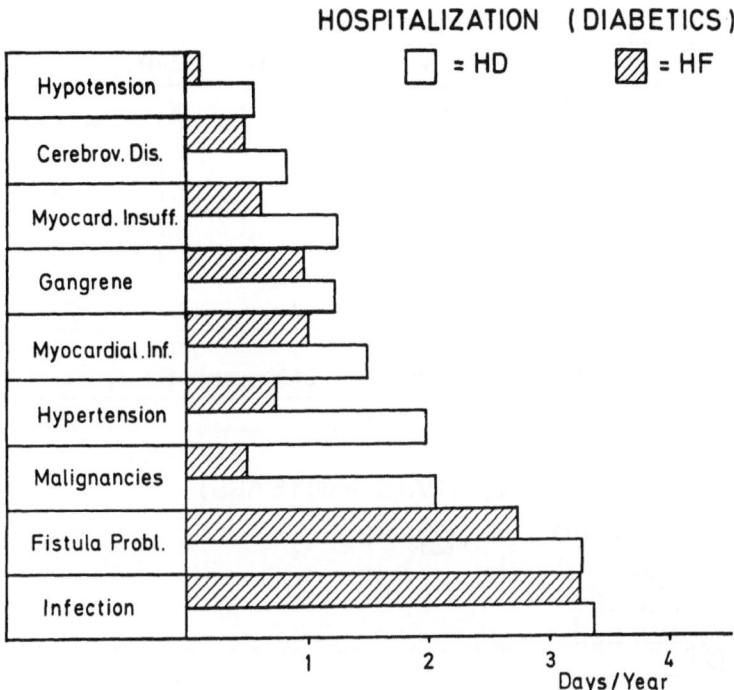

Fig. 5. Hospitalization in patients with diabetic nephropathy (HD, hemodialysis; HF, hemofiltration)

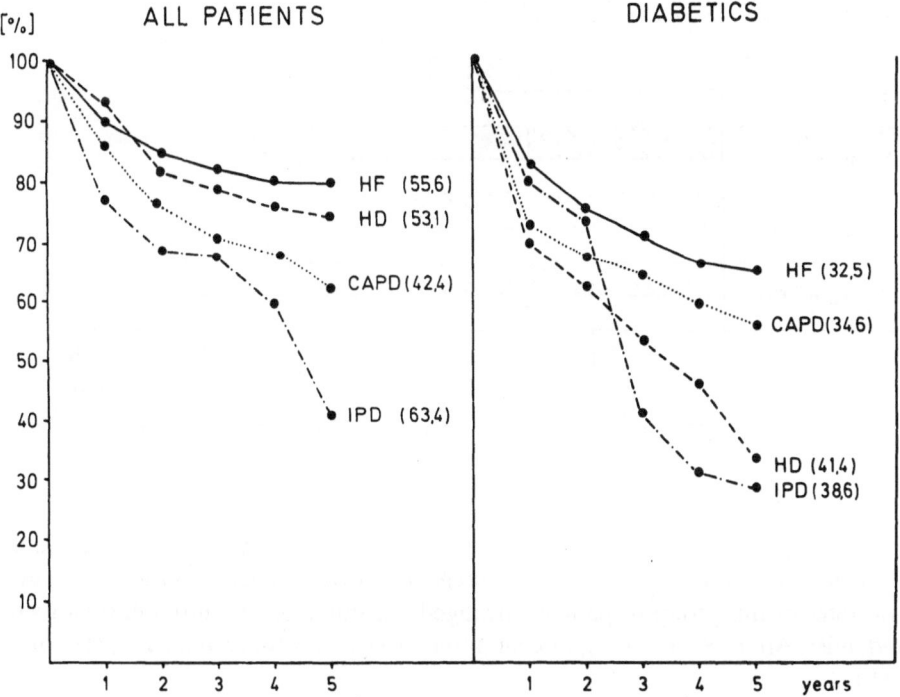

Fig. 6. Survival rates of patients with diabetic nephropathy depending on treatment modalities in comparison with survival rates of the whole group of dialysis patients; mean age in parentheses

Table 8. Causes of death in 31 patients with end-stage renal failure due to diabetic nephropathy

	HD	HF	CAPD	IPD
n =	32	28	16	23
Myocardial infarction	2	1	1	–
Myocardial insufficiency	2	1	1	1
Encephalomalacia	1	1	–	1
Pneumonia	1	1	–	2
Peritonitis	–	–	1	2
Gangrene	1	1	–	1
Unknown	4	–	2	3
Σ	11	5	5	10
%	34.4	17.9	31.3	43.5

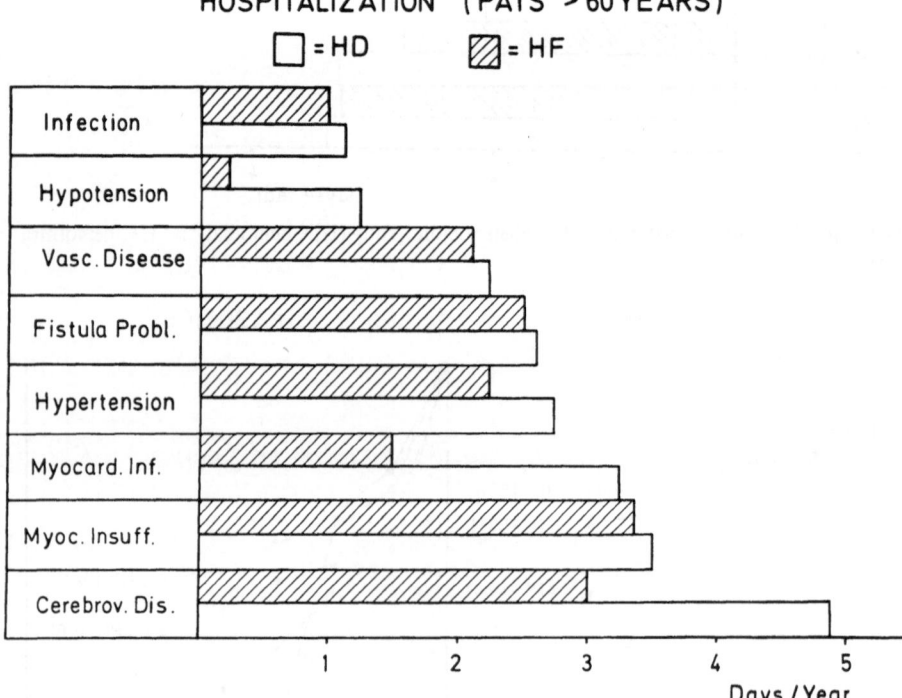

Fig. 7. Hospitalization in patients older than 60 years of age (HD, hemodialysis; HF, hemofiltration)

In this group, HD patients were hospitalized for 18 days per year of treatment and HF patients for 11.5 days per year on average. Figure 8 demonstrates the 5-year survival rates of this group of patients arranged according to the different treatment modalities. After 2 years, no significant difference can be observed for HF, HD, and CAPD.

However, the survival rate after 5 years demonstrates a significantly better outcome in the HF subgroup (75%) than in the HD and CAPD subgroups (60% and

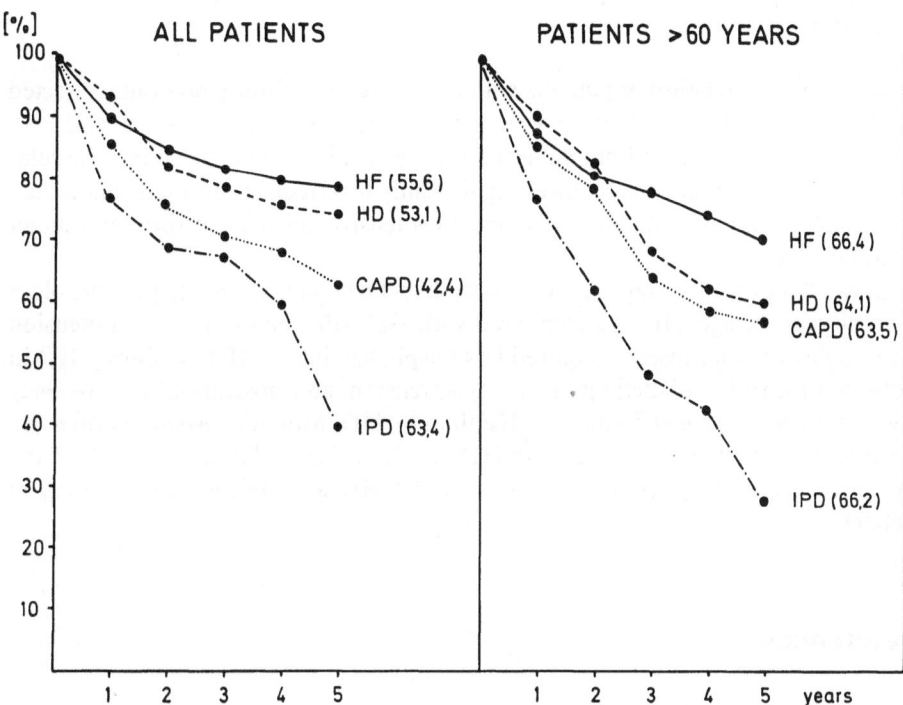

Fig. 8. Survival rates of patients older than 60 years of age with end-stage renal failure depending on treatment modalities in comparison with survival rates of the whole group of dialysis patients; mean age in parentheses

Table 9. Causes of death in 35 patients older than 60 years of age suffering end-stage renal failure

	HD	HF	CAPD	IPD
n=	32	41	18	22
Myocardial insufficiency	3	2	1	1
Myocardial infarction	1	1	–	2
Encephalomalacia	1	1	1	2
Malignancy	1	1	–	1
Pneumonia	1	1	1	2
Peritonitis	–	–	2	1
Unknown	4	1	2	1
Σ	11	7	7	10
%	34.4	17.1	38.9	45.5

57%, respectively). Again, IPD exhibits the poorest result with 60% at the 2-year and 27% at the 5-year level. It should be pointed out that for CAPD there is no difference in the survival rates when patients older than 60 years are compared with the whole group of dialysis patients. Among causes of death (Table 9), myocardial insufficiency and infarction predominate in all subgroups followed by encephalopathy. Sudden death, cause unknown, was registered in 8 of 35 cases (22.9%).

Summary

In a low-risk population of patients with end-stage renal failure randomly selected for intermittent HD or HF, the 5-year survival rate was the same for HF and HD. Main causes of death in both subgroups were cardiovascular or cerebrovascular complications. HF patients required significantly less frequent hospitalization than HD patients and exhibited less frequent hypotensive episodes in spite of a larger fluid removal.

In two "poor risk" groups, patients with diabetic nephropathy and patients older than 60 years of age, HF was compared with HD, IPD, and CAPD. Hypotension and cerebrovascular disease required less hospitalization in HF than during HD in both groups. In the diabetic patients, hypertension, and myocardial insufficiency were influenced more efficiently by HF than by HD. Mortality especially after the third year of treatment was higher in HD and IPD than in HF and CAPD for the diabetic group and higher in IPD than in CAPD, HD, and HF for the group of aged patients.

References

1. Frei U, Koch KM (1982) Fever and schock during haemofiltration. In: Baldamus CA, Koch KM, Schoeppe W (eds) Biocompatibility in Haemodialysis. Contrib Nephrol 36: 107-114
2. Schuenemann B, Quellhorst E, Kaiser H, Richter G, Mundt K, Weidlich E, Loeffler G, Zacha-riae M, Schunk O (1982) Regeneration of filtrate and dialysis fluid by electro-oxidation and ab-sorption. Trans Am Soc Artif Intern Organs 28: 49-53
3. Henderson LW, Beans E (1978) Successful production of sterile pyrogen-free electrolyte solu-tion by ultrafiltration. Kidney Int 14: 522-525
4. Quellhorst E, Schuenemann B, Doht B (1978) Haemofiltration – a new method for the treatment of chronic renal insufficiency. In: Frost T (ed) Technical aspects of renal dialysis. Pitman Medi-cal, London, pp 96-105
5. Popovich RP, Moncrief JW, Nolph KD, Ghods AJ, Twardowski ZJ, Pyle WK (1978) Continu-ous ambulatory peritoneal dialysis. Ann Intern Med 88: 449-455
6. Oreopoulos DG, Robson M, Izah S, Clayton S, de Veber GA (1978) A simple and safe technique for continuous ambulatory peritoneal dialysis (CAPD). Trans Am Soc Artif Intern Organs 24: 484-489
7. Cutler SJ, Ederer F (1958) Maximum utilization of the life table method in analyzing survival. J Chronic Dis 8: 699-712
8. Quellhorst E, Schuenemann B, Hildebrand U (1983) Morbidity and mortality in long-term hemo-filtration. ASAIO J 6: 185-191
9. Degoulet P, Reach I, Rozenbaum W, Aime F, Devries C, Berger C, Rojas P, Jacobs C, Lé-grain M (1979) Programme dialyse - informatique. VI: Survie et facteurs de risque. J Urol Néphrol 12: 909-916
10. Broyer M, Brunner FP, Brynger H, Donckerwolcke RA, Jacobs C, Kramer P, Selwood NH, Wing AJ (1982) Combined report on regular dialysis and transplantation in Europe, XI, 1980. Proc Eur Dial Transplant Assoc 19: 2-59
11. Baldamus CA (1983) Clinical value and technical feasibility of long-term hemofiltration. ASAIO J 6: 192-196

Continuous Arteriovenous Hemofiltration

J. P. BOSCH

Table of Contents

Definition

Continuous arteriovenous hemofiltration (CAVH) is an extracorporeal process in which fluid, electrolytes, small and medium-sized molecules (molecular weight less than 50000) are removed from the patient by ultrafiltration over an extended period (hours or days). Simultaneously, the blood volume is reconstituted by the administration of a fluid with an electrolyte composition similar to that of normal plasma. A small filter with a membrane highly permeable to water is used in this procedure. The patient's arterial-to-venous pressure gradient is usually sufficient to move the blood through the extracorporeal circuit.

In situations where neither hemodialysis nor peritoneal dialysis is possible, CAVH can be used as an effective alternative treatment. This technique is simple, can be initiated rapidly, and does not require complicated equipment or highly trained personnel.

Development

The clinical application of ultrafiltration for fluid removal dates from the advent of dialysis therapy. A modification of the standard hemodialysis circuit was proposed in 1974 by SILVERSTEIN and colleagues [1]. In their technique, they isolated ultrafiltration from the diffusive process by adding a filter for ultrafiltration to the standard dialysis apparatus. These authors also suggested the use of a separate system (filter, blood lines, and a pump) for ultrafiltration with patients with an intractable fluid overload. A technique based solely on the principle of convective solute transport (ultrafiltration) for the treatment of renal failure was proposed by HENDERSON and coworkers [2]. In this procedure, called hemofiltration, an ultrafiltrate of the plasma was produced by hydrostatic pressure exerted across a semipermeable membrane. A substitution fluid with a composition similar to that of the extracellular fluid was used to restore the blood volume. Hemofiltration was proposed as an alternative to hemodialysis.

This new methodology stimulated the development of new membranes and filters and, most importantly, opened the road to the understanding of the clinical consequences of in vivo ultrafiltration. In Germany, KRAMER et al. [3], using a filter originally designed for hemofiltration, eliminated the need for a blood pump by directly connecting an Amicon Dialfilter 20 (Amicon Corporation, Danvers, Mas-

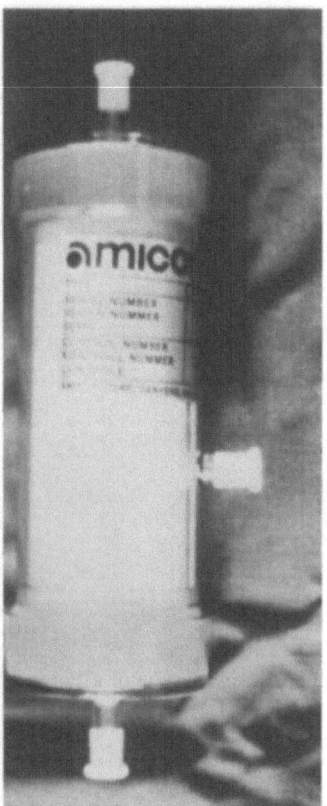

Fig. 1. Amicon 20 hemofilter

sachusetts; Fig. 1) to the femoral artery and vein. CAVH was intended to be a continuous form of therapy for renal failure as opposed to the intermittent nature of hemodialysis or hemofiltration. CAVH has been used by several investigators as the sole treatment for patients with acute renal failure or fluid overload [4, 5].

Equipment

Membrane

The first membranes used for ultrafiltration were made from the viscose cellulose employed in the manufacture of sausages. In the past decade improvements in membrane technology, spurred on by the clinical introduction of hemodialysis, have made possible greater ultrafiltration rates. The maximal rate of ultrafiltration in these earlier dialysis membranes was 10 ml/min/m². While these ultrafiltration rates were sufficient to remove fluid from patients on maintenance hemodialysis,

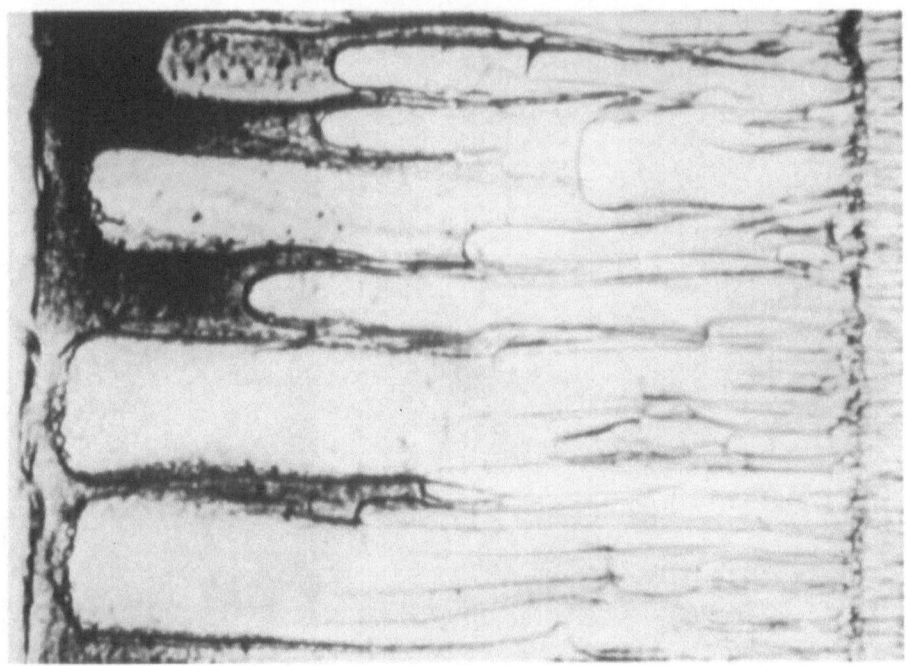

Fig. 2. Cross section of a Polysulphon membrane. Relationship between skin and stroma can be seen

they were inadequate for removal of significant quantities of solutes by ultrafiltration alone. The introduction of asymmetrical membranes made possible greater ultrafiltration rates (60 or more $ml/min/m^2$). These advances stimulated the development of hemofiltration and CAVH. Asymmetrical membranes used in CAVH are known by different names according to composition and manufacturer: Polysulphon-Amicon (Fig. 2), polyamide-Gambro, polyacrylonitrile-Hospal, etc. [6].

Filter

A small hollow-fiber filter with an asymmetrical membrane (Fig. 3) is most commonly used in CAVH. The inlet and outlet ports of the filter are connected to the blood lines. The ultrafiltrate is collected in a graduated bag linked to the ultrafiltrate port by a line. Several filters for CAVH are currently available. They vary as to membrane (Polysulphon, polyamide, etc.), number, and length of fibers used. A parallel-plate device with a polyacrylonitrile membrane is also commercially available. A pediatric filter has recently been introduced [7].

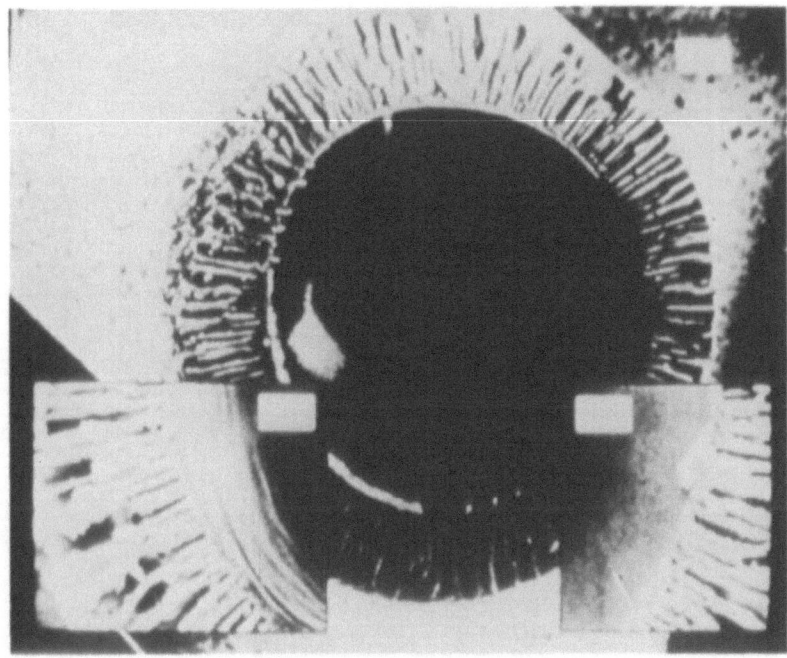

Fig. 3. Polysulphon hollow fiber. The complex nature of a typical asymmetrical membrane can be seen. The skin, or the portion of the membrane in contact with the blood, is smooth and thin. The stroma, or outer portion of the membrane, gives support and determines the water permeability of the membrane

Extracorporeal Circuit

The extracorporeal system is illustrated in Fig. 4. The arterial and venous lines are both 75 cm or less in length, with an internal diameter of 0.317 cm. Standard shortened hemodialysis lines or a custom-designed set can be used. Heparin is administered via the sleeve on the arterial line. The substitution fluid can be given systemically or through the sleeve in the venous line. The ultrafiltrate line, which connects the ultrafiltrate port and the collection bag, must be 40–60 cm long, with an internal diameter of 0.474 cm. In both blood lines, sampling ports are required.

Access

No special access is necessary for CAVH; percutaneous cannulation of an artery and a vein is adequate for access to the circulatory system. When a Scribner shunt is used, the arterial and venous branches of the shunt are connected to the arterial and venous line. In arteriovenous fistula access, the arterial and venous ends of the fistula are percutaneously cannulated with standard hemodialysis needles

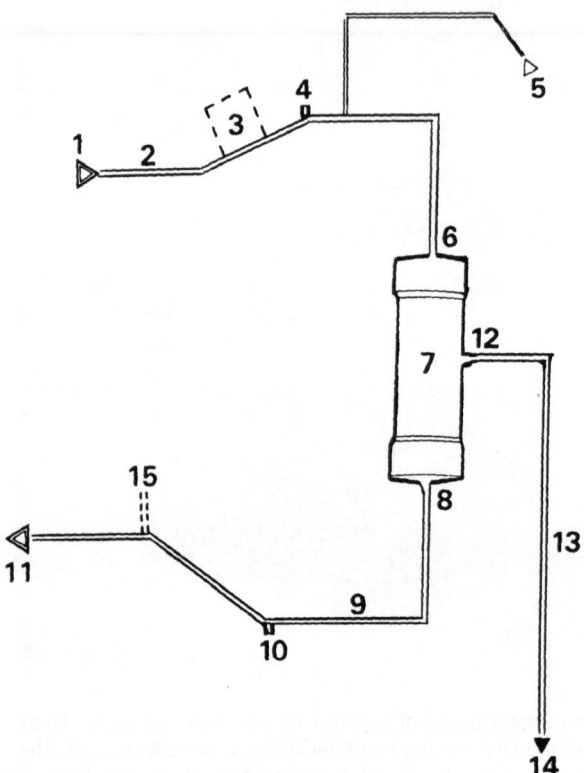

Fig.4. CAVH system. *1*, arterial access; *2*, arterial line; *3* optional blood pump segment; *4*, inlet sampling port; *5* heparin line; *6* inlet port; *7*, filter; *8*, outlet port; *9*, venous line; *10*, outlet sampling port; *11*, venous access; *12*, ultrafiltrate port; *13*, ultrafiltrate line; *14*, ultrafiltrate collection bag; *15*, substitution fluid line

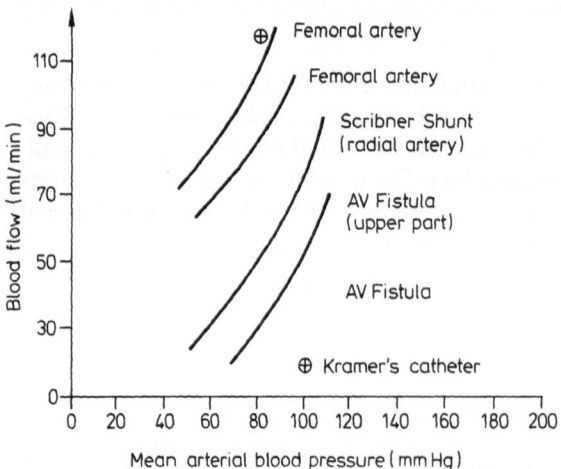

Fig.5. Effect of mean arterial pressure on blood flow rate with different types of vascular access (no pump). In these studies the length and internal diameter of blood lines are similiar. Cannulation was done via the femoral artery, with a 14-gauge catheter (indicated by *circled asterisk*) or a 16-gauge catheter; by radial-artery Scribner shunt; or by arteriovenous *(AV)* fistula in the lower arm. (C. Ronco)

(14–16 gauge). Femoral dialysis catheters (16 gauge) can be used to cannulate the femoral artery and vein, according to the Seldinger technique. In an arteriovenous vascular graft, arterial access is obtained by percutaneous cannulation of the graft with standard dialysis needles. The venous line must be attached to a peripheral vein.

The blood flow rate through the extracorporeal circuit is determined in part by the mean arterial blood pressure, the site and type of vascular access, and the internal diameter of the device used in arterial cannulation (Fig. 5). When the mean arterial pressure is less than 50 mmHg, the Scribner shunt and the arteriovenous fistula are inadequate. A femoral or other type of central catheter must be used.

Determinants of Ultrafiltration Rate

In a given filter for CAVH, the determinant factors of the ultrafiltration rate are

a) the hydrostatic pressure inside the filter, and
b) the oncotic pressure exerted by the plasma proteins [8].

The blood flow through the filter is a critical component in the production of the ultrafiltrate. It determines the hydrostatic pressure and influences the rise in the oncotic pressure inside the filter.

Blood Flow Rate

Measurement

To measure the blood flow through the extracorporeal system, blood samples are obtained from a sampling sleeve along the arterial (inlet) and venous (outlet) lines. Simultaneously, the ultrafiltration rate, Q_{Uf}, measured in milliliters per minute from timed volumetric collections, is recorded. Hematocrits are measured and the blood flow rate (milliliters per minute) at the inlet, Q_{Bi}, is calculated using the equation:

$$Q_{Bi} = \frac{(Q_{Uf} \times HCT \text{ outlet})}{(Hct \text{ inlet} - Hct \text{ outlet})}$$

where Hct is hematocrit.

Plasma flow (Q_{Pi}) in milliliters per minute is calculated from the equation:

$$Q_{Pi} = Q_{Bi} - \text{erythrocyte mass}$$

where erythrocyte mass (ml/min) at the inlet = $(Q_{Bi} \times Hct \text{ inlet})/100$.

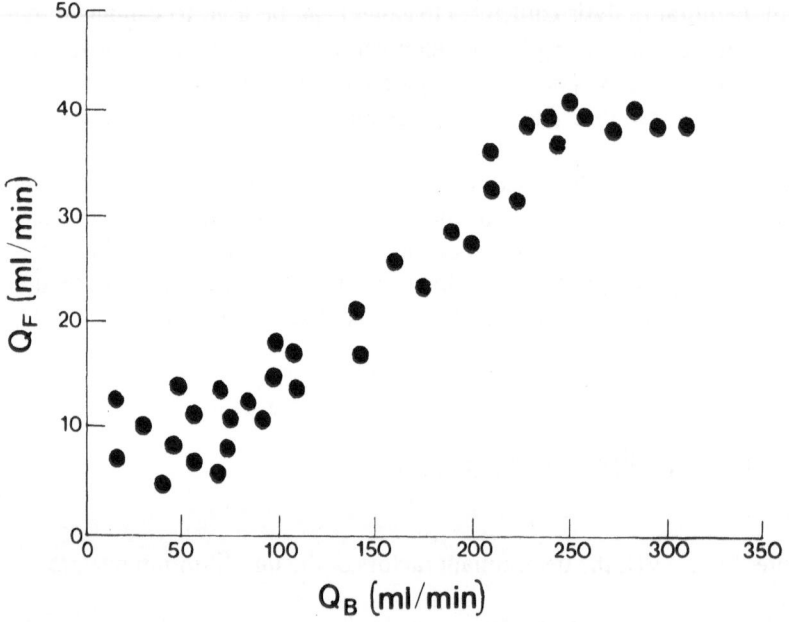

Fig. 6. Effect of blood flow rate (Q_B) on ultrafiltration rate (Q_F), with Amicon 20. Blood flow rates above 90 ml/min were obtained with the use of a blood pump

Effect

The blood is moved through the extracorporeal circuit by the patient's systemic arterial pressure, and the blood flow rate is dependent upon the mean arterial pressure. As pointed out earlier, other factors are also important - for example, size of the arterial cannulation, length of the blood lines, etc. - since they determine a drop in the pressure reaching the filter. In Fig. 6 the relationship between blood flow rate and ultrafiltration rate is depicted (Amicon 20). At blood flow rates below 90 or above 250 ml/min, the ultrafiltration rate was not flow-dependent. Between these two extremes, there was a direct relationship between blood flow and ultrafiltration rate. This effect of blood flow rate was explained in part by the pressure changes generated in the filter by differences in blood flow rate (Fig. 7). Augmentation of the blood flow rate above 90 ml/min caused a proportional increase in the filter pressure and, therefore, higher filtration rates. Blood flow rates less than 90 ml/min had no appreciable effect on the pressure in the filter or on the ultrafiltration rate. At flow rates greater than 250 ml/min, increases in the filter pressure also had no effect on the ultrafiltration rate. At this rate of blood flow the ultrafiltrate rate may have been membrane surface area limited.

At low blood flow rates, the hematocrit of the incoming blood becomes an important factor in determining the ultrafiltration rate. At these low flow rates, the higher the hematocrit, the lower the plasma flow rate, and hence the greater the rise in plasma protein concentration for a constant ultrafiltration rate. A plasma flow of 20-90 ml/min is sufficient to produce an ultrafiltrate [8].

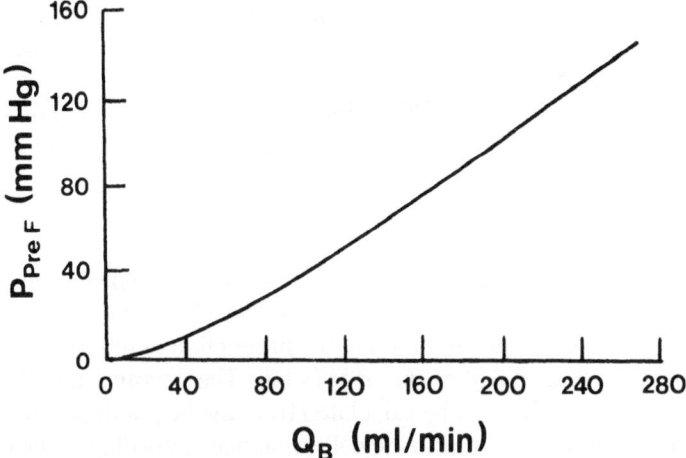

Fig. 7. Effect of blood flow rate (Q_B) on prefilter pressure (inlet pressure; P_{PREF}), with Amicon 20. An occlusive blood pump was used in these experiments to maintain the blood flow rate

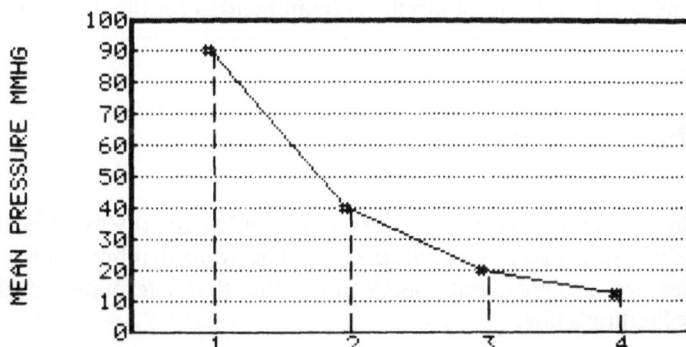

Fig. 8. Pressure drop in the CAVH circuit: pressure measurements in a typical case (Amicon 20). *1*, artery; *2*, prefilter; *3*, postfilter; *4*, vein

Hydrostatic Pressure

An ultrafiltrate is produced in the filter by a transmembrane pressure or net pressure gradient. The hydrostatic pressure favors the movement of water across the membrane. The oncotic pressure, generated by plasma proteins, tends to retain the fluid on the blood side of the membrane.

The hydrostatic pressure within the filter has two components: the arterial blood pressure and, on the ultrafiltrate side of the membrane, the negative pressure. The arterial pressure inside the filter is much lower than the patient's systemic blood pressure. Factors responsible for this pressure drop in the circuit (Fig. 8) are:

1) The type of access and the dimensions of the arterial cannulas. (The smaller the internal diameter of the needle, the greater the resistance)

2) The blood circuit: length and internal diameter of the blood lines. (The greater the length and the smaller the internal diameter of the arterial line, the greater the pressure drop.)
3) The resistance of the filter, which is determined by the filter design (number and length of the fibers), the filtration fraction obtained, and the viscosity of the blood.
4) The patient's venous pressure.

The negative pressure on the ultrafiltrate side of the membrane favors formation of the ultrafiltrate and is generated by the weight of the fluid column. This negative pressure is critically important in the production of ultrafiltrate, because the arterial pressure inside the filter can be very low. The pressure in the ultrafiltrate compartment, P_f, (mmHg) can be calculated from the height in centimeters of the line linking the ultrafiltrate port to the collection bag, according to the equation:

$$P_f = \text{height} \times 0.74 \, \text{mmHg}$$

If the filter is above the collection bag, the pressure in the ultrafiltrate compartment is negative. A length of 40 cm is recommended for the ultrafiltrate line.

Oncotic Pressure

The oncotic pressure at the inlet and outlet of the filter can be calculated from the measured protein concentration [8]. The transmembrane pressure (TMP) or net pressure gradient in millimeters of mercury that determines ultrafiltration is defined by Starling's law:

$$\text{TMP} = \text{hydrostatic pressure} - \text{oncotic pressure}$$

where hydrostatic pressure $= (\text{pre-} + \text{postfilter pressure})/2 + P_f$, and oncotic pressure is the oncotic pressure at the outlet.

Filtration Pressure

The oncotic pressure exerted by the plasma proteins inside the filter opposes the hydrostatic pressure. As plasma water is lost from the blood, the plasma protein concentration and, therefore, the oncotic pressure, rise. At some point along the filter, oncotic pressure equals the hydrostatic pressure, causing ultrafiltration to cease (Fig. 9). This equilibrium of pressures is always achieved in CAVH when an Amicon 20 or similar filter is used, and occurs because of the low hydrostatic pressure inside the filter and the low blood flow through the system. When a blood pump is used, and blood flow and hydrostatic pressure rise, pressure disequilibrium is achieved. The hydrostatic pressure in this case is greater than the oncotic pressure.

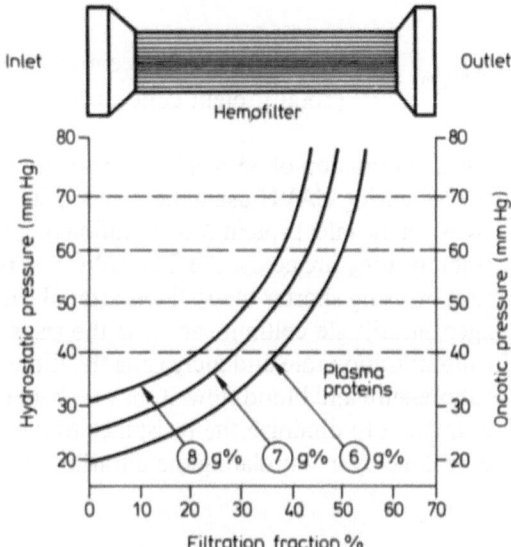

Fig. 9. Relationship between hydrostatic and oncotic pressure, total protein concentration, and filtration fraction, in the filter, assuming an equilibrium pressure of 77 mmHg. The *curved lines* denote oncotic pressure values for different inlet protein concentrations. *HP,* hydrostatic pressure in the filter. (C. Ronco)

The presence of filtration pressure equilibrium in CAVH has clinical implications. It is not possible to assert where in the filter this equilibrium of pressure takes effect. In the Amicon 20, it is probably closer to the inlet than to the outlet port. The remaining blood, now with a higher hematocrit and protein concentration and hence a greater viscosity, increases the resistance of the filter to the flow of blood. In patients with a low systemic arterial blood pressure and thus a low blood flow, this effect may further decrease the blood flow through the filter. A vicious circle is created, and eventually the filter clots.

CAVH is a low-blood-flow and low-pressure system. The low blood flow is in part a consequence of the high resistance of the filter. This resistance is only partially determined by the intrinsic design of the filter and is mainly a consequence of the filtration pressure equilibrium. The low pressure is due to the pressure drop that takes place in the circuit. Since this pressure drop can only be prevented to a certain extent (by shortening lines, etc.) the operator must rely on the negative pressure exerted by the ultrafiltrate column to maintain an adequate filtration pressure in the filter.

Filtration Fraction

The filtration fraction (FF) is that fraction of the plasma flowing through the filter that is ultrafiltered. It is calculated by the following formulas:

$$FF\ (\%) = \frac{Q_f}{Q_P}\ \text{inlet}$$

and

$$FF\,(\%) = 1 - \frac{\text{(Total protein concentration at the inlet)}}{\text{(Total protein concentration at the outlet)}}$$

A filtration fraction of 35%–40% appears to be the maximal efficiency that can be achieved during CAVH using the Amicon 20. A lower value may be the result of an increase in the inlet protein concentration or, more probably, a decrease in the trans-membrane pressure across the filter (filtration pressure). Altering the extracorporeal circuit by using shorter blood lines, arterial cannulas, with a larger diameter, and a longer ultrafiltrate column can raise the transmembrane pressure, thus improving the ultrafiltration rate and increasing the filtration fraction. In patients with low ar-terial pressure and blood flow, it may be better to accept a lower (15%–20%) filtra-tion fraction to diminish the resistance to the blood flow through the circuit. This can be done by manipulating the ultrafiltrate column.

Composition of the Ultrafiltrate

The fluid removed during CAVH has all the characteristics typical of an ultrafiltrate of plasma water:

1) It is protein-free. The membranes used in CAVH are impermeable to plasma pro-teins with a molecular weight of 50000 or more.
2) For nonelectrolyte solutes, including proteins with a molecular weight of less than 50000, the ultrafiltrate concentration progressively increases, reaching the same concentration as the plasma water, at molecular weights of 100 or less. As shown in rat glomeruli [9], the permeative capability of molecules with a sieving coefficient less than 1 but greater than 0 is dependent on plasma flow. In CAVH the influence of plasma flow on the permeative capability of solutes with these characteristics has not been determined.

Table 1. Composition of Ultrafiltrate. (From [10])

		Ultrafiltrate	Plasma water
Sodium	(mEq/l)	135.3 ±11.2	136.2±10.4
Potassium	(mEq/l)	4.1 ± 0.3	4.1± 0.7
Chloride	(mEq/l)	103.7 ± 9.6	99.3±10.8
Carbon dioxide	(mEq/l)	23.1 ± 5.1	19.8± 4.7
Blood urea nitrogen	(mg/dl)	82.9 ±38.4	79.1±36.1
Serum creatinine	(mg/dl)	6.6 ± 4.0	6.5± 3.9
Uric acid	(mg/dl)	7.5 ± 3.3	7.4± 3.0
Phosphorus	(mg/dl)	4.2 ± 1.3	3.9± 1.1
Calcium	(mg/dl)	5.1 ± 0.4	8.1± 0.6
Total bilirubin	(mg/dl)	0.44± 0.6	12.1± 9.5
Direct bilirubin	(mg/dl)	0.26± 0.3	7.4± 5.9

3) The concentration of the electrically charged electrolytes is affected by the negatively charged plasma proteins. Those which are negatively charged, such as chloride, have a concentration in the ultrafiltrate greater than in plasma water, while those with a positive charge have a concentration in the ultrafiltrate lower than their concentration in plasma water.

4) The physicochemical characteristics of the solute, such as protein binding or distribution in the red blood cell water, may result in lower concentration in the ultrafiltrate than in the plasma water (Table 1).

Improvements in Efficiency of CAVH

There have been attempts in four areas to improve the performance of CAVH:

a) pre-/postdilution mode;
b) use of a vacuum pump to increase the ultrafiltration pressure;
c) changes in the design of the filters used; and
d) the combination of diffusion and convection - continuous arteriovenous hemodiafiltration.

Pre-/postdilution Mode

Studies in hemofiltration have demonstrated that it is possible to increase the ultrafiltration rate, and thus solute removal, by diluting the blood before it enters the filter. The term pre-/postdilution mode in CAVH defines a system in which the substitution fluid is administered to the incoming blood as well as to the blood returning to the patient. In predilution a fraction of the substitution fluid is administered at the blood inlet (3-5 ml/min). In postdilution the majority of the substitution fluid is administered in the venous line or into the systemic circulation (8-10 ml/min [11]). The lowering by dilution of the incoming protein concentration will reduce the oncotic pressure inside the filter and thus increase the ultrafiltration rate for a constant hydrostatic pressure (Fig. 9). The benefits of this effect are offset by the lowering of the urea level, and other solute concentration levels in the ultrafiltrate. The predilution fluid is usually administered through the heparin line. The indication for using this substitution mode would be the case of patients in whom the blood flow through the circuit is very low or hematocrit very high and clotting of the filter frequent. The disadvantage of this system is that the computation of the fluid balance becomes more complicated.

Use of a Vacuum Pump

KAPLAN et al. [12] have shown that a vacuum suction attached to the filtrate port may be a useful adjunct to CAVH. The addition of suction increases the transmembrane pressure and, therefore, the ultrafiltration rate.

This modification to the original technique must be used with caution. Since increases in ultrafiltration pressure will result in the production of an ultrafiltrate even in the presence of very low blood flow, a filtration fraction in excess of 50% can be obtained. This may result in clotting, despite adequate heparin administration.

Changes in Filter Design

The filters currently used for CAVH were originally designed for machine-driven hemofiltration. With greater understanding of the determinants of ultrafiltration in CAVH, it is clear that design modifications may improve the performance of the technique. By shortening the length of the filter, it may be possible to avoid equilibrium pressure. This would produce a decrease in the resistance of the filter by avoidance of the dragging of the blood with a higher hematocrit and protein concentration through an area of membrane not used for filtration. By increasing the number of fibers, it may be possible to diminish the resistance of the filter and thereby increase the blood flow for a given systemic arterial pressure. This would also diminish the filtration fraction, while the ultrafiltration rate would remain unchanged.

Continuous Arteriovenous Hemodiafiltration

Several investigators have endeavored to improve solute clearance in CAVH by incorporating diffusive transport in to convective solute removal.

GERONEMUS and SCHNEIDER reported a modification called continuous arteriovenous hemodialysis (CAVHD) [13]. In this system a hemodialyzer was connected to the patient using a circuit comparable to that used in CAVH. In addition, dialysate was circulated through the dialyzer. Solute clearance was achieved by diffusion, and adequate urea clearances (10–15 ml) were obtained, with excellent cardiovascular stability. One disadvantage of this system was inadequate fluid removal. More recently, these investigators have performed similar studies using a 0.5^{-m2} flat-plate Polyacrylonitrile (PAN) membrane dialyzer. Dialysate was administered at 15 ml/min. Plasma urea clearance was 16.9 ml/min with an ultrafiltration rate of 5.4 ml/min. This treatment would be the equivalent of continuous arteriovenous hemodiafiltration (GERONEMUS 1985, personal communication).

C. RONCO (1985, personal communication) modified the standard Amicon 20 by adding an extra port to the ultrafiltrate compartment, so that solutes removed by Simultaneous diffusion and convection. The patients were treated with standard CAVH using this device, the added port being occluded. When increased solute removal was required, the added port was opened and a dialysate solution was circulated by gravity through the ultrafiltrate compartment of the filter. The addition of diffusion permitted the control of urea nitrogen levels even in patients in a severe by catabolic state.

Clinical Use of CAVH

The clinical value of CAVH depends on the ability of this therapy to maintain acceptable levels of urea nitrogen and fluid and electrolyte balance.

Urea Nitrogen Levels

The level of urea nitrogen in plasma during CAVH depends on the rates of production and removal of urea nitrogen and the amount of substitution fluid administered. In patients who produce approximately 10 g or less of urea nitrogen per day, an exchange of 10-12 l in 24 h is sufficient to maintain a blood urea nitrogen level below 90 mg/dl. In severely catabolic patients who produce more than 10 g of urea nitrogen per day, CAVH may be used in conjunction with hyperalimentation. This combination of therapies may promote anabolism and a decrease in the rate of urea nitrogen production. Anabolism, or an increase in the number of liters of substitution fluid exchanged per day, or both, may permit the maintenance of an acceptable level of plasma urea nitrogen in severely catabolic patients on CAVH.

When no substitution fluid is administered, as in continuous slow ultrafiltration (SCUF) [14], plasma urea nitrogen will remain unchanged or increase rather than decrease, as would be expected, since urea is being removed in the ultrafiltrate. The concentration of urea in the ultrafiltrate is equal to its concentration in the plasma water therefore only when substitution fluid is administered; a dilution of the plasma water will take place and plasma water concentration will fall [9].

Fluid Balance

One of the advantages of CAVH is that it offers almost complete control of the patient's fluid balance. Under most operating conditions 5-10 ml/min of ultrafiltrate are obtained. By administering a smaller amount of substitution fluid - 2-5 ml/min, for example - a negative fluid balance can easily be established. Most studies have demonstrated that a negative fluid balance induced in this fashion does not result in hemodynamic changes; blood pressure is maintained and cardiac output may even increase with time. For a given patient it would appear that the rapidity with which the negative fluid balance is attained and the total volume of fluid removal are important. Hypotension is usually not observed at negative fluid losses of 0.5 ml/min/kg body weight if volume overload exists clinically. It has been our experience that it is better to achieve the negative fluid balance over an extended period of time. In patients with severe fluid overload we prescribe that only 50% of the ultrafiltrate obtained in the previous hour should be replaced with substitution fluid.

Electrolyte Balance

The electrolyte losses during CAVH will depend on (a) the concentration in the ultrafiltrate and (b) the volume of ultrafiltrate obtained. The gain of a given electrolyte will depend on (a) the concentration in the substitution fluid and (b) the volume of fluid administered:

$$\text{Electrolyte balance} = V_{uf} \times [\quad]_{uf} - V_{sf} \times [\quad]_{sf}$$

where V_{uf} is the volume of ultrafiltrate; V_{sf} is the volume of substitution fluid; $[\quad]_{uf}$ is the electrolyte concentration of the ultrafiltrate; and $[\quad]_{sf}$ is the electrolyte concentration of the substitution fluid.

For example, the sodium balance during CAVH in a patient who has a weight loss of 2 l (plasma Na, 140 mEq/l; ultrafiltrate Na, 140 mEq/l; substitution fluid Na, 130 mEq/l), will be different depending on the volume of substitution fluid used (Table 2).

This feature of the treatment permits the administration or removal of a particular electrolyte with ease and allows dissociation of electrolyte loss or gain from changes in total body water. It is also useful in the treatment of acidosis (to administer bicarbonate), alkalosis (to remove alkali), or in patients with congestive heart failure (to remove water with or without sodium).

Table 2. Sodium balance during CAVH

	Volume of Ultrafiltrate	
	2000 ml	10000 ml
Na losses	280 mEq	1400 mEq
Substitution fluid administered	0	8000 ml
Na gain	0	1040 mEq
Na balance	-280 mEq	-360 mEq

Heparin Usage

There are several ways to adjust the dosage of heparin during CAVH. Whatever schedule is used, a priming dose of 2000 IU is required, and during the treatment close monitoring of the systemic partial thromboplastin time (PTT) is essential. For example, at a heparin dosage of 10 IU/kg/h, which must be adjusted according to the blood flow through the filter, the objective of this regimen is to achieve a heparin concentration of 0.5-1.0 IU per ml of blood in the filter. At blood flows of less than 80 ml/min, using this schedule, it may be possible to avoid systemic anticoagulation.

Heparin dose $IU/h = 0.5-1.0 \times Q_B \times 60$

Substitution Fluid

In the United States there are no commercially available substitution fluids for hemofiltration or CAVH. We have used Ringer's solution, composed of sodium (130 mEq/l), potassium (4 mEq/l), calcium (3 mEq/l), chloride (109 mEq/l), and lactate (28 mEq/l).

A similar composition is available with acetate instead of lactate. No problems in metabolizing the acetate or lactate have been observed by us. It must be pointed out that the amount of acetate administered is far below the quantity at which acetate intolerance has been described (300 mEq/h).

It is better to modify the replacement solution as needed than to use a fixed substitution fluid.

Indications

CAVH is a treatment that permits access to the extracellular fluid of patients with a variety of diseases. It thus gives the nephrologist the possibility to modify the composition and volume of extracellular fluid. It should be used in patients with altered extracellular fluid composition and renal failure in whom hemodialysis or peritoneal dialysis cannot be performed or are contraindicated.

It has been our experience that in patients with acute renal failure it is preferable to initiate the treatment early in the course of the developing uremia. General indications for CAVH are:

Fluid Overload
1) Hemodialysis patients with preexisting access
   a) Acute pulmonary edema
   b) Hemodynamic instability
2) Patients with acute renal failure
   a) Hemodynamic instability
   b) Postoperative cardiac surgery
   c) Recent myocardial infarct
   d) Sepsis
3) Patients with pump failure
   a) Diuretic fast
   b) Oliguria despite inotropic support

4) Oliguric states in patients who require large quantities of fluid
   a) Hyperalimentation
   b) Medications, etc.
5) Chronic fluid overload
   a) Ascites
   b) Nephrotic edema

Solute Removal
Alternative therapy to hemodialysis or peritoneal dialysis in patients with chronic or acute renal failure and
a) Hypotension
b) Hemodynamic instability
c) Need for parenteral fluids
d) Associated medical comolications

Electrolyte Disturbances
a) Metabolic alkalosis
b) Metabolic acidosis
c) Hyponatremia, etc.

Contraindications

CAVH should not be performed in patients who are severely hypotensive and/or catabolic despite hyperalimentation. In patients with systemic bleeding the advantages and the risks must be carefully weighed up. It is clear that in subjects with generalized bleeding the combination of low blood pressure, low blood flow through the filter, and the need for high ultrafiltration rates makes CAVH a difficult technique to apply.

Acknowledgement

The author wants to thank the following coworkers and friends, whose contributions have made these studies possible: Dr. BEAT VON ALBERTINI, Dr. R. GERONEMUS, Dr. A. LAUER, Dr. C. RONCO, and Dr. S. GLABMAN.

References

1. Silverstein ME, Ford CA, Lysaght MJ, Henderson LW (1974) The treatment of intractable fluid overload. N Engl J Med 291: 747
2. Henderson L, Besarab A, Michaels A, Bluemle LW Jr (1967) Blood purification by ultrafiltration and fluid replacement (diafiltration). Trans Am Soc Artif Intern Organs 13: 216

3. Kramer P, Wigger W, Rieger J, Matthaei D, Scheler F (1977) Arteriovenous haemofiltration: a new and simple method for treatment of over-hydrated patients resistant to diuretics. Klin Wochenschr 55: 1121
4. Synhaivsky A, Kurtz SB, Wochos DN, Schniepp J, Johnson WJ (1983) Acute renal failure treated by slow continuous ultrafiltration. Mayo Clin Proc 58: 729
5. Kramer P, Kaufhold C, Grone HJ, Wigger W, Rieger D (1980) Management of anuric intensive-care patients with arteriovenous hemofiltration. Int J Artif Organs 3: 225
6. Gohl H, Konstantin P, Gulberg CA (1982) Hemofiltration membranes. Contrib Nephrol 32: 20
7. Lieberman KV, Nardi L, Bosch JP (1985) Treatment on an infant with acute renal failure using continuous arteriovenous hemofiltration. J Pediatr (In press)
8. Lauer A, Saccaggi A, Ronco C, Belledonne M, Glabman S, Bosch JP (1983) Continuous arteriovenous hemofiltration in the critically ill patient. Ann Intern Med 99: 455
9. Chang RL, Ueki IF, Troy JL, Deen WM, Robertson CR, Brenner BM (1975) Permselectivity of the capillary wall to macromolecules. II. Experimental studies in rat using neutral dextran. Biophys J 15: 887
10. Kaplan AA, Longnecker RE, Folkert VW (1984) Continuous arteriovenous hemofiltration: a report of six months' experience. Ann Intern Med 100: 359
11. Geronemus R, von Albertini B, Glabman S, Lysaght M, Kahn T, Bosch JP (1978) Enhanced molecular clearance in hemofiltration. Proc Clin Dial Transplant Forum 8: 147
12. Kaplan AA, Longnecker RE, Folkert VW (1983) Suction-assisted continuous arteriovenous hemofiltration. Trans Am Soc Artif Intern Organs 29: 408
13. Geronemus R, Schneider W (1984) Continuous arteriovenous hemodialysis: a new modality for treatment of acute renal failure. Trans Am Soc Artif Intern Organs 30: 423
14. Paganini EP, Nakamoto S (1980) Continuous slow ultrafiltration in oliguric acute renal failure. Trans Am Soc Artif Intern Organs 26: 201

Nutritional Aspects of Hemofiltration

J. R. MAULT and R. H. BARTLETT

Table of Contents

The metabolic management of renal failure patients requires special consideration due to the nature of the disease. Nutritional support must be designed to provide adequate energy and protein substrates without exacerbating protein catabolism. In addition, fluid restrictions may preclude administration of optimal therapy.

Acute and chronic renal failure are distinct diseases with regard to nutritional management. In chronic renal failure (CRF), a patient's energy requirements differ little from those of a normal individual and are easily met per os. Protein intake is required only for metabolic turnover and therefore is restricted to minimize urea generation and other products of protein catabolism.

In contrast to CRF patients, the energy requirements of acute renal failure (ARF) patients are typically elevated due to soft tissue injury, sepsis, and multisystem failure. Endogenous carbohydrate stores are rapidly depleted and proteins and lipids are catabolized for energy production. Protein utilization is further increased for anabolic wound healing and sustained immune function. Administration of adequate nutrition may be limited by volume concerns and inability to perform hemodialysis (HD) due to the hemodynamic instability often encountered in these patients. Studies of energy metabolism and balance have suggested that the high mortality of ARF patients may be due, in part, to malnutrition [1, 2].

Continuous arteriovenous hemofiltration (CAVH) is a modality of treatment of ARF patients that permits administration of unlimited quantities of energy and protein substrates [3]. KRAMER [4] and others [5, 6] have demonstrated that CAVH is effective in the management of uremia and fluid balance with little incidence of hemodynamic instability.

Given the potential to supply unlimited nutrition to these patients, the clinician must determine the "optimal" therapy. Grossly exceeding caloric requirements is not recommended. Carbohydrate supplied in great excess of metabolic expenditure is converted to fatty acids, leading to fatty infiltration of the liver and increased carbon dioxide production which may exacerbate respiratory failure [7]. As the clinical course of ARF is extremely variable, assessment of nutritional requirement on an individual basis is necessary.

This chapter will discuss the nutritional management of ARF patients through the use of CAVH. The general principles of energy metabolism and nutritional assessment will be reviewed first.

Measurement of Energy and Protein Requirements

The original work of HARRIS and BENEDICT in 1919 first described the amount of energy required to maintain the most basic bodily functions [8]. This quantity of energy, expressed as kilocalories per day, is known as the basal metabolic rate or BMR. The BMR has a precise relationship with age, body size, and gender, and can be estimated from nomograms based upon these parameters [9]. Although nomograms may accurately predict the energy requirements of healthy, normal subjects, the metabolic rate of any given patient may significantly differ according to clinical circumstances. Because the metabolic rate has been shown to correlate with injury, sepsis, and HD, in addition to the type and severity of disease [10, 11, 1], actual measurement of energy requirement will enhance clinical judgement. The parameter which accounts for the changes described above is the resting energy expenditure (REE).

While direct measurement of REE is not possible in the clinical setting, caloric expenditure can be accurately determined through the measurement of oxygen consumption. This is known as indirect calorimetry. From the stoichiometry of aerobic pathways, a caloric equivalent has been derived for each class of foodstuffs. The caloric equivalent of a given energy substrate is amount of heat (in calories) produced per liter of oxygen burned. Similarly, each class of foodstuffs has a unique respiratory quotient (RQ); see Table 1. The RQ is the ratio of carbon dioxide pro-

Table 1. Energy equivalents and respiratory quotients of foodstuffs

Foodstuff	Caloric value (kcal/g)	Caloric equivalent (kcal/LO_2)	Respiratory quotient
Carbohydrate	4.1	5.1	1.00
Protein	4.1	4.6	0.82
Fat	9.3	4.7	0.71

LO_2, liter of O_2

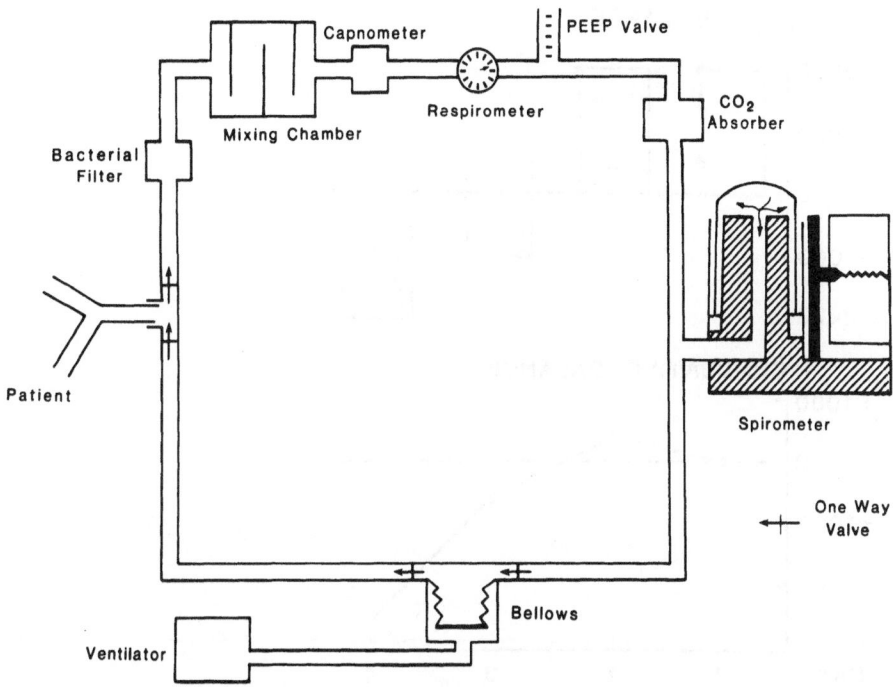

Fig. 1. Schematic diagram of a closed-circuit rebreathing spirometer

duced to oxygen consumed in the stoichiometric oxidation of a particular substrate. By measuring the RQ and the nitrogen excretion, it is possible to determine the ratio of fat, protein, and carbohydrate substrates catabolized and assign the caloric expenditure from oxygen consumption using the caloric equivalents listed above. Since the value of nitrogen excretion is generally not available for same-day calculation of energy requirements, a conversion factor of 5 kilocalories per liter oxygen consumed is used. This will result in an overestimation of the energy expenditure by about 4% under normal energy metabolism.

Routine measurement of oxygen consumption in the clinical setting can be accomplished by closed-circuit rebreathing spirometry, mixed-exhaled gas analysis, or calculated using the Fick equation. The closed-circuit rebreathing method utilizes a spirometer filled with oxygen and a carbon dioxide scrub. With inspiration, oxygen flows from the spirometer to the subject where a portion of the oxygen is consumed. The unused oxygen and carbon dioxide produced is expired through a calcium hydroxide scrub which removes carbon dioxide from the circuit while the remaining gas returns to the spirometer. Assuming no air leaks within the closed rebreathing circuit, the net volume loss as recorded by the spirometer, divided by the time of the study, equals the oxygen consumption. Carbon dioxide production is also measured by placing a capnometer in-line before the gas is removed. We have developed a system of this type which can be used for spontaneously breathing or mechanically ventilated patients at any inspired oxygen concentration [10] (Fig. 1).

Mixed-exhaled gas analysis is another method which provides for measurement of both oxygen consumption and carbon dioxide production. In this technique, the volume and concentration of oxygen and CO_2 are measured in the exhaled gas.

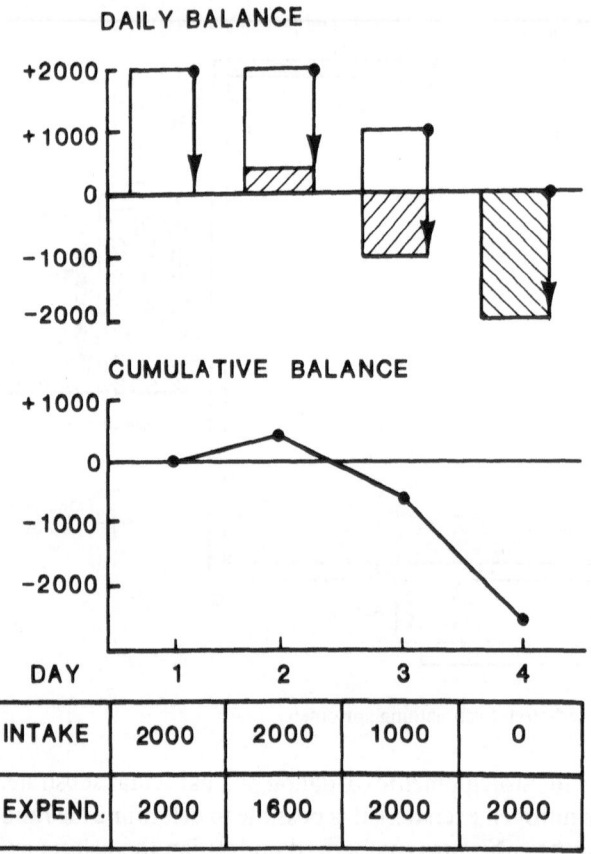

DAILY BALANCE

CUMULATIVE BALANCE

DAY	1	2	3	4
INTAKE	2000	2000	1000	0
EXPEND.	2000	1600	2000	2000

Fig. 2. Calculation of daily and cumulative caloric balance. Intake is plotted from the baseline up, and caloric expenditure is plotted from the top of the intake line down. Positive or negative balance is seen as a deviation above or below the baseline, respectively. Cumulative balance is the sum of the consecutive daily balances

Oxygen consumption is then determined by subtracting the amount of expired oxygen from the amount inspired. This method is simple and accurate for study of relatively healthy subjects breathing room air. However, this technique is unsuitable for study of patients on supplemental oxygen or those mechanically ventilated due to slight fluctuations in the inspired oxygen concentration and volume of ventilating gas.

The Fick equation may also be utilized for calculation of oxygen consumption by measuring arterial and mixed-venous oxygen content and cardiac output (usually by thermal dilution). However, with the numerous assumptions necessary for determination of cardiac output and oxygen content, an oxygen consumption value obtained through the Fick equation should be considered only as an approximation of the metabolic rate. This method does not allow for measurement of carbon dioxide production.

Assessment of protein balance should also be conducted to evaluate the overall nutritional status of the patient. A reasonable approximation of protein catabolism in the oliguric patient is accomplished through calculation of the urea generation rate [12]. In this calculation, changes in blood urea nitrogen and fluid balance are recorded over a 24-h period. Urea nitrogen content must also be measured from collections of ultrafiltrate (from CAVH), wound drains, etc., obtained during the same time interval. Assuming that the urea produced by protein catabolism is not reutilized and that it is contained within the extracellular space, the urea generation rate is calculated from the above values. The rate of protein catabolism can be derived from the urea generation rate.

Having determined the rate of energy and protein catabolism, the daily and cumulative caloric balance can be tabulated. Daily caloric and protein balances are calculated by subtracting the amount catabolized from the amount given. Cumulative balances result from the addition of the daily balances (Fig. 2). It is important to note that one of the objectives of nutritional therapy in these patients is to prevent the breakdown of endogenous protein while at the same time maintain adequate immune function and anabolic wound healing. Therefore, protein should not be considered an energy substrate when tabulating the caloric balance.

Energy and Protein Metabolism in Acute Renal Failure

Renal failure, by itself, has no effect on the metabolic rate. Anephric patients, or stable patients on chronic treatment modalities are characterized by a normal metabolic rate. ARF is typically one component of a multiple organ failure syndrome often accompanied by a systemic septicemia. The hypermetabolism observed in ARF patients is not a consequence of the renal failure, but of the underlying disease processes which may be responsible for the renal failure. Similarly, the high mortality of ARF patients is not so much the renal failure, but rather the severity of the underlying medical or surgical disorder.

The need to provide plentiful amounts of energy and protein to the hypermetabolic multiple organ failure patient is precluded by concerns of overhydration and urea generation when ARF is encountered. This paradox in nutritional therapy usually results in a state of malnutrition and may be a contributing factor to mortality of these patients.

When contemplating nutritional therapy for normal, healthy individuals, it is accurate to assume that protein catabolism has a linear relationship with energy expenditure. Therefore, assessment of one metabolic parameter (REE or nitrogen balance) will allow for calculation of the other. However, in the disease state, energy metabolism is not directly correlated to protein metabolism and conclusions drawn regarding nitrogen balance do not necessarily apply to energy balance.

While resting energy expenditure can increase 50%-100% above normal under maximum physiological stress [2], net protein catabolism can double or even triple in magnitude [13]. The difference occurs because energy metabolism and protein metabolism respond differently to various chemical messengers. The control of normal energy metabolism is mediated primarily by catecholamines and thyroxine [14], whereas the initiation of fever by the brain is signaled by a protein named endogenous or leukocytic pyrogen (interleukin-1) [15]. Leukocytes or macrophages appear to release interleukin in response to tissue damage or infection. Recently, this same human leukocytic pyrogen has been implicated as the mediator for abnormal muscle protein catabolism in sepsis and trauma [16, 17].

Interestingly, the hemodynamic instability encountered during HD may be due, in part, to the phenomenon described above [19]. Complement activating properties of cellulose-based dialysis membranes may trigger monocytes to release interleukin. The production of interleukin increases the metabolic rate through the initiation of fever. We have observed an acute and sustained increase in oxygen consumption during HD that is likely due to this mechanism [1]. This increase in systemic oxygen requirement places a demand on the cardiovascular system to deliver additional oxygen at a time when cardiac reserve may be limited by the underlying disease. To further confound these difficulties in the oxygen delivery-uptake process, complement and leukocyte-mediated acute pulmonary dysfunction has also been demonstrated during HD [20].

Energy Balance

In energy balance studies of critically ill patients with multiple organ failure [10] and chest trauma [18], we have observed a direct correlation between mortality and negative cumulative caloric balance. In multiple organ failure patients studied, a caloric deficit of 10000 kilocalories or greater was associated with an 86% mortality, whereas the mortality of patients in positive cumulative balance was only 27% ($P < 0.01$).

Study of energy balance and outcome of ARF patients resulted in similar findings [2]. In this study, resting energy expenditure was measured daily in 29 ARF patients characterized by multiple organ failure and extended mechanical ventilation. Daily and cumulative caloric balances were tabulated and related to survival of the acute episode.

HD was performed as needed to treat hypervolemia and uremia and no specific nutritional protocol was followed. The results of this investigation identified a direct correlation between cumulative caloric balance and survival of the acute episode. Of the 29 patients studied, 20 completed the study in negative caloric balance and two survived (10%); whereas, nine patients finished the study in positive cumulative caloric balance and five survived (56%, $P < 0.01$ using chi-square analysis); see Fig. 3). Also, the mean cumulative caloric balance of survivors ($+1800$ kcal) was greater than of nonsurvivors (-6000 kcal; $P < 0.05$). Each group received the same amount of calories and protein. The REE of all patients studied was 40% above normal and was significantly higher in nonsurvivors.

Others have also observed this relationship between caloric intake and survival of ARF patients. In a controlled double-blind study of parenteral nutrition in ARF patients, Feinstein and associates [13] found that energy intake was significantly greater in those who recovered renal function or survived ($P < 0.005$).

Cause and effect cannot be implied in either of the above studies. It is reasonable to suggest that the severity of disease dictated the ability (or inability) to provide nu-

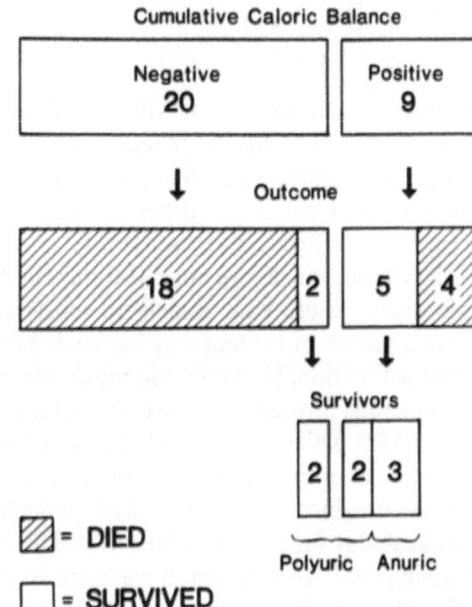

Fig. 3. Relationship between cumulative caloric balance (CCB) and outcome. Survival of patients in positive CCB was 56%, while survival of patients in negative CCB was 10% ($P < 0.01$). Of the seven survivors, four were polyuric and three were anuric (required hemodialysis)

trition and maintain positive caloric balance. Conversely, a malnourished state may lead to decreased immune function, respiratory distress, and impaired tissue healing, which all may contribute to the mortality of these patients. Nevertheless, a strong correlation certainly exists between energy balance and survival of ARF patients.

Positive energy balance may also make management of uremia less difficult. If a patient receives fewer calories than his resting energy expenditure, the difference is covered by utilization of endogenous energy stores. In a well-nourished individual, carbohydrate stores rarely exceed 2500 kilocalories. After this has been used, lipid and protein stores are mobilized. In the disease state, endogenous protein may be catabolized preferentially as an energy substrate in the absence of readily available glucose [16]. Maintenance of positive energy balance by supplying glucose calories in excess of metabolic expenditure should minimize the amount of protein catabolized and hence limit the urea generation rate. Several investigators have concluded that the degree of protein catabolism in ARF can be reduced by increasing caloric intake [13, 20, 21, 22].

As mentioned previously, grossly exceeding caloric requirements is not recommended. Instead, energy requirements should be met by providing glucose and lipids at a rate of REE plus 200–400 kilocalories per day. The optimum ratio of glucose to lipid calories has yet to be studied.

Finally, the timing of nutritional support may be equally important. In a study of general critical illness, including ARF, early feeding (1–2 days after admission to the intensive care unit, or ICU) was compared with conventional feeding (5–7 days). The mortality of patients in positive cumulative caloric balance on day 7 was 27%, compared with 54% for patients in negative balance on day 7 ($P < 0.05$) [23].

Protein Balance

The protein management of ARF is often confused with that of CRF. As stated previously, CRF patients are generally healthy individuals who require only enough protein to maintain basic chemical pathways. Therefore, protein restriction is indicated for these patients in order to minimize urea generation and possibly slow the progression of their renal disease [24].

The circumstances are much different in ARF. These are often patients with multiple organ failure with associated sepsis and they are generally hypermetabolic. Large amounts of protein may be needed for proper wound healing and sustained immune function. However, too much protein may worsen uremic effects.

Numerous investigators have studied the potential benefits of administering protein to ARF patients. In one of the earlier studies of this type, Abel and colleagues compared an intravenous solution of hypertonic glucose and essential amino acids (EAA) with glucose alone in 53 ARF patients [25]. Energy intake averaged 1426 and 1641 kcal/day for the two solutions and amino acid intake was 16 g/day in patients receiving the EAA solution. It was reported that recovery of renal function was significantly more frequent in patients receiving the EAA solution, but overall survival was not significantly different between the two groups. However, in patients whose ARF was classified as severe (associated pneumonia, sepsis, hemorrhage, or requiring HD) survival was significantly greater in those receiving the solution containing EAA.

More recently, Feinstein and associates conducted a study of total parenteral nutrition in ARF patients that compared three solutions:

a) glucose alone;
b) glucose and 21 g/day EAA; and
c) glucose and 21 g/day EAA and 21 g/day nonessential amino acids (NEAA) [13].

Thirty patients with ARF and unable to receive nutrition enterally were randomized into the three groups. Energy intake averaged approximately 2500 kcal/day and did not differ between the three regimens. Overall survival was 37% and did not differ between the groups. Urea nitrogen appearance was significantly greater in patients receiving EAA and NEAA as compared with only EAA. Nitrogen balance was negative in all patients and did not differ between groups. While energy balance was not measured, energy intake was significantly greater in survivors than nonsurvivors. The authors concluded that greater amounts of energy and both EAA and NEAA may be beneficial to ARF patients.

The two most important concerns regarding protein in ARF are how much to administer and what type. Most studies such as those above report that the protein catabolic rate of ARF patients (as assessed through measurement of urea generation rate) can range from 70 to as much as 200 g/day. However, few, if any, studies have administered enough protein to achieve positive balance. Most provide 30–60 g/day and the effects of providing larger amounts have yet to be studied in these patients.

The answers are equally unclear with regard to the type of protein to administer. Several studies contend that a solution of only essential amino acids should be given [26, 27], while others suggest benefit in providing a solution of mixed amino acids (both essential and nonessential) [28, 29]. In addition, solutions containing a high ratio of branch-chained amino acids may enhance positive nitrogen balance [30].

The current consensus [31] about protein nutrition in ARF patients is as follows:

a) In order to minimize the amount of protein that is catabolized for energy production, enough calories (carbohydrate and/or lipid) must be supplied to maintain positive caloric balance
b) Protein (amino acids) should be infused at a rate to achieve positive nitrogen balance
c) In the absence of conclusive evidence supporting the use of specialized formulations (i. e., essential or branched-chain solutions), administration of mixed amino acids is recommended.

Nutritional Management with CAVH

In nearly all of the studies of nutrition in ARF presented above, the patients who demonstrated the greatest benefit from parenteral nutrition were the most severe cases, with complications such as sepsis, pneumonia, and/or peritonitis. It is also these patients who experience the most hemodynamic instability when treated with conventional HD. Administration of fluids, colloid, and inotrops is often necessary to maintain blood pressure during the treatment period. Fluid restrictions are instituted to prevent hypervolemia and minimize the need to perform this destabilizing procedure except only when required to remove solutes. These circumstances place extreme limits on the amount of nutrition that can be supplied to the very patients who need it most.

Continuous arteriovenous hemofiltration (CAVH) is a modality of treatment of ARF that permits excellent control of fluid volume without hemodynamic instability and eliminates the need for restriction of fluids [4, 5, 6]. Using this therapy, optimal amounts of nutrition can be administered freely without concerns for overhydration. Therefore, a primary indication for the use of CAVH is the need to provide nutrition to ARF patients [3].

The nutritional course of a typical ICU patient with ARF treated with CAVH is illustrated in Fig. 4. This patient was a 67-year-old woman who underwent a segmental aortic replacement, right nephrectomy, and left aortorenal bypass. Nonoliguric renal failure developed postoperatively, and progressed to anuria. The patient also suffered a brain-stem infarction and developed Candida sepsis. CAVH was initiated 2 weeks after operation due to fluid overload and uremia, (serum BUN and creatinine were 117 and 11.0 mg/dl, respectively), and the need to provide greater nutritional support. No episodes of hemodynamic instability directly attributable to CAVH were encountered. The ultrafiltration rate averaged 12.1 liters per day while mean hemofilter life was 5 days. Mean resting energy expenditure was ap-

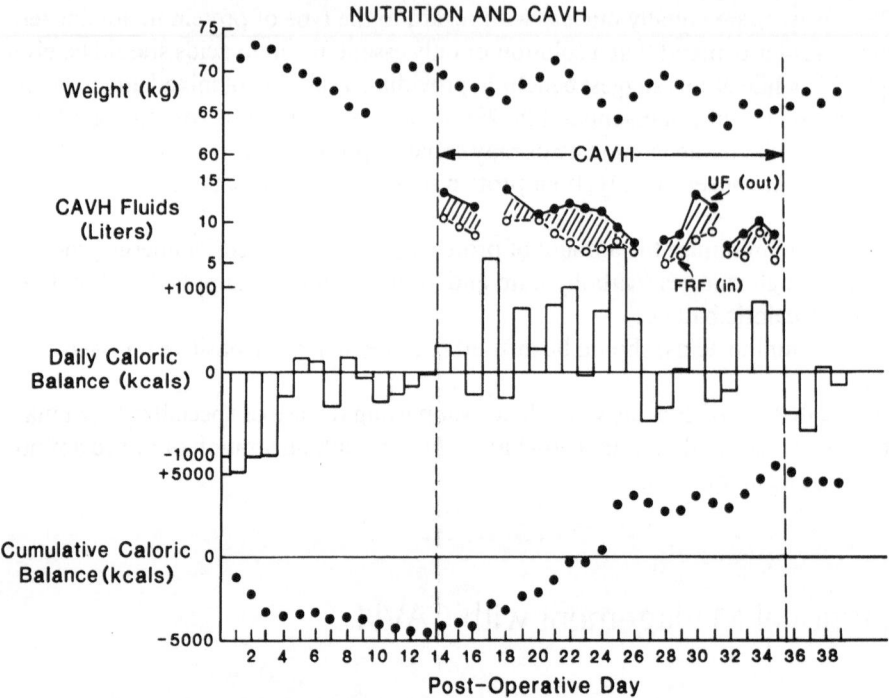

Fig. 4. Nutritional course of a typical critically ill ARF patient treated with CAVH. Fluid restrictions resulted in negative cumulative caloric balance reaching − 5000 kcal by postoperative day 13. Use of CAVH permitted positive caloric balance to be achieved

proximately 2500 kcal/day. Prior to initiation of CAVH, a negative cumulative caloric balance of − 5000 kilocalories was reached due to ensuing fluid constraints. Once CAVH was initiated, positive daily and eventually positive cumulative caloric balance was accomplished. Protein catabolic rate as derived from measurement of urea nitrogen appearance averaged 74.6 g/day. After 3 weeks of CAVH, urine output returned to normal and CAVH was discontinued. Despite relative metabolic stabilization, no neurological recovery was gained and the patient died 7 weeks postoperatively.

As demonstrated by this patient's medical course, CAVH is an ideal kidney replacement therapy for treatment of critically ill ARF patients. One of the unique advantages of CAVH over conventional HD is the relative hemodynamic stability of patients undergoing this procedure. This may be due to a lack of the blood activation properties common to cellulose-based HD membranes. KRAMER and colleagues reported that little complement and leukocyte activation occurs with the polysulfone membrane of the hemofilter [32]. Our preliminary studies confirm this and also indicate that oxygen consumption does not change with CAVH.

When utilizing the nutritional potential of CAVH, several considerations must be kept in mind. First, nutrition should be administered enterally if possible. When this is contraindicated, parenteral nutrition may be utilized.

Hyperconcentrated parenteral solutions are no longer necessary when CAVH is utilized. As the rate of filter replacement fluid is changed according to fluid balance, parenteral nutrition should be infused at a site independent of the filter replacement fluid. Hyperglycemia is commonly encountered in these patients and use of insulin may be necessary to provide the level of nutrition desired. Measurement of urea generation and calculation of protein catabolism is simple to perform with CAVH and was discussed previously in this chapter. Finally, significant loss of nutrition does not accompany CAVH and is not a concern for this procedure [33].

References

1. Mault JR, Dechert RE, Bartlett RH, Swartz RD, Ferguson SK (1982) Oxygen consumption during hemodialysis for acute renal failure. Trans Am Soc Artif Intern Organs 28: 510-515
2. Mault JR, Bartlett RH, Dechert RE, Clark SF, Swartz RD (1983) Starvation: A major contributor to mortality in acute renal failure? Trans Am Soc Artif Intern Organs 29: 390-395
3. Mault JR, Kresowik TF, Dechert RE, Arnoldi DK, Swartz RD, Bartlett RH (1984) Continuous arteriovenous hemofiltration: The answer to starvation in acute renal failure? Trans Am Soc Artif Intern Organs 30: 203-206
4. Kramer P, Kaufhold G, Grone HJ, Wigger W, Rieger J, Matthaei D, Stokke T, Buchardi H, Scheler F (1980) Management of anuric intensive care patients with arteriovenous hemofiltration. Int J Artif Organs 3: 225-230
5. Lauer A, Saccaggi A, Ronco C, Belledonne M, Glabman S, Bosch JP (1983) Continuous arteriovenous hemofiltration in the critically ill patient. Ann Intern Med 99: 450-460
6. Kaplan AA, Longnecker RE, Folkert VW (1984) Continuous arteriovenous hemofiltration. Ann Intern Med 100: 358-367
7. Askanazi J, Nordenstrom J, Rosenbaum SH, Elwyn DH, Hyman AI, Carpontier YA, Kinney JM (1981) Nutrition for the patient with respiratory failure: Glucose vs fat. Anesthesiology 54: 1373-1377
8. Harris JA, Benedict FG (1919) Biometric studies of basal metabolism in man. Carnegie Institute of Washington, Washington, DC (publication 279)
9. Willmore DW (1977) The metabolic management of the critically ill. Plenum Medical, New York
10. Bartlett RH, Dechert RE, Mault JR, Ferguson SK, Kaiser AM, Erlandson EE (1982) Measurement of metabolism in multiple organ failure. Surgery 92: 771-778
11. Siegel JH, Cerra FB, Coleman B, Giovannini I, Shetye M, Border JR, McMenamy RH (1979) Physical and metabolic correlations in human sepsis. Surgery 86: 163-193
12. Sargent J, Gotch F, Borah M, Piercy L, Spinozzi N, Schoenfeld P, Humphreys M (1978) Urea kinetics: A guide to nutritional management of acute renal failure. Am J Clin Nutr 31: 1696-1702
13. Feinstein EI, Blumenkrantz MJ, Healy M, Koffler A, Silberman H, Massry SG, Kopple JD (1981) Clinical and metabolic responses to parenteral nutrition in acute renal failure. Medicine 60: 124-137
14. Guyton AP (1981) Textbook of medical physiology. Saunders, Philadelphia, pp 882-885
15. Dinarello CA, Wolff SM (1982) Molecular basis of fever in humans: Am J Med 72: 799-819
16. Clowes GH Jr, Goerge BC, Villee CA Jr, Saravis CA (1983) Muscle proteolysis induced by a circulating peptide with sepsis or trauma. N Engl J Med 308: 545-552
17. Baracos V, Rodemann HP, Dinarello CA, Goldberg AL (1983) Stimulation of muscle protein degradation and prostaglandin E_2 release by leukocytic pyrogen (interleukin-1). N Engl J Med 308: 553-558
18. Bartlett RH, Dechert RE, Mault JR, Clark SF (1984) Metabolic studies in chest trauma. J Thorac Cardiovasc Surg 87: 503-508
19. Henderson LW, Koch KM, Dinarello CA, Shaldon S (1983) Hemodialysis hypotension: The interleukin hypothesis. Blood Purification 1: 3-8
20. Craddock PR, Fehr J, Brigham KL, Kronenberg RS, Jacob HS (1977) Complement and leukocyte-mediated pulmonary dysfunction in hemodialysis. N Engl J Med 296: 769-774

21. Sprieter SC, Myers BD, Swenson RS (1980) Protein-energy requirements in subjects with acute renal failure receiving hemodialysis. Am J Clin Nutr 33: 1433-1437
22. Asbach HW, Stoeckel H, Schuler HW, Conradi R, Wiedmann K, Mohring K, Rohl L (1974) The treatment of hypercatabolic acute renal failure by adequate nutrition and hemodialysis. Acta Anaesthiesiol Scand 18: 225-260
23. Kresowik TF, Dechert RE, Mault JR, Arnoldi DK, Whitehouse WM Jr, Bartlett RH (1984) Does nutritional support affect survival in critically ill patients? Surg Forum 35: 108-109
24. Brenner BM, Meyer TW, Hostetter TH (1982) Dietary protein intake and the progressive nature of kidney disease: The role of hemodynamically mediated glomerular injury in the pathogenesis of progressive glomerular sclerosis in aging, renal ablation, and intrinsic renal disease. N Engl J Med 307: 652-659
25. Abel RM, Clyde HB Jr, Abbott WM, Ryan JA, Barnett GO, Fischer JE (1973) Improved survival from acute renal failure after treatment with intravenous essential amino acids and glucose. N Engl J Med 288: 695-699
26. Kopple JD, Feinstein EI (1983) Current problems in amino acid therapy for acute renal failure. Proc Eur Dial Transplant Assoc 19: 129-140
27. Freund H, Atamian S, Fisher J (1980) Comparative study of parenteral nutrition in renal failure using essential and nonessential amino acid containing solutions. Surg Gynecol Obstet 151: 652-656
28. Blackburn GL, Etter G, Mackenzie T (1978) Criteria for choosing amino acid therapy in acute renal failure. Am J Clin Nutr 31: 1841-1853
29. Mirtallo JM, Schneider PJ, Mavko K, Ruberg RL, Fabri PJ (1982) A comparison of essential and general amino acid infusions in the nutritional support of patients with compromised renal function. JPEN 6: 109-113
30. Cerra FB, Mazuski JE, Chute E, Nuwer N, Teasley K, Jolynn L, Shronts EP, Konstantinides FN (1984) Branched chain metabolic support: A prospective, randomized, double-blind trial in surgical stress. Ann Surg 199: 286-291
31. Teschan PE, Abel RM, Conger JD, Kopple JD, Kramer P, Snider MT (1983) Acute renal failure versus nutrition: No free lunch in the ICU. Trans Am Soc Artif Intern Organs 29: 764-769
32. Kramer P, Bohler J, Kehr A, Grone HJ, Schrader J, Matthaei D, Scheler F (1982) Intensive care potential of continuous arteriovenous hemofiltration. Trans Am Soc Artif Intern Organs 28: 28-32
33. Paganini EP, Flaque J, Whitman G, Nakamoto S (1982) Amino acid balance in patients with oliguric acute renal failure undergoing slow continuous ultrafiltration (SCUF). Trans Am Soc Artif Intern Organs 28: 615-620

Hemodiafiltration

M. SCHMIDT

Table of Contents

Nomenclature

A	Membrane area (cm^2)	V	Distribution volume (l)
C	Concentration (mol/ml)	σ_s	Staverman reflection coefficient
Cl	Clearance (ml/min)	π	Osmotic pressure (bar)
D	Diffusion coefficient (cm^2/min)		
Dl	Dialysance (ml/min)		
K	Mass transfer coefficient	**Subscripts**	
N	Removal rate (mol/min)		
P	Permeability (cm/min)	B	Blood
Q	Flow rate (ml/min)	D	Dialysate
d	Wall thickness (μm)	E	Extracellular space
l_p	Specific hydrostatic permeability	F	Filtrate
	(cm^2/bar × min)	I	Intracellular space
n	Solute flux (mol/cm^2 × min)	IE	Intra- to extracellular transfer
p	Hydrostatic pressure (bar)	R	Kidney
q	Solvent flux (ml/cm^2 × min)	i	Value at the inlet port
t	Time	o	Value at the outlet port
$x, y\, z$	Cartesian coordinates	s	Solute

Introduction

Terminology

Hemodialysis eliminates solutes from the body by predominantly diffusive mass transfer, while hemofiltration is based on convective mass transfer. Hemodiafiltration is a method of blood purification which combines aspects of hemodialysis and hemofiltration. Solute removal occurs by both diffusion and convection across a selectively permeable membrane. The driving force for diffusion is the difference in concentration of the permeating substances in the blood and in the dialysate. The driving force for convection is the pressure gradient across the membrane, resulting in transport of water and permeating solutes from the blood to the dialysate. The fluid removed by this procedure is replaced by a sterile and nonpyrogenic substitution fluid of appropriate composition.

The actual term hemodiafiltration predates the technique with which it is associated today. Originally, the terms "hemodiafiltration," "diafiltration," and "hemofiltration" were used synonymously for the process which is now known as hemofiltration [1–3]. At a meeting in Braunlage, Federal Republic of Germany, in 1976, BURTON suggested that the terminology associated with hemofiltration be standardized, as summarized in [4]. Following a meeting in Gstaad, Switzerland, in 1977, a consensus was reached which called for the total abandonment of the term "hemodiafiltration." The process of combining features of hemodialysis and hemofiltration was to be called simultaneous hemofiltration/hemodialysis [5, 6]. Once "hemofiltration" had become universally accepted as the term for the process of solute removal via predominantly convective mechanisms, "hemodiafiltration" was reintroduced [7] with its current definition: simultaneous hemodialysis and hemofiltration with the use of replacement fluid [8].

However, care still has to be taken when using this term. For example, when reviewing literature one needs to clarify whether "hemodiafiltration" refers to hemofiltration (which it almost certainly does in work published prior to 1978) or to simultaneous hemofiltration/hemodialysis. In publications from the USSR, in some cases the term "hemodiafiltration" even refers to all kinds of hemodialysis with simultaneous ultrafiltration [9].

History

Dialysis with some concomitant ultrafiltration to achieve the required patient fluid loss during treatment has been used since the inception of dialysis. As early as 1929, HAAS in Gießen, (FRG) observed that his first patient to undergo hemodialysis lost 20% of his blood volume during the procedure [10], which was a consequence of ultrafiltration [11]. In the mid-1970s, with the advent of membranes of higher hydraulic permeability, interest arose in studying the effect of higher ultrafiltration rates during dialysis on both the efficiency of the technique with respect to solute removal and on potential procedural side effects. This was motivated by the "middle molecule hypothesis," which advocated enhanced clearance for solutes of a size between 300 and 3000 daltons [12, 13], and by the observation that hemodynamic stability was higher in procedures with mainly convective fluid removal, such as hemofiltration [14-16] or sequential ultrafiltration and hemodialysis [17].

The concept of hemodiafiltration in the sense of the definition given above was already realized in 1969 by SHINABERGER et al. [18], who used saline infusions to limit the concentration polarization occurring at high ultrafiltration rates. Seven years later, KUNITOMO started to advocate hemodiafiltration, which he at that point called "pre-dilution dialysis" [19,20]. In 1977, he reported his first clinical experiences [21, 22]. Almost simultaneously, two West German groups presented their initial in vitro and in vivo results [23, 24]. From 1978 on, results of long-term experiences with the new technique have been available from the Federal Republic of Germany and Japan [25, 26].

According to statistics collected by the European Dialysis and Transplantation Association, the total number of patients on hemodiafiltration in Europe on 31 December, 1983 was 1127, in comparison to 1740 on hemofiltration, 76179 on some form of hemodialysis, and 6695 on variants of peritoneal dialysis [27]. In April 1979, the estimated number of patients on hemodiafiltration in Japan was 134, compared to 182 on hemofiltration [28]. In the United States, the treatment has not yet received official clinical approval and is therefore limited to experimental procedures.

Theoretical Aspects

Clearance Determination

A schematic diagram of mass transfer in a dialyzer is given in Fig. 1. Nomenclature is defined at the beginning of this chapter.

Clearance in hemodiafiltration, as in any other form of blood-purifying process, is defined as the ratio of the solute removal rate (N_s) to the concentration of the solute at the inlet of the device (C_{s_i}). Solute clearance (Cl_s) in the device shown in Fig. 1 can be expressed as:

$$Cl_s = \frac{N_s}{C_{s_i}} \tag{1}$$

This is an exact analogy to the clearance concept in renal physiology [29] and can be visualized as the total volume of blood which is completely cleared of the respective solute per unit of time.

Assuming steady-state conditions, N_s can be calculated as:

$$N_s = Q_{B_i} \times C_{B_i} - Q_{B_o} \times C_{B_o} = Q_{D_o} \times C_{D_o} - Q_{D_i} \times C_{D_i} \tag{2}$$

The filtration rate (Q_F) is given by:

$$Q_F = Q_{B_i} - Q_{B_o} = Q_{D_o} - Q_{D_i} \tag{3}$$

By combining Eqs. 1, 2, and 3, the expression for whole-blood clearance in hemodiafiltration can be rewritten as:

$$Cl_s = Q_{B_i} \times \frac{C_{B_i} - C_{B_o}}{C_{B_i}} + Q_F \times \frac{C_{B_o}}{C_{B_i}} \tag{4}$$

In systems where dialysate is being recirculated, the dialysance (Dl_s) is a more useful parameter for determining dialyzer performance:

$$Dl_s = \frac{N_s}{C_{B_i} - C_{D_i}} \tag{5}$$

For hemodiafiltration, dialysance can be expressed as:

$$Dl_s = Q_{B_i} \times \frac{C_{B_i} - C_{B_o}}{C_{B_i} - C_{D_i}} + Q_F \times \frac{C_{B_o}}{C_{B_i} - C_{D_i}} \tag{6}$$

Clearance and dialysance for a specific solute can be determined by methods analogous to those used to measure clearance and dialysance in conventional hemodialysis. Solute concentrations and flow rates can be determined at blood and dialysate

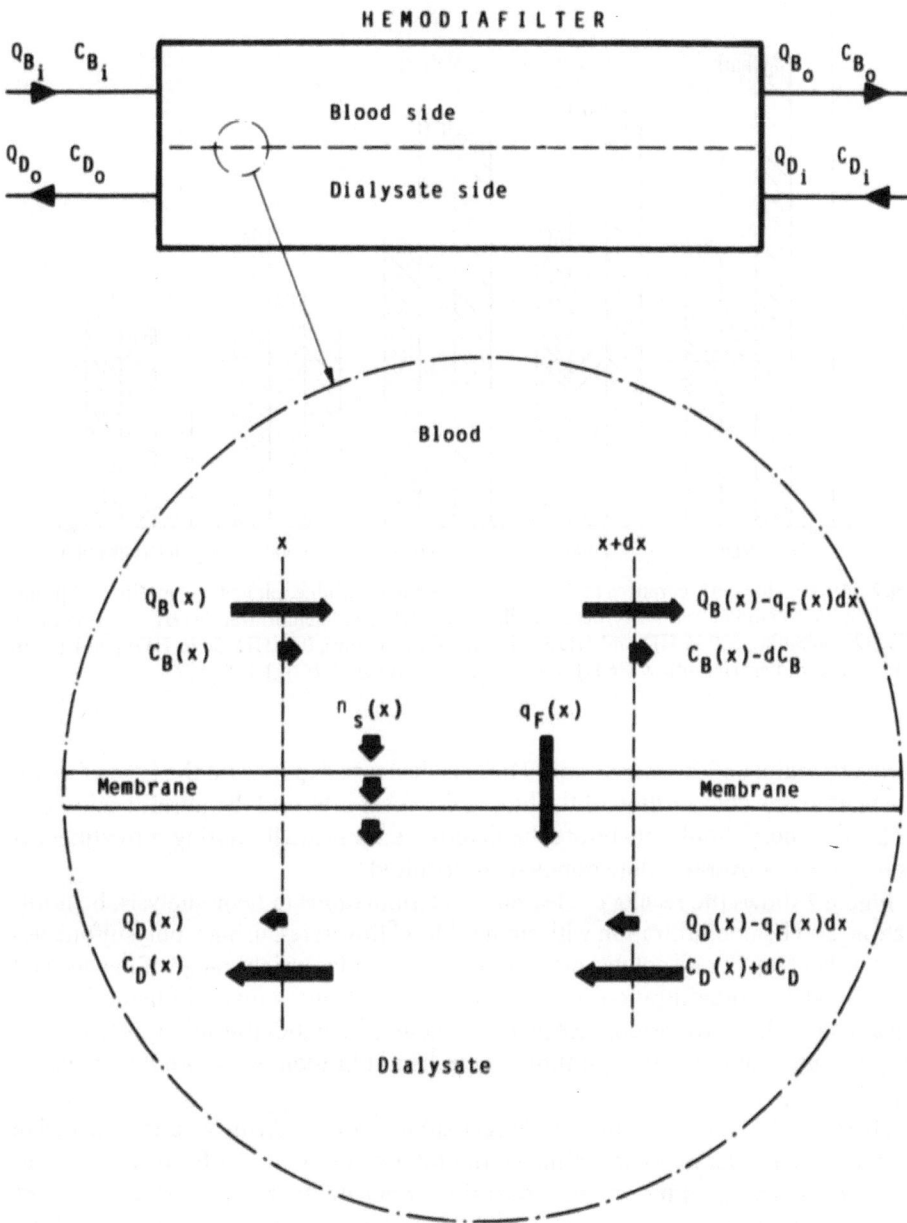

Fig. 1. Schematic diagram of mass transfer in a dialyzer

inlet and outlet ports, either in steady state for smaller molecules (below 300 daltons) or in a recirculating system for substances of higher molecular weight [30–32].

Under certain assumptions, solute clearance can also be calculated from the change in mean arterial concentration of the solute during the treatment [33].

In the course of a hemodiafiltration procedure clearance values can decrease, primarily as a result of a decline in the filtration rate and sieving coefficients with time,

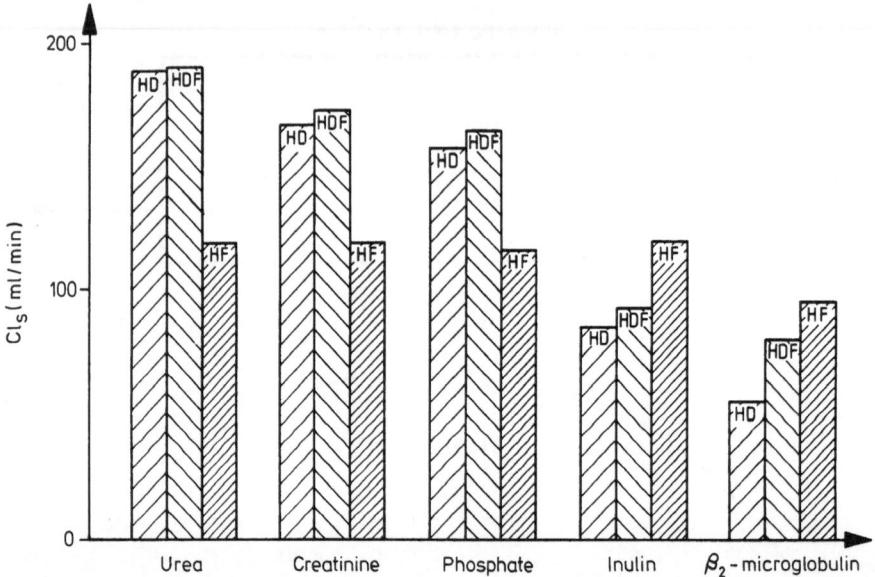

Fig. 2. Average in vivo clearances in 12 patients for urea, creatinine, phosphate, inulin, and β_2-microglobulin in hemodialysis *(HD)*, hemodiafiltration *(HDF)*, and hemofiltration *(HF)*. Q_B (ml/min), 200; Q_D (ml/min), 500 in HD and HDF, 0 in HF; Q_F (ml/min), 0 in HD, 50 in HDF, and 120 in HF; hemodiafilter: Hemoflow F 60 (Fresenius AG, Oberursel, FRG) [36]

owing to fouling of the membrane [34]. This decrease depends on the type of membrane used, the composition of the blood, the shear rate, and the ultrafiltration rate [35]. Clearances should, therefore, be determined repeatedly during a treatment if exact values of overall solute removal are required.

Figure 2 shows the results of clearance determinations in hemodialysis, hemofiltration, and hemodiafiltration with similar blood flow rates, using a polysulfone hemodiafilter [36]. For all solutes measured in a molecular weight range of between 60 and 13 000, hemodiafiltration resulted in higher clearances than did hemodialysis. Clearance in hemofiltration exceeded the value in hemodiafiltration only for the larger solutes, although the filtration rate in hemofiltration was more than twice as high.

These results also show that the direct summation of diffusive and convective clearances considerably overestimates the total solute removal by hemodiafiltration. For dialyzers with very high diffusive permeability, the additional effect of high ultrafiltration rates on the clearance is almost negligible for molecules of the size of urea or creatinine [37, 38].

Diffusive and Convective Solute Transport

In discussing the interaction between diffusion and convection in more detail, it is helpful to consider first the general transport equations across a selectively permeable membrane separating two homogeneous, isothermal solutions. On this basis the situation in a typical dialyzer, in which flow rates, pressure gradients, and concentration gradients vary along the length of the device, can be elaborated.

Assuming a homogeneous membrane with the area A, the thickness d, and well-mixed solutions on both sides, transport processes across it can be described using the laws of thermodynamics of irreversible processes [39-42].

The driving force for diffusive solute flux is the concentration gradient across the membrane. Solute flux, defined as rate of solute transport per unit of area, can be expressed as:

$$n_s = D_s \times \frac{\partial c}{\partial y} \tag{7}$$

Integrating Eq. 7 across the membrane and over the entire membrane area to obtain the solute removal rate results in:

$$N_s = P_s \times (C_B - C_D) \tag{8}$$

where (P_s) is the diffusive permeability of the membrane for the respective solute.

The driving force for convective transport is the pressure gradient, resulting in a local solvent (water) flux of

$$q_F = l_p \times \frac{\partial p}{\partial y} \tag{9}$$

where l_p ist the specific hydrostatic permeability characterizing the local ultrafiltration coefficient of a membrane. The pressure gradient across the selectively permeable membrane is the result of both hydraulic and osmotic pressures. The total filtration rate across the membrane can be expressed as:

$$Q_F = l_p \times A \times \{(P_B - P_D) - \sigma_s \times (\pi_B - \pi_D)\} \tag{10}$$

where σ_s is the reflection coefficient, which takes values of 1 for solutes to which the membrane is impermeable and 0 for solutes which are not rejected by the membrane at all (compare OFSTHUN and COLTON, this volume). It was introduced by STAVERMAN [43] to describe the difference between an ideally semipermeable membrane (no permeability for solutes, only for the solvent) and real, selectively permeable membrane (permeable to both solvent and, in varying degrees, to some solutes).

The reflection coefficient can be defined as the ratio of the actual hydrostatic pressure required to stop volume flow across a selectively permeable membrane to the osmotic pressure as calculated theoretically using van't Hoff's equation for the osmotic pressure across an ideally semipermeable membrane:

$$\sigma_s = \lim_{q_F \to 0} \frac{(P_B - P_D)}{(\pi_B - \pi_D)} \tag{11}$$

The total solute flow (N_s) resulting from the water flow across the membrane can be written as:

$$N_s = Q_F \times (1 - \sigma_s) \times C_B \tag{12}$$

If diffusion and convection occur simultaneously, the laws of thermodynamics of irreversible processes allow the summation of the local contributions of diffusion and convection to give overall solute transfer [44]. One might intuitively assume that this also allows Eqs. 8 and 11 to be combined, resulting in

$$N_s = P_s \times (C_B - C_D) + Q_F \times (1 - \sigma_s) \times C_B \tag{13}$$

However, in membranes used for blood purification Eq. 13 is not valid. Diffusion and convection occur simultaneously within the same membrane pores and not independently in different pores, as one would have to assume by integrating both contributions separately. An appropriate expression for solute flux with combined diffusion and convection has been suggested by VILLAROEL et al. [45]:

$$N_s = P_s \times (C_B - C_D) + Q_F \times (1 - \sigma_s) \times \hat{C}_B, \text{ where } \hat{C}_B = \frac{(C_B - C_D)}{\ln(C_B / C_D)} \tag{14}$$

$\hat{C}_B$ is an appropriately defined mean concentration within the membrane. The difference between the concepts of macroscopic and local additivity is reflected in the difference between Eqs. 13 and 14. For the same boundary conditions, a lower rate of solute flux is predicted by Eq. 14 than by Eq. 13. This can be attributed to a reduction in the rate of diffusion across the membrane owing to the reduced residence time for a volume element traversing the membrane. Thus, increasing the convective contribution results in a decreased diffusive contribution.

Thus far, a homogeneous membrane separating any two well-mixed and isothermal solutions has been considered. When analyzing dialyzer performance, the concept of adding diffusive and convective mass transfer components is further invalidated. In dialyzers with counter-current blood and dialysate flows, the assumption of constant concentrations along the length of the membrane is not valid. As solutes diffuse from blood to dialysate their blood concentration diminishes, so that the amount of solute convectively removed near the blood outlet is significantly decreased when compared to convective solute removal near the blood inlet. Also, with high ultrafiltration rates and imperfect dialysate flow patterns, the concentration of the solute at the membrane surface on the dialysate side may increase, reducing the driving force for diffusive transport. Furthermore, with coil-type dialyzers and parallel-plate dialyzers, an increase in transmembrane pressure can result in a decrease in diffusive clearance. The latter is caused by loss of total membrane area owing to expansion of the blood channels, masking of the membrane surface, and channeling of the dialysate flow [46–48]. Concentration polarization and the decrease in hydraulic permeability during the process further complicate the situation [6, 49, 50].

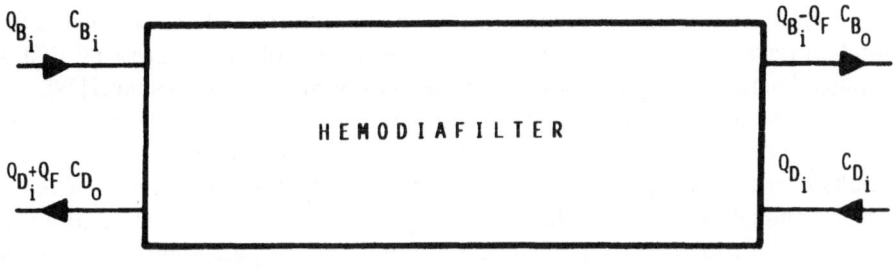

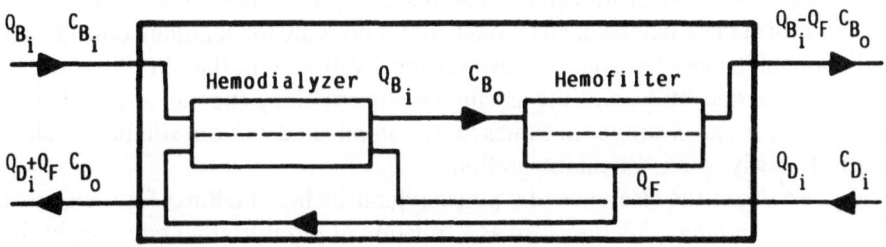

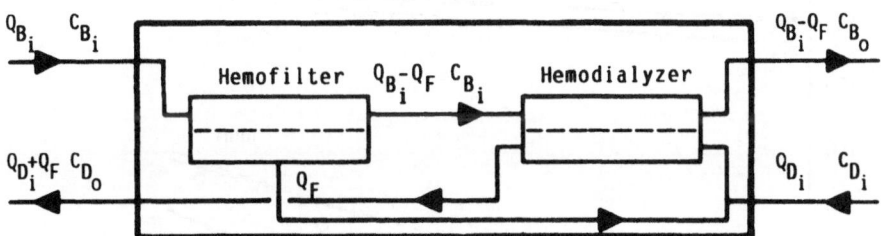

Fig. 3. Schematic diagram of a black-box approach toward hemodiafiltration, where the convective and the diffusive processes are assumed to occur not simultaneously, but in two separate devices (model of Granger et al. [66] and Vantard [79])

Clearance Prediction

Neither Eqs. 4 and 5 nor the basic transport equation (14) are of any use in predicting solute clearance of a specific hemodiafilter with a membrane of known area, geometry, and permeabilities under given operating conditions.

For hemodialysis, a wide variety of theoretical models are available which describe the relationship between the operating parameters, design criteria, characteristic membrane properties, and solute clearance of a hemodialyzer [51–58]. None of these models can be used in the case of hemodiafiltration, as they all neglect the convective term in their basic transport equations.

Therefore, most groups studying systems which combine dialysis with high ultra-filtration rates have developed their own model to describe the process [59–78]. A detailed description of many of these models has been given by VANTARD [79].

One of the simplest models was suggested by GRANGER et al. [66], who treat the hemodiafilter as a black box, in which hemodialysis and hemofiltration occur not simultaneously, but separately, in two different filters. Their model is depicted in Fig. 3. Although these assumptions certainly oversimplify the process and are in sharp contradiction to the arguments discussed in the last paragraph of the section on diffusive and convective solute transport, the model allows a surprisingly good first approximation of the effect of ultrafiltration on total solute clearance.

A theoretically more appropriate approach has been introduced by SIGDELL [77], who integrates the local transport equation along the length of the dialyzer (see Fig. 1 for local mass balance). His model allows not only for simultaneous diffusive and convective mass transfer, but also for local variation in the ultrafiltration, the membrane permeability, and the sieving coefficient along the membrane. His expression for solute clearance becomes more complicated, but can still be calculated relatively easily by numerical integration.

Figure 4 shows the clearance of a polyacrylonitrile hemodiafilter for urea, creatinine, inulin, and myoglobin in vitro as a function of ultrafiltration rate. The broken

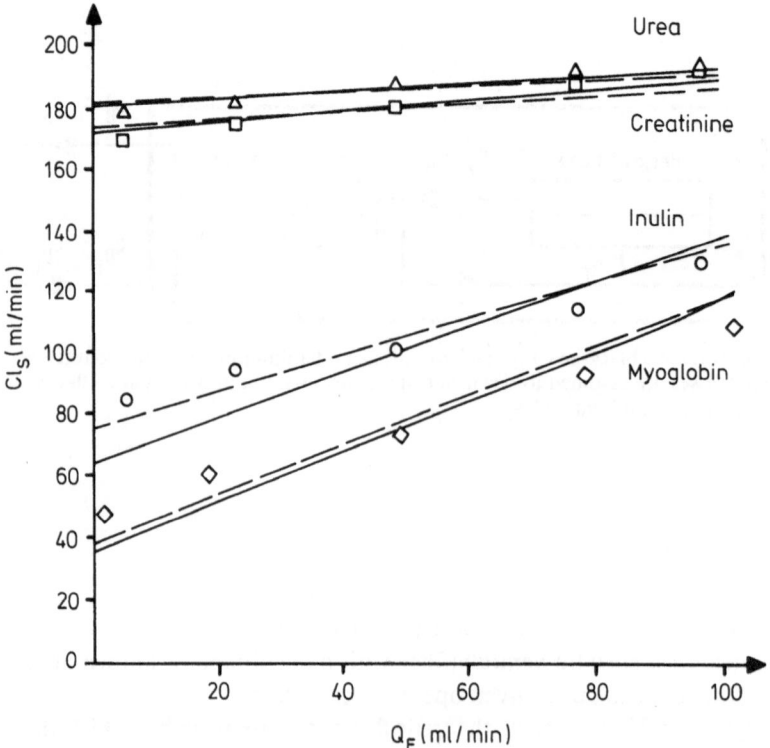

Fig. 4. Average in vitro clearances in five parallel experiments for urea, creatinine, inulin, and myoglobin (daltons) as a function of ultrafiltration rate. Q_B (ml/min), 200; Q_D (ml/min), 500; hemodiafilter: PAN 250 (Asahi Medical, Tokyo, Japan); *broken line*, clearance prediction from [66]; *continuous line*, clearance prediction from [77]

line shows the prediction of Granger's model, the continuous line that of SIGDELL's model.

Variation of dialyzer performance with different production lots is sometimes far greater than the differences in the values predicted by the different models. In addition, in the actual in vivo situation, especially with high-flux hemodiafiltration, clearance varies not only from patient to patient, but has also a time dependency during the treatment [80]. Therefore, the question as to what degree of precision has to be achieved by these models under clinical conditions remains to be answered. If the removal rates of different solutes need to be precisely known, for example for the kinetic modeling of hemodiafiltration, it is recommended that the clearance of a hemodiafilter as a function of time be determined again for each patient under the operating conditions of the treatment [81].

Kinetic Modeling of Hemodiafiltration

One of the arguments in favor of hemodiafiltration is its potential for optimal individualization of therapy by the achievement of appropriate clearances for the different solutes, varying the composition of dialysate and substitution fluid and choosing the operating parameters according to the patient's needs and the technical feasibility (blood flow, etc.). As in standard hemodialysis, an individualized prescription of doses of "hemodiafiltration" requires not only a model of solute removal through the hemodiafilter, but also information about intake, generation rates, intracompartmental transfer and distribution coefficients, distribution volumes, and residual renal clearance for the different solutes in question in the individual patient.

Although the clinical benefits of kinetic modeling remain controversial, it is of great importance in evaluating the possibilities for high-performance hemodiafiltration with reduced treatment times [82]. The lower time limit for any such procedure is presented by the maximal physiological transfer rates between the different compartments, as a fast clearing of the extracellular volume does not necessarily imply sufficient removal of toxic substances from the intracellular pool [83]. Kinetic modeling could thus help in determining the minimal dialysis time for sufficient treatment.

An overview of the existing literature, the different models available, and the necessary transport parameters has recently been published by SPRENGER et al. [84]. They differentiate between sophisticated models which are used as a research tool to evaluate the quantitative validity of proposed physiological mechanisms, and models for routine clinical application which need to achieve a satisfactory predictive value with a minimum of variables to be measured.

Single-pool models assume a uniform distribution of the marker solute in one homogenous compartment, normally of the size of total body water [85, 86]. The time change of the solute concentration in this pool can then be calculated by solving the differential equation

$$\frac{d}{dt}\{V(t) \times C_B(t)\} = -Cl_s(t) \times C_B(t) - Cl_R \times C_B(t) + G \tag{15}$$

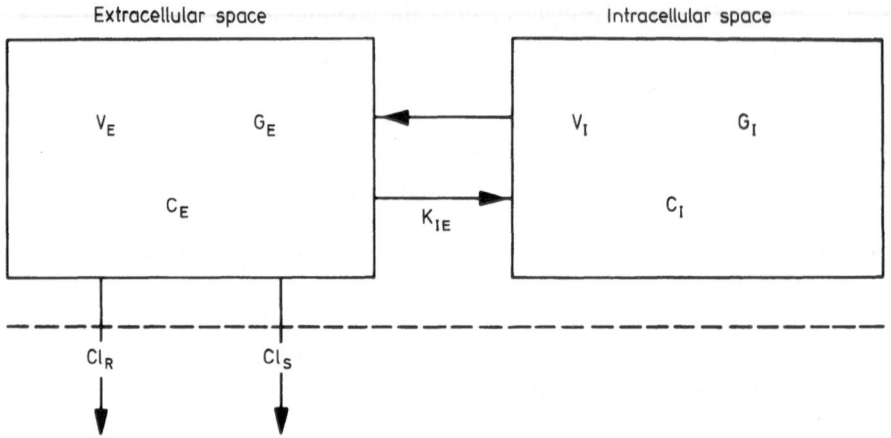

Extracellular space   Intracellular space

Fig. 5. Schematic diagram of a two-pool model for describing solute kinetics during hemodiafiltration [85]

The generation rate *(G)* is generally used not as a measurable quantity, but as a parameter to fit the concentration changes to the actual measurements.

For a more exact description of the rebound of the concentration of different solutes after the end of the treatment, two-pool or even multiple-pool models have been suggested [87-89]. The latter have not yet gained clinical importance, as lack of data on transport and distribution coefficients and other parameters limits their applicability [84].

KUNITOMO et al., the first group to apply kinetic modeling in hemodiafiltration [90], used a two-pool model [87] for the calculation of the weekly profile of intra- and extracellular concentrations of urea, vitamin B_{12}, and inulin, both in the transition period from 3×5 h standard hemodialysis to 3×3 h of hemodiafiltration, and in the steady state of hemodiafiltration. The model predicts a significant lowering of intracellular concentrations of inulin and vitamin B_{12} as a marker for "middle molecules" when the patient is transferred from hemodialysis to hemodiafiltration. A steady state is reached after about 4 weeks.

Figure 5 shows a schematic representation of a two-pool model. The equations in this case under certain assumptions can be written as:

$$V_I \frac{dC_I}{dt} = G_I - K_{IE} \times (C_I - C_E) \tag{16a}$$

$$V_E \frac{dC_E}{dt} = G_E + K_{IE} \times (C_I - C_E) - (Cl_s + Cl_R) \times C_E \tag{16b}$$

with the solutions:

$$C_I = R_I \times \exp\{-(\alpha-\beta)t\} + S_I \times \exp\{-(\alpha+\beta)t\} + T_I \tag{17a}$$

$$C_E = R_E \times \exp\{-(\alpha-\beta)t\} + S_E \times \exp\{-(\alpha+\beta)t\} + T_E \tag{17b}$$

where R, S, and T are constants derived from the integration of the respective differential equation. While for the description of urea kinetics a single-pool model is sufficient [91], a two-pool model should be chosen for modeling creatinine, uric acid, vitamin B_{12}, and inulin [84].

Technical Aspects

Monitoring Systems

The first clinical experience with hemodiafiltration was gathered using a wide variety of equipment, which in general was based on conventional dialysis machines to which some modification had been made to allow ultrafiltration control and delivery of a substitution fluid.

Figure 6 shows the simplest method of performing hemodiafiltration. The patient's fluid loss can be controlled by manually adjusting the negative pressure on the dialysate side of the dialyzer and the rate of infusion of substitution fluid. Such a system has been used for a short clinical study [92]. LEBER et al. used a similar set-up in their initial studies [93], where transmembrane pressure was controlled using a double-pump system which increased the pressure on the blood side within the dialyzer.

A necessary prerequisite for routine clinical application of hemodiafiltration was the availability of automated monitoring devices to minimize user intervention and maximize patient safety.

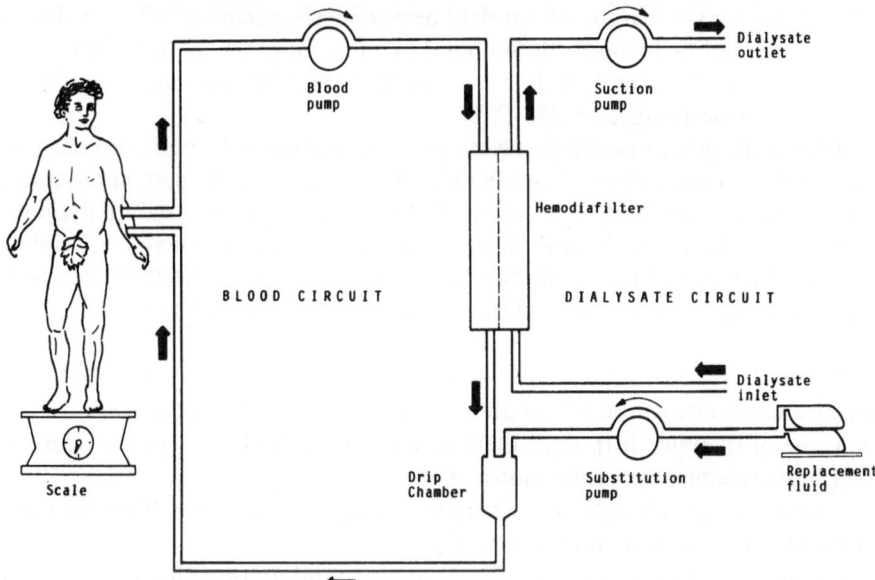

Fig. 6. Schematic diagram of a simple circuit for performing hemodiafiltration

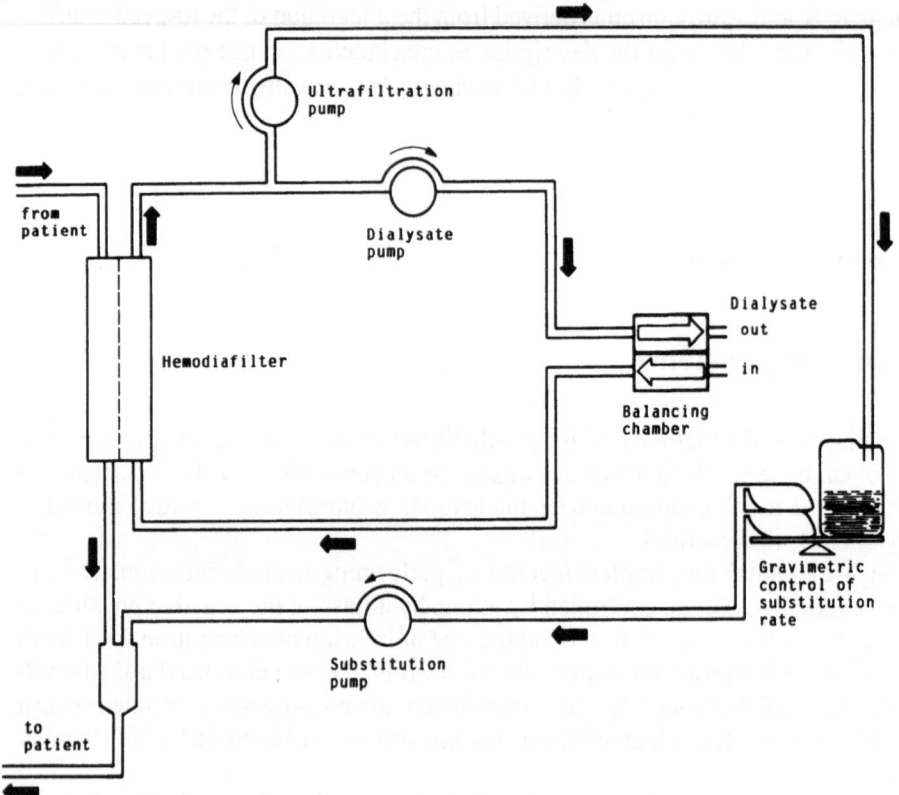

Fig. 7. Schematic diagram of a monitor for automatic control of hemodiafiltration (A 2008 HDF, Fresenius AG, Oberursel, FRG)

In addition to the features of standard hemodialysis machines [94], a machine capable of monitoring hemodiafiltration has to allow for exact control of the rates of ultrafiltration and substitution. For the control of ultrafiltration rate, many different methods have been suggested [95–97].

Many of the groups investigating the possible benefits of hemodiafiltration have used the Cotral controller (Rhone-Poulenc, Paris, France). The system has a dialysate reservoir containing 1200 ml of dialysate; 1000 ml of used dialysate are replaced by 1000 ml of fresh dialysate at a rate which is a function of dialysate flow rate. The replenishment of dialysate takes place every 2 min if the device dialysate flow rate is 500 ml/min. Ultrafiltration rates of 7200 ml/h can be achieved [98].

The disadvantages of this system are the periodic mixing of "used" with fresh dialysate and the interruption of all transport processes across the dialyzer during the exchange of dialysate [81]. Both these factors diminish efficacy of treatment and complicate clearance determination [99].

Single-pass dialysate delivery systems providing controlled ultrafiltration may be preferable to the recirculating system [35].

As a function of the desired fluid loss and the ultrafiltration rate, the rate of substitution of infusion fluid can be calculated from:

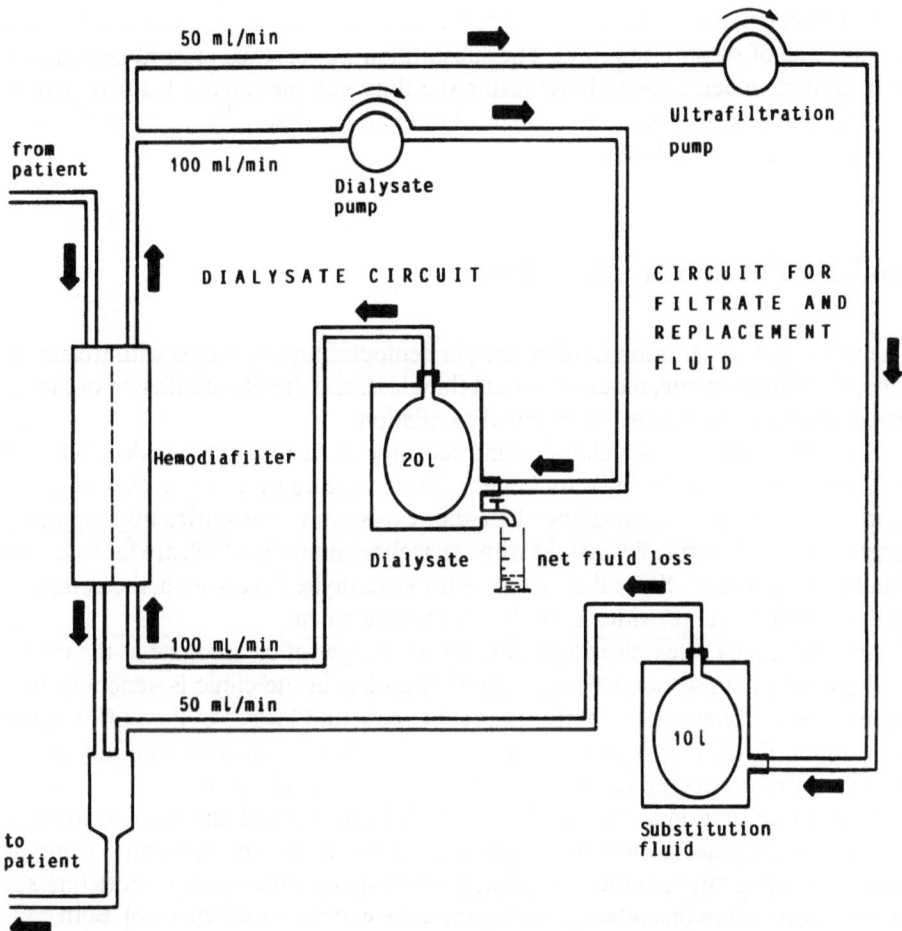

Fig.8. Schematic diagram of a closed circuit for low-flow hemodiafiltration, as devised by Van Geelen et al. [102]

$$\text{Infusion rate} = \text{Filtration rate} - \left(\frac{\text{Total fluid loss}}{\text{Treatment time}}\right) \tag{18}$$

Exact control of fluid substitution rates is generally based on a gravitational method borrowed from hemofiltration. A microprocessor is used to calculate the fluid substitution rate as a function of the chosen ultrafiltration rate, net fluid loss, and treatment time. Figure 7 shows a schematic diagram of a typical clinical monitor for hemodiafiltration with volumetric control of ultrafiltration rate and gravimetric control of substitution rate.

A completely different approach was chosen by VAN GEELEN to achieve low-flow hemodiafiltration [100, 101]. He devised a closed-volume system with two airtight tanks; a schematic diagram is given in Fig.8. At the beginning of treatment, 20 l of dialysate float in a PVC bag in liquid in one tank, and 10 l of sterile and nonpyrogenic substitution fluid float in another PVC bag in liquid in the second tank. Dialysate is pumped from the PVC bag through the dialyzer into the tank containing the bag. Another pump draws liquid from the dialysate into the tank containing the floating bag of substitution fluid. The substitution fluid is thus pressed into the venous drip chamber, accurately replacing the fluid volume removed. If the patient should have a net fluid loss, additional volume can be withdrawn from the dialysate circuit through a valve [103].

Dialysis and Substitution Fluid

The volume of substitution fluid needed in hemodiafiltration varies with treatment time, ultrafiltration rate, required patient fluid loss, and the site of infusion of the replacement fluid into the extracorporeal circulation.

The composition of both dialysate and substitution fluid can vary widely between different centers (see Table 1). As in hemofiltration, care needs to be exercised not to induce an electrolyte imbalance by either excessively or insufficiently replacing large volumes of extracellular fluid with electrolyte solutions which are far from optimal in composition. Since the clearance for electrolytes is very high, the composition of the dialysate provides a baseline for the treatment.

Although many researchers agree on the advantages of bicarbonate as the buffer in dialysate or substitution fluid, hemodiafiltration in the clinic is generally performed using acetate as the buffer in the dialysate and lactate as the buffer in the substitution fluid. This is partially due to registration regulations, partially to the complexity of producing stable i. v. fluids containing bicarbonate.

As in hemofiltration and hemodialysis, the influence of sodium concentration on vascular stability has aroused great interest, with some groups suggesting hemodiafiltration using "hypertonic" solutions [110–114] and other groups modeling sodium concentration (osmolarity) during the course of the treatment [115]. Both concepts have recently also been realized with a commercial industrial monitor for hemodiafiltration [116].

The site of administration of the substitution fluid can be either before (predilution) or after (postdilution) the hemodiafilter. In some cases, substitution fluid has been given between two hemodiafilters. The same arguments for (more efficient removal of substances of high molecular weight [117]) and against (the need for more substitution fluid [118]) pre-dilution pertain in hemodiafiltration as in hemofiltration. In clinical practice with the current automated monitors, postdilution is almost exclusively used.

Because of the cost of the substitution fluid, both for hemodiafiltration and for hemofiltration, interest has arisen in on-line production of the substitution fluid [119–124]. If such a procedure were risk-free and inexpensive, then predilution could again be of clinical interest. On-line production of substitution fluid can be achieved by the filtration of unsterile dialysate through bacterial and pyrogen filters [115, 126].

A recently developed system for on-line substitution fluid production is shown in Fig. 9. This system is based on bicarbonate-containing dialysate and has been successful in achieving very high clearance rates [128, 129]. However, long-term clinical experience is still lacking. Although less substitution fluid is needed in hemodiafil-

Table 1. Constitution of dialysate and substitution fluid

		Reference							
		Cambi et al. 1981 [104]	Kohnle et al. 1979 [98]	Kunitomo et al. 1978 [90]	Leber et al. 1978 [105]	Ota et al. 1978 [106]	Sprenger et al. 1981 [107]	Von Albertini et al. 1984 [108]	Wizemann et al. 1983 [109]
Dialysate									
Sodium	(mmol/l)	130.0	140.0	131.0	138.0	132.0	143.0	140.0	143.0
Potassium	(mmol/l)	2.0	33.0	1.5	2.0	2.0	2.5	2.0	2.0
Calcium	(mmol/l)	2.0	1.5	1.6	1.8	1.9	1.8	2.3	1.8
Magnesium	(mmol/l)	0.8	0.5	0.5	0.5	0.8	1.0	0.4	1.0
Chloride	(mmol/l)	112.5	111.0	103.8	112.5	105.0	116.0	108.2	115.0
Bicarbonate	(mmol/l)	–	–	–	–	–	–	35.0	–
Acetate	(mmol/l)	25.0	36.0	33.0	32.0	33.0	35.0	4.0	35.0
Glucose	(mmol/l)	5.5	–	–	16.7	11.1	–	5.6	11.1
Osmolarity	(mosm/l)	282.0	292.0	273.5	304.0	286.0	299.0	297.5	309.0
Substitution fluid									
Sodium	(mmol/l)	275.0	142.0	142.0	135.0	138.0	142.0	Filtered dialysate	140.0
Potassium	(mmol/l)	–	–	2.0	2.0	2.0–3.0	1.0		2.0
Calcium	(mmol/l)	–	2.0	1.5	1.9	1.9	2.0		2.1
Magnesium	(mmol/l)	–	0.8	–	1.0	0.8	0.8		0.8
Chloride	(mmol/l)	150.0	103.0	131.5	102.7	107.5	103.0		112.0
Bicarbonate	(mmol/l)	125.0	–	–	–	–	–		–
Lactate	(mmol/l)	–	44.5	14.0	40.0	34.0	44.5		35.8
Glucose	(mmol/l)	–	–	–	30.5	3.8	–		8.3
Osmolarity	(mosm/l)	550.0	300.5	289.0	310.0	289.0	302.5		301.0

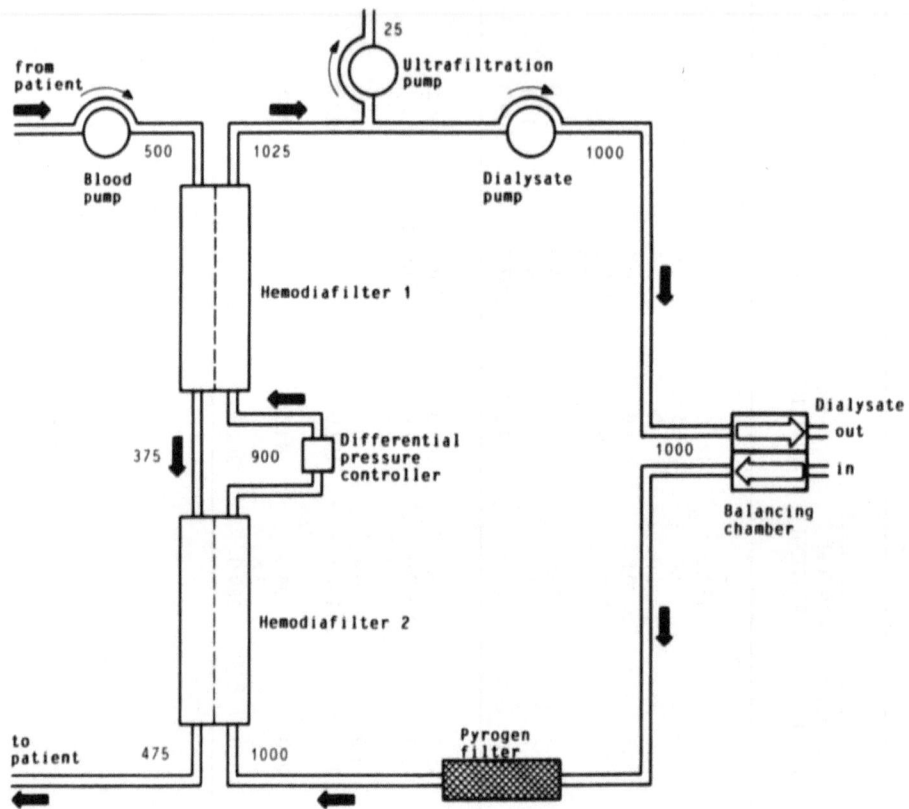

Fig. 9. Schematic diagram of a system for on-line production of bicarbonate-containing substitution fluid showing flow rates, as suggested by Miller et al. [127]

tration than in hemofiltration, the same precautions and safety aspects have to be observed (see EISENBACH and SHALDON, this volume).

Hemodiafiltration is defined as a combination of hemodialysis with ultrafiltration and substitution of replacement fluid. As it was shown that under certain operating conditions an internal backfiltration of dialysate into the patient's blood occurs [130], there has recently been discussion as to whether hemodialysis with highly permeable membranes should be considered to be some form of hemodiafiltration with on-line production of substitution fluid [131]. All publications dealing with this subject agree that for low net ultrafiltration rates some backfiltration can occur within every highly permeable dialyzer. The quantity of the effect remains controversial. Estimations vary between 4 ml/min and 20 ml/min at zero net ultrafiltration rate with conventional two-needle dialysis [132–139]. In certain single-needle systems, the amount of backfiltration can be estimated to be above these values, owing to pressures on the dialysate side being above the pressures on the blood side of the dialyzer [140, 141].

According to the definitions of terms given at the beginning of this chapter, some modifications of the hemofiltration technique could also be called hemodiafiltration [142], such as "hemofiltration without substitution fluid" [143] and "hemofiltration with dialysis-regeneration of ultrafiltrate" [144].

Membranes

An optimal membrane for hemodiafiltration has to combine high hydraulic with good diffusive permeability. From a purist's point of view, most of the membrane materials used for the production of hemofilters are not ideal, as large inner pores, asymmetry, and too great a wall thickness affect diffusive transport negatively (stagnant layers, large diffusive barrier). Homogeneous, highly permeable materials might therefore be advantageous; examples are Cuprophan, which can be produced with sufficient hydraulic permeability for the purposes of hemodiafiltration [145], or synthetic polymers such as certain polysulfone membranes (Fig. 10).

On the other hand, most of today's devices for "high-flux" dialysis with ultrafiltration coefficients above 10 ml/h/mmHg can be and have been used for hemodia-

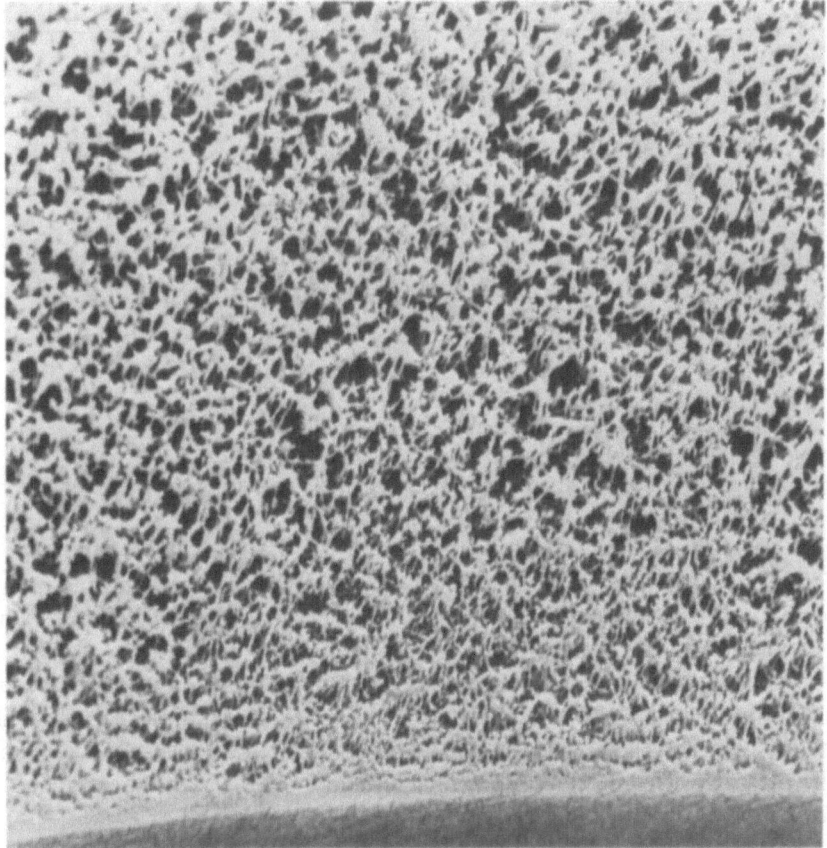

Fig. 10. Raster electron-microscopic photograph of a cross section of a polysulfone hollow-fiber membrane used in hemodiafilters (Fresenius AG, Oberursel, FRG)

Table 2. Technical specifications of different hemodiafilters (manufacturer's information)

1. Capillary dialyzers

Manu-facturer	Filter type	Membrane material	Effective surface area (m²)	Inner diameter (µm)	Wall thickness (µm)	Ultra-filtration coefficient (ml/ h × mmHg)
Asahi Medical	HFD 30	Polyacrylo-nitrile	1.3	200	50	9
	HFD 40	nitrile	1.4	200	50	18
	PAN 150		1.1	200	55	14
	PAN 200		1.4	200	55	21
	PAN 250		1.8	200	55	27
CD Medical	Duo-Flux	Cellulose acetate	1.4	220	30	15
Fresenius	Hemoflow D 6	Cuprophan	2.0	150	8	15
	Hemoflow F 40	Polysulfone	0.7	200	40	20
	Hemoflow F 60	Polysulfone	1.3	200	40	40
Secon	212 E	Cuprophan	1.6	150	8	16
Toray	Filtryzer B-1-L	Polymethyl-	2.1	240	32	20
	Filtryzer B-1-M	methacrylate	1.4	240	40	11

2. Plate dialyzers

Manu-facturer	Filter type	Membrane material	Effective surface area (m²)	Membrane thickness (µm)	Ultra-filtration coefficient (ml/h × mmHg)
Gambro	Lundia Major high-flux	Cuprophan	1.4	19–20	11
	5 HF		1.0	16	14
	6 HF		1.4	16	20
Hospal	RP 6	AN 69	1.0	30	12
	RP 610		1.0	30	12
	Biospal 1200 S		0.5	22	22
	Biospal 1800 S		0.7	22	29
	Biospal 2400 S		1.0	22	42
	Biospal 3000 S		1.2	22	50

filtration (see Table 2). Some of the producers of hemofilters limit their market by supplying their devices in a housing with only one outlet for the filtrate, so that they cannot be used in a dialysis mode.

Although many of the initial studies on hemodiafiltration were done using flat-sheet membranes, there are some arguments in favor of the use of hollow-fiber he-modiafilters [146]. One reason is the increase in channel width in a plate dialyzer as the pressure difference across the membrane rises, along with the potential risk of formation of channels on the dialysate side [47, 147, 148].

Table 3. Operating parameters and clearances in hemodiafiltration

	Low-flow hemodiafiltration			Standard hemodiafiltration						
Reference	Granger et al. 1978 [66]	Vantelon 1979 [149]		Van Geelen et al. 1983 [150]	Kirkwood et al. 1978 [151]	Leber et al. 1978 [105]	Ota et al. 1978 [106]	Kohnle et al. 1979 [98]		
Hemodiafilter	RP6	RP6		RP610	Filtryzer B-1-M	RP-6	Filtryzer B-1	RP-6		
Treatment/week (min)	3 × 240	3 × 240	3 × 240	3 × 210	3 × 180	3 × 180	3 × 180	3 × 210	3 × 210	3 × 210
Flow rates (ml/min)										
Blood				200	200	200	200	200	200	300
Dialysate	83	80	42	100	500	900	500	500	1000	1000
Filtrate	21	20	62	50–60	50	55	55	60–70	60–70	60–70
Clearances (ml/min)										
Urea	87	88	93	91	159	140	139	140	155	182
Creatinine	80			74		138	122	125	137	155
Uric Acid						100	108	117	120	138
Phosphate						73		105	110	120
Vitamin B	48	52	65		87.7					
Inulin	26	37	52		39.2	88		75	82	95
β_2-microglobulin									below 5	

Tabelle 3. Fortsetzung

High-flow hemodiafiltration

Reference	Ahrenholz et al. 1981 [37]	Chapman et al. 1982 [152]	Shinzato et al. 1982 [153]	Streicher and Schneider 1983 [154]	Wizemann et al. 1983 [145]	Wizemann et al. 1983 [155]		Von Albertini et al. 1984 [156]		
Hemodiafilter	Duoflux 1.8 m	Nipro F1	2 × PAN 15	F60	Hemoflow D6	PAN 20	Filtryzer B 1-L	Hemoflow F 60 (2×)	Filtryzer B 1-L (2×)	DuoFlux (2×)
Treatment/week (min)	3 × 180–240	3 × 300				3 × 105	3 × 105	Below 3 × 120	Below 3 × 120	Below 3 × 120
Flow rates										
Blood	200	200	200	200	250	400	400	630	630	630
Dialysate	500	500	500	500	500	500	500	1006	1008	992
Filtrate	50	25–30	65–70	50	50	90–140	90–140	146	127	111
Clearances (ml/min)		recirculating dialysated	single-pass dialysis system							
Urea	166	123	141 183	191	220	237	227	514	480	446
Creatinine		99	122 172	173	190	212	205	432	377	366
Uric Acid			163							
Phosphate				165	165			399	373	357
Vitamin B$_{12}$	103		101							
Inulin	69		53		30	31	58	171	163	148
β$_2$-microglobulin			33	93				(Plasma clearance)		

Modes of Therapy

When hemodiafiltration is used as a research tool for achieving shorter treatment times or optimizing solute removal, the operating conditions chosen by the different groups vary over a wide range. Table 3 compiles some of the operating parameters in different studies.

In clinical routine, values of 250 ml/min or more are generally chosen for the blood flow rate and 500 ml/min for the dialysate flow rate. Treatment time depends on the patient's interdialytic weight gain, but is rarely below 3×3 h per week. Substitution volume is in the range between 9 and 18 l [35].

Cost of Treatment

Some authors see the higher cost of hemodiafiltration as the sole disadvantage of a technique which otherwise offers only benefits [81]. As an automated device is preferred for routine clinical application, the cost difference in comparison to conventional hemodialysis comes about by the higher investment in hardware plus disposables such as a dialyzer with a highly permeable membrane, substitution solution, and special tubing. The price for the extra module for controlling filtration and substitution rate (Fresenius AG, Oberursel, FRG) is about DM 15000 (US$ 5000) as of May 1985. Extra disposable cost per treatment is about DM 50-DM 75 (US$ 15-US$ 25). An industrial system with integrated production of substitution fluid and consequent reuse of disposables could reduce these extra expenses considerably. However, as long as the replacement fluid is not produced on site, but has to be purchased from industrial companies, hemodiafiltration will remain significantly more expensive than traditional hemodialysis. Hemofiltration is still even approximately 10% more expensive than hemodiafiltration, owing to the larger volumes of substitution fluid required.

On the other hand, if a shortening in treatment time could be achieved without increasing the complication rate and thus the need for staff intervention, the economics of performing hemodiafiltration could be justified on the basis of total cost analysis [157].

Clinical Aspects

Long-term Studies

Numerous technical and clinical studies on hemodiafiltration have been undertaken [158-170], but a large number of them are still limited in a) duration and b) patient numbers. The motivation in the early days of the procedure was to show the feasibility of hemodiafiltration in principle; and later on to show the advantages of different modifications of the basic procedure, such as maximizing solute clearances or minimizing treatment times. However, only a few studies have been conducted over a long period under controlled conditions.

The longest experiences with hemodiafiltration were published by LEBER et al. [105, 171], who compared ten patients who had been treated by 3×3 h of hemodiafiltration per week for between 2.5 and 3 years, to ten other patients who had been on 3×4 h of hemodialysis per week for the same length of time. Although total treatment time was reduced by 25% and the surface area of the hemodiafilter was only 60% of the area of the dialyzer, they could not find significant differences in clinical chemistry between the two patient groups. As indicated by a similar number of therapeutic interventions and a lower frequency of complications, hemodiafiltration seemed to be better tolerated than hemodialysis. However, the interdialytic weight gain was higher in the hemodiafiltration group (1.9 kg vs 1.5 kg).

Clinical signs of polyneuropathy or increased uremic osteopathy could not be found; however, neurophysiological and histological examination failed to show any improvement in comparison to the patients on hemodialysis [172]. Objective and subjective tolerance to fluid removal seemed to be better with hemodiafiltration than with hemodialysis and was comparable to the complication rate in hemofiltration. Serum osmolarity and intraocular pressure remained stable during hemodiafiltration, in contrast to hemodialysis [173].

SPRENGER et al. studied six patients over a period of 1 year in an ABA study, where six months of hemodiafiltration (B) were preceded and followed by 3 months of hemodialysis (A) [174]. Although hemodiafiltration treatment time was only two-thirds of hemodialysis treatment time, no deterioration of the patient's well-being as indicated by the occurrence of discomfort syndrome and disturbance of blood chemistry was observed. The velocity of nerve conduction improved, although this was not statistically significant. The acid–base status was better controlled in hemodiafiltration than in hemodialysis.

Another long-term cross-over study was undertaken by CHAPMAN et al. [152], who compared hemodiafiltration (C) and sorbent membrane dialysis (B) with conventional hemodialysis (A) over a period of a year in an ABACA study. They chose identical treatment times in hemodialysis and hemodiafiltration, but as the ultrafiltration rates chosen were low, solute removal in hemodiafiltration was not significantly higher than in hemodialysis. Some of the results found on hemodiafiltration could even be interpreted as signs of under-dialysis. Consequently, they could not find any practical advantages of hemodiafiltration over hemodialysis.

Biochemical Data, Acid-Base Status, and "Middle Molecules"

In the ABA study of SPRENGER et al. the reduction in treatment time caused the removal rates of smaller molecules such as urea and creatinine to fall below those in conventional hemodialyzers with a large surface area; this resulted in a 15% increase in concentrations of urea, creatinine, and anorganic phosphate during the hemodiafiltration period in comparison to the hemodialysis period.

Today's hemodiafilters, which have highly permeable membranes combining good hydraulic with adequate diffusive permeability, allow removal rates which are sufficient for controlling serum concentrations of both small and larger molecules. In some of the high-flux procedures, care even has to be taken to avoid any depletion of essential metabolites [175, 176].

Loss of amino acids during hemodiafiltration is comparable to that in hemofiltration: using a membrane of polymethylmetacrylate, OTA et al. found a total amino acid loss of 3 g during a 3 h treatment period (with clearances between 27 ml/min for glutamic acid and 88 ml/min for β-alanine) [106].

The enhancement of "middle molecule clearances," which was one of the reasons for the introduction of hemodiafiltration [177], is still the aim in some approaches to the technique [50, 104, 114]. However, there is as yet no controlled study showing the benefits of the potentially higher clearance of the yet to be identified "middle molecules" during hemodiafiltration [178]. On the contrary, in the long-term study by LEBER et al., with a tenfold increase in "middle molecule clearance" by hemodiafiltration in comparison to conventional hemodialysis over more than 2.5 years, no improvement in renal anemia or polyneuropathy was observed [177].

Newly developed membranes show higher permeabilities in the range of solute sizes up to albumin [146, 176]. Beneficial effects of the removal of hormones, complement factors, and other mediator substances have been hypothesized, but not proven [180-182]. SAITO et al. have even suggested protein-permeating hemodiafiltration [183-188].

Cardiovascular Stability

Several groups reported a significant reduction in dialysis-associated side effects during hemodiafiltration in comparison to hemodialysis [8, 189-192]. This observation was substantiated by investigation of the acute hemodynamic effects of hemodiafiltration as compared with hemodialysis and hemofiltration.

WIZEMANN et al. demonstrated in six patients with acute renal failure that patients on hemodiafiltration react to fluid removal by increasing total peripheral resistance as cardiac output decreases [193]. This effect was less marked than during hemofiltration, however. Standard acetate hemodialysis resulted in a drop in peripheral resistance, often accompanied by symptomatic hypotension. Bicarbonate or high-sodium (above 150 mmol/l) hemodialysis could not stabilize cardiovascular reaction as much as could hemodiafiltration and hemofiltration [194].

On the basis of experiments in five patients with chronic renal failure, SCHNEIDER et al. found the same pattern of hemodynamic response to fluid removal with acetate as the buffer. Total peripheral resistance increased and cardiac output decreased in acetate hemofiltration and hemodiafiltration, whereas total peripheral resistance decreased in acetate hemodialysis. However, they did not observe an adequate reduction in pulmonary pressures with any of these forms of treatment [195]. In this study the effect of using bicarbonate as the buffer was more substantial: cardiac output increased in all bicarbonate procedures, usually because of a higher stroke volume, while total peripheral resistance fell slightly. Mean arterial pressures remained constant. No hypotensive episodes were observed with the bicarbonate procedures, while symptomatic hypotension occurred in four cases during the treatments with acetate as buffer (three times during hemodialysis, once during hemodiafiltration). Epinephrine and norepinephrine levels decreased during all acetate-related treatment procedures, whereas they remained unchanged or even increased in the bicarbonate-related procedures.

JAHN et al. demonstrated that in ten patients with a normal predialysis pulmonary wedge pressure (PWP), hemofiltration and hemodiafiltration did not result in a decrease in PWP. Hemodialysis caused a drop in PWP, which can have a negative effect on left ventricular performance [196].

A noninvasive study in 14 patients with end-stage renal failure was unable to show significant differences in the change of mean arterial pressure and several echocardiographic parameters (e.g., contractility, mean velocity of circumferential fiber shortening, ejection fraction) when hemodialysis and hemodiafiltration were compared to hemofiltration using a synthetic, highly permeable membrane under very standardized conditions [197]. Conventional hemodialysis, however, resulted in a significant drop in mean arterial pressure during treatment in comparison to the other three methods.

The sometimes conflicting results from different investigations on hemodynamic effects of varying treatment modalities can be partially attributed to differences in patient selection [198]. All studies demonstrate, however, that vascular stability in hemodiafiltration is greater than that in conventional hemodialysis treatment and is comparable to that in hemofiltration. The reasons for this phenomenon remain unclear, as is the case for hemofiltration [199, 200]. Biocompatibility has been suggested as one factor. An as yet unknown effect of convective transport has also been discussed and could, in principle, also explain the results of the above-mentioned echocardiographic study [197]. A positive sodium balance might also contribute to the increased vascular stability [201–203]. In some studies, the main benefit of hemodiafiltration is related to the advantages of exact balancing methods for fluid removal [35].

Treatment Time

As solute removal can be enhanced by hemodiafiltration in comparison to hemodialysis and hemofiltration, the concept of decreasing treatment time without diminishing the quantity of solutes removed has attracted a lot of attention, especially in recent years.

With experimental hemodiafiltration, V. WIZEMANN and A. WIZEMANN were able to eliminate 30–35 g of urea within 45 min at a blood flow rate of 600 ml/min using a 4 m^2 dialyzer, without neurological disturbances or changes in intraocular pressure [204]. KRAMER et al. reported the results of a 6-month period of observation of six patients on "ultrashort hemodiafiltration" with a mean duration of $3 \times 105 \pm 14$ min/week [205]. They used acetate as the buffer in the dialysate and lactate in the substitution fluid. Dialysate flow was 500 ml/min. Using this method, they were able to achieve the same removal of urea as by 240 min of conventional hemodialysis, and a slightly smaller removal of creatinine. They did not find a deterioration in the biochemical data of the patients, despite a 56% reduction in treatment time. With a fluid loss of 1.3 ± 0.2 kg/h during hemodiafiltration in contrast to 0.5 ± 0.1 kg/h during hemodialysis, hemodynamic tolerance was adequate, with a normalization of stroke volume and rise in total peripheral resistance.

The average interdialytic weight gain of the patients rose from 2.1 ± 0.7 kg during the preceding hemodialysis period to 2.8 ± 0.7 kg after 6 months of hemodiafiltration. As the further increases in fluid removal rates were not generally tolerated, ultrashort hemodiafiltration had to be discontinued after the 6-month study period [8].

Recently introduced systems for high-efficiency short-time hemodiafiltration, where 2.6 kg are removed within 115 min by the kind of system shown in Fig. 9, must therefore be carefully judged in respect of their long-term effect. The choice of buffer certainly plays an important role in the acute tolerance of these procedures; the long-term consequences of chronic large shifts in the hydration state of a dialysis patient have to be watched carefully [206].

WIZEMANN suggested a list of contraindications for short-duration dialysis (below 3×3 h), which includes presence of cardiac arrhythmias, arterial hypertension or drug-induced normotension, or weight gain above 3% of dry weight between dialysis treatments [8].

Conclusions

Comparison of Hemodiafiltration with Other Forms of Treatment
For the removal of small molecule substances, there is no difference in the efficiency of hemodiafiltration and hemodialysis with dialyzers of high hydraulic permeability ("high-flux hemodialysis") [37, 139]. There is still a lack of controlled, long-term studies comparing the two treatment modalities with respect to dialysis-associated symptoms, patient well-being, and objective hemodynamic stability, but some reports seem to indicate that the effects of the buffer and of controlled ultrafiltration play a much bigger role than does the additional fluid removal by convection in hemodiafiltration.

In comparison to hemofiltration, hemodiafiltration has the advantage of achieving comparable removal rates of solutes with molecular weights above 1000 without requiring extremely high blood flow rates. Whether the hypothesis of the potential benefit of removing unknown solutes pertains depends on a future proof of "middle molecule" toxicity.

The frequently quoted argument that hemodiafiltration combines the advantages of both hemodialysis and hemofiltration might, however, turn out to be too mechanistic. If some of the assumptions of the recently introduced interleukin-1 hypothesis [206, 207] can be supported by measurements, then the contrary could be true: hemodiafiltration may be a combination of the disadvantages of hemofiltration (need for a sterile and nonpyrogenic substitution fluid) and hemodialysis (contact of monocytes with pyrogen-containing dialysate via a permeable membrane, which would result in production of interleukin-1) [198]. However, owing to the more pronounced solvent drag of the higher filtration rates in hemodiafiltration, the permeation of low-molecular-weight endogenous pyrogens would be hampered far more than during conventional hemodialysis.

Indications for Hemodiafiltration

It is not yet possible to come to a final conclusion on the indications for hemodiafiltration and its differential indication when compared to hemofiltration or "high-flux hemodialysis" [208–210].

The discussion as to whether hemodiafiltration should be used to reduce treatment time or, keeping treatment time constant, to optimize solute removal, is far from settled [146, 176]. Hemodiafiltration as a method of drastically reducing treatment time in the long run is probably acceptable for only a small percentage of patients with end-stage renal failure. As hemodiafiltration is the only routinely applicable method in which the removal of molecules of different size can be influenced selectively by appropriate choice of hemodiafilter and operating conditions, it plays an important role as a research tool.

Owing to the proven hemodynamic tolerance of hemodiafiltration, it can be indicated in the treatment of patients with cardiovascular problems, such as coronary heart disease and hypotension, and of patients with symptomatic hypertension, especially if they have inadequate vascular access for effective hemofiltration [178]. Children and elderly people can also benefit from treatment by hemodiafiltration [210, 211]. Whereas for the elderly hemofiltration is an adequate alternative, children profit more from hemodiafiltration (better vascular access, shorter treatment time) [213].

Future Prospects for Hemodiafiltration

Monitors for hemodiafiltration might incorporate the on-line preparation of the substitution fluid, thus allowing a cost reduction, as well as the routine application of pre- or mid-dilution for the replacement of lost fluid.

The greater cost of hemodiafiltration over costs of conventional forms of treatment will nevertheless limit its widespread use. It will be reserved for a limited number of patients, for whom the factors of efficient removal of fluid and solute without stress as well as individualized therapy are important.

With the advent of membranes possessing sieving characteristics analogous to those of the human glomerulus, it might become possible in the future to imitate more closely the total excretory function of the kidney. Long-term studies will be necessary to prove or disprove the beneficial effects of such procedures on all kinds of uremic complications, such as myocardiopathy and osteopathy.

References

1. Colton CK, Henderson LW, Ford CA, Lysaght MJ (1975) Kinetics of hemodiafiltration I. In vitro transport characteristics of a hollow fiber blood ultrafilter. J Lab Clin Med 85: 355
2. Henderson LW, Colton CK, Ford CA (1975) Kinetics of hemodiafiltration II. Clinical characterization of a new blood cleansing modality. J Lab Clin Med 85: 372
3. Streicher E, Schneider H, v Mylius U, Mahler B (1976) Haemodiafiltration mit asymmetrischen Kapillarmembranen. Nieren Hochdruckkr 5: 191
4. Henning HV (1976) Arbeitstagung über Hämofiltration, Braunlage/Harz, 25 September 1976 Wiss. Inform. Fresenius Nephrologie 4: 85
5. Leber H-W, Wizemann V, Goubeaud G, Rawer P, Schütterle G (1978) Hemodiafiltration: A new alternative to hemofiltration and conventional hemodialysis. In: Inou T, Atsumi K, Ohta K (eds) Proc Int Soc Artif Organs, Tokyo 1977. Artif Organs 2 (suppl): 408
6. Henderson LW (1983) Biophysics of ultrafiltration and hemofiltration. In: Drukker W, Parsons FM, Maher JF (eds) Replacement of renal function by dialysis. Nijhoff, Boston, p 242
7. Schütterle G, Wizemann V, Seyffart G (eds) (1982) Hemodiafiltration. Hygieneplan, Oberursel
8. Wizemann V (1985) Hemodiafiltration - an avenue to shorter dialysis? In: Lysaght MJ, Wetzels E, Gurland HJ (eds) Disputed issues in renal failure therapy. Contrib Nephrol 44: 49
9. Kulakov GP, Konovalov GA, Melikyan AM, Makarova KM (1983) Consecutive ultrafiltration with hemodialysis in the treatment of patients with chronic renal failure. Urol Nefrol (Mosk) 34 (in Russian)
10. Haas G (1928) Über Blutwaschung. Klin Wochenschr 7. 1356
11. Drukker W (1983) Haemodialysis: a historical review. In: Drukker W, Parsons FM, Maher JF (eds) Replacement of renal function by dialysis. Nijhoff, Boston, p 3
12. Babb AL, Farrell PC, Uvelli DA, Scribner BH (1972) Hemodialyzer evaluation by examination of solute molecular weight spectra: implications for the square-meter-hour hypothesis. Trans Am Soc Artif Intern Organs 18: 98
13. Klinkmann H, Bergström J, Dzurik R, Funck-Brentano JL (eds) (1980) Middle molecules in uremia and other diseases. Proc symp of present status and future orientation of middle molecules in uremia and other diseases, Nov 1980, Avignon. Artif Organs 4 [suppl]
14. Hampl H, Paeprer H, Unger V, Kessel MW (1979) Hemodynamics during hemodialysis, sequential ultrafiltration and hemofiltration. J Dial 3: 51
15. Shaldon S, Deschodt G, Beau MC, Claret G, Mion H, Mion C (1979) Vascular stability during high flux haemofiltration (HF). Proc Eur Dial Transplant Assoc 16: 695
16. Baldamus CA, Ernst W, Fassbinder W, Koch KM (1980) Differing haemodynamic stability due to different sympathetic response: comparison of ultrafiltration, haemodialysis and haemofiltration. Proc Eur Dial Transplant Assoc 17: 205
17. Bergström J, Asaba M, Fürst P, Oules R (1976) Dialysis, ultrafiltration and blood pressure. Proc Eur Dial Transplant Assoc 13: 293
18. Shinaberger JH, Miller JH, Rubini ME, Gardner PW, Martin FE (1969) Initial clinical evaluation of 'diafiltration'. Trans Am Soc Artif Intern Organs 15: 97
19. Kunitomo T, Lowrie EG, O'Brien M, Lazarus JM, Gottlieb MN, Kumazawa S, Merrill JP (1976) Performance and clinical use of a convertible hemodialysis (HD) - ultrafiltration (UF) system. Proc Dial Transplant Forum 6: 120
20. Lowrie EG, Kunitomo T, Kirkwood RG, Kumazawa S (1978) Dilution dialysis: controlled ultrafiltration (UF) with optimal dialysis (HD). Proc assoc advance med inst 13th ann meeting, p 177
21. Kunitomo T, Lowrie EG, Gottlieb MN, Lazarus JM, Kumazawa S, Merrill JP (1977) Clinical performance of a convertible hemodialysis (HD) - ultrafiltration (UF) system. Proc assoc advance med inst 12th ann meeting, p 146
22. Kunitomo T, Lowrie EG, Kumazawa S, O'Brien M, Lazarus JM, Gottlieb MN, Merrill JP (1977) Controlled ultrafiltration (UF) with hemodialysis (HD): analysis of coupling between convective and diffusive mass transfer in a new HD-UF system. Trans Am Soc Artif Intern Organs 23: 234
23. Leber HW, Wizemann V, Goubeaud G, Rawer P (1977) Hemodiafiltration, an effective alternative to hemofiltration and conventional hemodialysis in the treatment of uremic patients. Opuscula Medicotechnica Lundensia 18: 107

24. Dieter K, Franz HE, Breitig D, Meyer C, Schmidt-Wiederkehr P (1977) Blutdetoxikation durch simultane Dialyse und Diafiltration. Biomed Tech (Berlin) 22: 277
25. Leber H-W, Wizemann V, Goubeaud G, Rawer P, Schütterle G (1978) Simultaneous hemofiltration/hemodialysis: An effective alternative to hemofiltration and conventional hemodialysis in the treatment of uremic patients. Clin Nephrol 9: 115
26. Ota K, Suzuki T, Ozaku Y, Era K, Agishi T, Sugino N, Haraguchi M, Mitani N, Kumazawa S (1978) Clinical evaluation of a pre-set ultrafiltration rate controller available for single pass and hemodiafiltration systems. Artif Organs 2: 141
27. Kramer P, Broyer M, Brunner FP, Brynger H, Challah S, Oules R, Rizzoni G, Selwood NH, Wing AJ, Balas EA (1984) Combined report on regular dialysis and transplantation in Europe. Proc Eur Dial Transplant Assoc 21: 5
28. Maekawa M, Kishimoto T, Ohyama T, Tanaka H (1980) Present status of hemofiltration and hemodiafiltration in Japan. Artif Organs 4: 85
29. Smith HW (1951) The kidney: structure and function in health and disease. Oxford University Press, New York, p 39
30. Sprenger KBG (1982) Measurement of mass transport during hemodiafiltration. In: Schütterle G, Wizemann V, Seyffart G (eds) Hemodiafiltration. Hygieneplan, Oberursel, p 49
31. Bass OE, Nolph KD, Maher JF (1975) Dialysance and clearance measurements during clinical dialysis – A plea for standardization. J Lab Clin Med 86: 378
32. Klein E, Autian J, Bower JD, Buffaloe G, Centella LJ, Colton CK, Darby TD, Farrell PC, Holland FF, Kennedy RS, Lipps B Jr, Mason R, Nolph KD, Villaroel F, Wathen RL (1977) Evaluation of hemodialyzers and dialysis membranes. Report of a study group for the artificial kidney – chronic uremia prog. DHEW Pub no 77-1294. NIH, Bethesda
33. Van Geelen JA, Flendrig JA, Carpay WM (1985) Evaluation of in vivo solute clearances during hemodialysis and hemodiafiltration. Dial Transplant 14: 85
34. Sprenger KGB, Kratz W, Stadtmüller U, Junginger E, Franz HE (1981) Massenbilanzierung und kinetische Modelle bei Hämodiafiltration. Biomed Tech (Berlin) 26: 236
35. Sprenger KBG, Franz HE (1983) Hämodiafiltration. In: Franz HE (ed) Blutreinigungsverfahren – Technik und Klinik. Thieme, Stuttgart, p 433
36. Streicher E, Schneider H (1983) Polysulphone membrane mimicking human glomerular basement membrane. Lancet II: 1136
37. Ahrenholz P, Falkenhagen D, Roy T, Esther G, Klinkmann H (1982) Effektivitätsuntersuchungen bei der Hämodiafiltration im Vergleich zur Hämodialyse, High-Flux-Single-Pass-Dialyse, Hämofiltration und Hämodialyse/Hämoperfusion unter besonderer Berücksichtigung mittelmolekularer Substanzen. In: Schütterle G, Wizemann V, Seyffart G (eds) Hemodiafiltration. Hygieneplan, Oberursel, p 37
38. Schmidt M, Baldamus CA, Schoeppe W (1984) In vitro evaluation of solute clearances and sieving coefficients in hemodiafiltration (Abstract). Artif Organs 8: 117
39. Meixner J, Reik H (1959) Thermodynamik der irreversiblen Prozesse. In: Handbuch der Physik III/2. Springer, Berlin Göttingen Heidelberg, p 413
40. Kedem O, Katchalsky A (1958) Thermodynamic analysis of the permeability of biological membranes to non-electrolytes. Biochim Biophys Acta 27: 229
41. Schlögl R (1964) Stofftransport durch Membranen. Steinkopff, Darmstadt
42. Pusch W (1985) Measurement techniques of transport through membranes. In: Lior N (ed) Measurement and control in desalination. Elsevier, Amsterdam (in press)
43. Staverman AJ (1951) The theory of measurement of osmotic pressure. Rec Trav Chim Pays-Bas 70: 344
44. Bresler EH, Groome LJ (1981) On equations for combined convective and diffusive transport of neutral solute across porous membranes. Am J Physiol 241: F469
45. Villaroel F, Klein E, Holland F (1977) Solute flux in hemodialysis and hemofiltration membranes. Trans Am Soc Artif Intern Organs 23: 225
46. Nolph KD, New DL (1976) Effects of ultrafiltration on solute clearances in hollow fiber kidneys. J Lab Clin Med 88: 593
47. Nolph KD, Hopkins C, Van Stone J (1977) Effects of ultrafiltration on solute clearances in parallel plate dialyzers. Clin Nephrol 8: 453
48. Nolph KD, Hopkins CA (1978) Effects of ultrafiltration on diffusion and convection in two newer coils. Nephron (Basel) 22: 153

49. Schneider H, Nagel W, Streicher E (1982) Is hemodiafiltration really an advantage? A study based on kinetic considerations. Abstr Eur Dial Transplant Assoc 127

50. Maeda K, Shinzato T, Sezaki R, Yamada K, Saito A, Ohta K (1984) Decreased sieving coefficient for middle molecules during hemofiltration and infusion-free hemodiafiltration (Abstract). Blood Purif 2: 54

51. Grimsrud L (1965) A theoretical and experimental investigation of the performance of a parallel-plate dialyzer in the laminar flow regime, with application to hemodialyzer design. Ph D-thesis, University of Washington, Seattle

52. Wolf L, Zaltzman S (1968) Optimum geometry for artificial kidney dialyzers. Chem Eng Prog Symp Ser 64: 104

53. Colton CK (1969) Permeability and transport studies in batch and flow dialyzers with application to hemodialysis. Ph D-thesis, Massachusetts Institute of Technology

54. Davis HR, Parkinson GV (1970) Mass transfer from small capillaries with wall resistance in the laminar flow regime. Appl Sci Res 22: 20

55. Colton CK, Smith KA, Stroeve P, Merril EW (1971) Laminar flow mass transfer in a flat duct with permeable walls. Am Inst Chem Eng J 17: 773

56. Cooney DO, Kim SS, Davis EJ (1974) Analysis of mass transfer in hemodialysers for laminar blood flow and homogeneous dialysate. Chem Eng J Sci 29: 1731

57. Sigdell J-E (1974) A mathematical theory for the capillary artificial kidney. Hippokrates, Stuttgart

58. Walker G, Davis T (1974) Mass transfer in laminar flow between parallel permeable plates. Am Inst Chem Eng J 20: 881

59. Popovich RP, Christopher TG, Babb AL (1971) The effects of membrane diffusion and ultrafiltration properties on hemodialyzer design and performances. Clin Eng Prog Symp Ser No 114, 67: 105

60. Blatt WF, Nelson L, Zipilivan EM, Porter MC (1972) Rapid salt exchange by coupled ultrafiltration and dialysis in anisotropic hollow fibers. Separat Science 7: 271

61. Popovich RP, Ng JS, Moncrief JW, Decherd JF, Morris S (1977) The effects of ultrafiltration on the clearance of a hemodialyzer with a recirculating single pass dialysate mode. Proc 2nd Australian conference on heat and mass transfer

62. Ross SM, Uvelli DA, Babb AL (1973) A one-dimensional mathematical model of transmembrane diffusional and convective mass transfer in a hemodialyzer. Am Soc Mech Eng Paper No 73-WA/Bio-14

63. Ross SM (1974) A mathematical model of mass transport in a long permeable tube with radial convection (part 1). J Fluid Mech 63: 157

64. Dieter K, Franz HE, Mayer G, Schmidt-Wiederkehr P, Breitig D (1976) Blutreinigungsverfahren. DFG-Projekt Fr 200/13

65. Jagannathan R, Shettigar UR (1977) Analysis of tubular haemodialyser - effect of ultrafiltration and dialysate concentration. Med Biol Eng Comp 15: 134

66. Granger A, Vantard G, Vantelon J, Perrone B (1978) A mathematical approach of simultaneous dialysis and filtration (SDF). Proc Eur Soc Artif Intern Organs 5: 174

67. Zelman A, Gisser D (1979) In vitro characterization of the R.P. 6 dialyzer: co-current and counter-current clearance as a function of ultrafiltration. J Dial 3: 237

68. Werynski A (1979) Evaluation of the impact of ultrafiltration on dialyzer clearance. Artif Organs 3: 140

69. Jaffrin MY, Malbrancq JM (1980) Prédictions de la clearance de l'urée en hémofiltration-dialyse simultanée. Rapport U.T.C. 79-7

70. Jaffrin MY, Malbrancq JM, Vantard G (1980) Coupling between diffusive and convective transport in simultaneous dialysis and hemofiltration. Proc 2nd int conf on mechanics in medicine and biology, p 60

71. Jaffrin MY, Gupta BB, Kovalesky O, Vanhoutte C (1981) Factors governing clearance in simultaneous dialysis and hemofiltration. Artif Organs 5 (suppl): 642

72. Lewis AED, Sprenger KBG, Stephan HG, Franz HE (1981) Practical method for prediction of clearances for hemodiafiltration, hemodialysis and hemofiltration (Abstract). Abstr Eur Dial Transplant Assoc 18: 86

73. Jaffrin MY, Gupta BB, Malbrancq JM (1981) A one-dimensional model of simultaneous hemodialysis and ultrafiltration with highly permeable membranes. J Biomech Eng 103: 261

74. Timmermann M, Keller H-J, Walitza E, Chmiel H (1981) Numerische Simulation zum Hämo-dialyse- und Hämofiltrationsvorgang. Biomed Tech (Berlin) 26 (suppl): 106
75. Dieter K (1982) Stofftransport bei Hämodialyse, Hämofiltration und Hämodiafiltration. In: Schütterle G, Wizemann V, Seyffart G (eds) Hemodiafiltration. Hygieneplan, Oberursel, p 7
76. Lewis AED (1982) Mathematical modelling of hemodiafiltration with particular reference to prediction of clearance. In: Schütterle G, Wizemann V, Seyffart G (eds): Hemodiafiltration. Hygieneplan, Oberursel, p 63
77. Sigdell JE (1982) Calculation of combined diffusive and convective mass transfer. Int. J Artif Organs 5: 361
78. Sargent JA, Gotch FA (1983) Principles and biophysics of dialysis. In: Drukker W, Parsons F M, Maher JF (eds) Replacement of renal function by dialysis. Nijhoff, Boston, p 53
79. Vantard G (1981) Analyse de l'épuration extra-rénale par hémodialyse hémofiltration simulta-nées. Doctor thesis, Compiègne
80. Sprenger KBG, Kratz W, Stadtmüller U, Franz HE (1982) Mass balance and kinetic modelling of haemodiafiltration. In: Klinkmann H, Ahrenholz P, Biester F-D, Courtney JM, Falkenha-gen D, Gaylor JD (eds) Proc int symp on kinetic modelling in artificial organs. Rostock-War-nemünde, GDR, p 141
81. Sprenger KBG (1983) Review article: hemodiafiltration. Life Support Systems 1: 127
82. Albertini B von, Miller JH, Gardner PW, Shinaberger JH (1984) High-flux hemodiafiltration: under six hours/week treatment. Trans Am Soc Artif Intern Organs 30: 227
83. Farrell PC (1984) Discussion of Manuscript # 73. Trans Am Soc Artif Intern Organs 30: 381
84. Sprenger KBG, Kratz W, Lewis AE, Stadtmüller U (1983) Kinetic modelling of hemodialysis, hemofiltration, and hemodiafiltration. Kidney Int 24: 143
85. Wideroe T-E, Grimsrud L, Berg KJ, Godal A, Jensen R, Jörstad S (1974) A mathematical sin-gle-pool model for short-time hemodialysis. Proc Eur Dial Transplant Assoc 11: 136
86. Schindhelm K, Farrell PC (1978) Patient-hemodialyzer interactions. Trans Am Soc Artif Intern Organs 24: 357
87. Dombeck DH, Klein E, Wendt RP (1975) Evaluation of two-pool model for predicting serum creatinine levels during intra- and interdialytic periods. Trans Am Soc Artif Intern Organs 21: 117
88. Popovich RP, Hlavinka DJ, Bomar JB, Moncrief JW, Decherd JF (1975) The consequences of physiological resistance on metabolite removal from the patient-artificial kidney system. Trans Am Soc Artif Intern Organs 21: 108
89. Stiller S, Mann H, Higashi F (1977) Berechnung von Stoff- und Wasseraustausch zwischen den Körper-Kompartimenten während der Dialyse durch ein mathematisches Modell. Projekt-trägerschaften-Bericht: Materialien und Systeme zur Organunterstützung, Munich GSF con-tract DVM 136 (in German)
90. Kunitomo T, Kirkwood RG, Kumazawa S, Lazarus JM, Gottlieb MN, Lowrie EG (1978) Clini-cal evaluation of postdilution dialysis with a combined ultrafiltration (UF) – hemodialysis (HD) system. Trans Am Soc Artif Intern Organs 24: 169
91. Lewis AED (1978) Optimization of dialysis treatment conditions using a programmable calcu-lator. Proc Eur Soc Artif Organs 5: 182
92. Schmidt R, Ivanovich P, Klinkmann H, del Greco F (1981) A simplified method of hemodiafil-tration for treatment of chronic renal failure. Artif Organs 5 (suppl): 675
93. Leber H-W, Wizemann V, Goubeaud G, Rawer P, Schütterle G (1978) Hemodiafiltration: a new alternative to hemofiltration and conventional hemodialysis. Artif Organs 2: 150
94. Keshaviah PR, Shaldon S (1983) Haemodialysis monitors and monitoring. In: Drukker W, Parsons FM, Maher JF (eds) Replacement of renal function by dialysis. Nijhoff, Boston, p 223
95. Flendrig J, Carpay W, Dekkers W (1978) The accurate control of ultrafiltration. Artif Organs 2: 144
96. Roy T, Ahrenholz P, Falkenhagen D, Klinkmann H (1982) Volumetrically controlled ultrafil-tration. Current experiences and future prospects. Int J Artif Organs 5: 131
97. Polaschegg HD (1985) Methoden und Geschichte der Ultrafiltrationskontrolle in der Hämodi-alyse. Wiss Informationen Fresenius, Nephrologie 1: 135
98. Kohnle W, Sprenger KBG, Spohn B, Franz HE (1979) Haemodiafiltration using readily avail-able equipment. J Dialysis 3: 27
99. Chapman GV, Hone PWE, Bolton W, Blogg A, Stokoe C, Cahill T, Mahony JF, Farrell PC

(1982) Evaluation of hemodiafiltration and sorbent membrane dialysis. I. in vivo and in vitro dialyzer performance. Dial Transpl 11: 758

100. Van Geelen JA (1983) Hemodiafiltration – the simultaneous application of hemodialysis and hemofiltration. Doctor Thesis, Maastricht, Netherlands

101. Van Geelen JA, Carpay W, Flendrig JA (1984) Clinical experience with a closed-volume hemodiafiltration apparatus (Abstract). Blood Purif 2: 50

102. Van Geelen JA, Carpay W, Dekkers W, Fiers H-A, Mulder AW, Flendrig JA (1979) Simultaneous hemodialysis and hemofiltration, a simple, safe and effective treatment of uremic patients. ASAIO J 2: 50

103. Shettigar UR (1984) Hemodiafiltration thesis by JA Van Geelen. Dial Transpl 12: 762

104. Cambi V, Buzio C, Arisi L, Calderini C, David S, Manari A, Bono F, Zanelli P (1981) Vascular stability and middle-molecule removal in hypertonic hemodiafiltration. Artif Organs 5 (suppl): 59

105. Leber H-W, Wizemann V, Techert F (1980) Simultaneous hemofiltration/hemodialysis (HF/HD): short- and long-term tolerance. Introduction of a system for automatic fluid replacement. Artif Organs 4: 108

106. Ota K, Suzuki T, Ozaku Y, Hoshino T, Agishi T, Sugino N (1978) Short-time hemodiafiltration using polymethylmethacrylate hemodiafilter. Trans Am Soc Artif Intern Organs 24: 454

107. Sprenger KBG, Bundschu D, Figueroa P, Franz HE (1980) Comparison of hemodialysis with controlled ultrafiltration and hemodiafiltration in an ABA manner performed as a longterm study. ASAIO J 3: 64

108. Albertini B von, Miller JH, Gardner PW, Shinaberger JH (1985) Performance characteristics of the Hemoflow F 60 in high-flux hemodiafiltration. In: Streicher E, Seyffart G (eds) Highly permeable membranes. Contrib Nephrol 46: 169

109. Wizemann V, Kramer W, Knopp G, Rawer P, Mueller K, Schütterle G (1983) Ultrashort hemodiafiltration: efficiency and hemodynamic tolerance. Clin Nephrol 19: 24

110. Basile C, Di Maggio A, Longo S, Coviello F, Scatizzi A (1982) Simultaneous haemofiltration-haemodialysis (SHH) with iso-osmotic dialysate and hypertonic diluting fluid with bicarbonate: 15-month experience (Abstract). Abstr Eur Dial Transplant Assoc 11

111. Basile C, Di Maggio A, Longo S, Orbello G, Scatizzi A (1982) Simultaneous haemofiltration-haemodialysis (SHH) with iso-osmotic dialysate and hypertonic diluting fluid with bicarbonate. A kinetic study (Abstract). Abstr Eur Dial Transplant Assoc

112. Basile C, Di Maggio A, Scatizzi A (1983) Emofiltrazione-emodialisi simultanea con dialisato iso-osmotico e reiniezione ipertonica con bicarbonato. Minerva Nefr 30: 93

113. Basile C, Granger A, Scatizzi A (1983) Sodium kinetics in hypertonic hemodiafiltration. Proc 4th Congr Int Soc Artif Organs, pp 575

114. Cambi V, Buzio C, Arisi L, Calderini C, David S, Manari A, Bono F, Zanelli P (1981) Vascular stability and middle molecules removal in hypertonic haemodiafiltration. Proc Eur Dial Transplant Assoc 18: 681

115. Maeda K, Saito A, Kawaguchi S, Asada A, Niwa T, Ohta K, Kobayashi K (1980) Hemodiafiltration with sodium concentration-controlled dialysate. Artif Organs 4: 121

116. Fresenius AG, Oberursel, FRG, Product Information, 1984

117. Streicher E, Schneider H (1977) Asymmetric polyamide hollow-fiber filters in the haemofiltration system. J Dial 1: 727

118. Quellhorst E (1983) Ultrafiltration and haemofiltration, practical applications. In: Drukker W, Parsons FM, Maher JF (eds) Replacement of renal function by dialysis. Nijhoff, Boston, p 265

119. Shinzato T, Sezaki R, Usuda M, Maeda K, Toyota T, Ohbayashi S (1981) Infusion-free hemodiafiltration: simultaneous hemofiltration and dialysis with no need for infusion fluid. Int J Artif Organs 4: 250

120. Cheung AC, Kato Y, Leypoldt JK, Henderson LW (1982) Hemodiafiltration using a hybrid membrane system for self-generation of diluting fluid. Trans Am Soc Artif Intern Organs 28: 61

121. Shinzato T, Sezaki R, Maeda K, Asada H, Kawaguchi S, Usuda M (1982) Infusion-free hemodiafiltration. Jpn J Nephrol 24: 71–77 (in Japanese)

122. Usuda M, Shinzato T, Sezaki R, Kawanishi A, Maeda K, Kawaguchi S, Shibata M, Toyoda T, Asakura Y, Ohbayashi S (1982) New simultaneous HF and HD with no infusion fluid. Trans Am Soc Artif Intern Organs 28: 24

123. Shinzato T, Maeda K, Usuda M, Yoshida F, Sezaki R, Tsuruta Y, Yamada K, Atsumi H, Toyo-da T, Ohbayashi S, Saito A, Ohta K (1983) Clinical application of a new infusion-free HDF system. Blood Purif 1: 58

124. Canaud B, N'Guyen QV, Lagarde C, Stec F, Polaschegg HD, Mion C (1985) Clinical evaluation of a multipurpose dialysis system adequate for hemodialysis or for postdilution hemofiltration/hemodiafiltration with on-line preparation of substitution fluid from dialysate. In: Streicher E, Seyffart G (eds) Highly permeable membranes. Contrib Nephrol 46: 184

125. Henderson LW, Beans E (1978) Successful production of sterile pyrogen-free electrolyte solution by ultrafiltration. Kidney Int 14: 522

126. Henderson LW, Sanfelippo ML, Beans E (1978) "On line" preparation of sterile pyrogen-free electrolyte solution. Trans Am Soc Artif Intern Organs 24: 465

127. Miller J, Albertini B von, Gardner P, Hercz G, Shinaberger J (1984) Technical aspects of high-flux hemodiafiltration for adequate short (under 2 hours) treatment. Trans Am Soc Artif Intern Organs 30: 377

128. Albertini B von, Shinaberger J, Gardner P, Miller J (1984) Performance characteristics of high flux hemodiafiltration (Abstract). Blood Purif 2: 44

129. Albertini B von, Miller JH, Gardner PW, Norris KC, Roberts CE, Shinaberger JH (1984) High flux hemodiafiltration (Abstract). Am Soc Nephrology 76 A

130. Schmidt M, Baldamus CA, Schoeppe W (1984) Characterization of solute and solvent kinetics in hemodialyzers with highly permeable membranes. Abstr Am Soc Artif Intern Organs 13: 55

131. Schmidt M, Baldamus CA, Schoeppe W (1984) Hemodialysis (HD) with highly permeable membranes (HPM): an advanced form of hemodiafiltration (HDF)? (Abstract). Blood Purif 2: 62

132. Sigdell JE (1984) A new operational principle for blood treatment with highly permeable membranes. Int J Artif Organs 7: 193

133. Streicher E, Schneider H (1985) The next generation of dialysis membranes – barriers or pathways? In: Lysaght MJ, Wetzeles E, Gurland HJ: Disputed issues in renal failure therapy. Contrib Nephrol 44: 127

134. Stiller S, Mann H, Brunner H (1985) Rückfiltration von Dialysierflüssigkeit bei der Dialyse mit hochpermeablen Membranen. Nieren-Hochdruckkrk 14: 41

135. Bosch T, Schmidt B, Samtleben W, Gurland HJ (1985) Effect of protein absorption on diffusive and convective transport through polysulfone membranes. In: Streicher E, Seyffart G (eds) Highly permeable membranes. Contrib Nephrol 46: 14

136. Stiller S, Mann H, Brunner H (1985) Backfiltration in hemodialysis with highly permeable membranes. In: Streicher E, Seyffart G (eds) Highly permeable membranes. Contrib Nephrol 46: 23

137. Streicher E, Schneider H (1985) The development of a polysulfone membrane. A new perspective in dialysis? In: Streicher E, Seyffart G (eds) Highly permeable membranes. Contrib Nephrol 46: 1

138. Schmidt M, Baldamus CA, Schoeppe W (1984) Backfiltration in hemodialyzers with highly permeable membranes. Blood Purif 2: 108

139. Schneider H, Streicher E (1985) Mass transfer characterization of a new polysulfone membrane. Artif Organs 9: 180

140. Vanholder R, Billiouw JM, Liu J-D, Clippele M de, Ringoir S (1985) Single-needle hemodiafiltration. Artif Organs (in press)

141. Wizemann V, Techert F, Weber N, Brüning S (1983) Single-needle hemodialysis and hemofiltration in an extremely open membrane. Int J Artif Organs 6: 21

142. Koch KM, Minetti L, Shaldon S, Zucchelli P (1984) Second annual workshop of the international society of hemofiltration, July 6–7 1984, Milan. Artif Organs 8: 502

143. Bosticardo GM, Alloatti S, Comune L, Gianoli P, Pellerey M, Belardi P, Giachino G, Piccoli G (1983) Hemofiltration with dialysis-regeneration of ultrafiltrate (HF-DR). Proc 10th ann meet ESAO, Bologna, 1983. Life Supp Syst 1 (Suppl 1): 297

144. Civati Guastoni C, Teatini U, Perego A, Scorza D, Minetti L (1984) Haemofiltration without substitution fluid. Proc Eur Dial Transplant Assoc 21: 441

145. Wizemann V, Gödel G, Rawer P, Schütterle G (1983) Hämodiafiltration mit Cuprophan-Membranen? Nieren-Hochdruckkr 12: 142

146. Sprenger KBG, Stephan H, Kratz W, Huber K, Franz HE (1985) Optimising of hemodiafiltra-

tion with modern membranes? In: Streicher E, Seyffart G (eds) Highly permeable membranes. Contrib Nephrol 46: 43

147. Stephan H-G (1982) Hämodiafiltration and Hämodialyse: Klinischer Test mit vier Dialysatoren. M D thesis Ulm

148. Nagel W, Schneider H, Streicher E (1983) Untersuchungen zur Eliminationscharakteristik von Hämodiafiltrationsmembranen. 17 Jahrestagung der Deutschen Ges für Biomed Technik, Erlangen 8: 28

149. Vantelon J (1979) Traitement de l'insuffisance rénale chronique par filtration et dialyse combinée. Report contrat DGRST No 78.70, p 146

150. Van Geelen JA, Carpay W, Dekkers WE, Fiers H-A, Mulder AW, Flendrig JA (1979) Simultaneous hemodialysis and hemofiltration, a simple safe and effective treatment of uremic patients. Proc 2nd symp int soc artif organs, p 119

151. Kirkwood RG, Kunitomo T, Lowrie EG (1978) High rates of controlled ultrafiltration combined with optimal diffusion: recent advances in hemodialysis technique. Nephron (BASEL) 22: 175

152. Chapman GV, Hone PWE, Shirlow MJ, Bolton W, Blogg A, Stokoe C, Cahill T, Mahony JF, Farell PC (1982) Evaluation of hemodiafiltration and sorbent membrane dialysis. II. clinical, nutritional, and middle molecule assessment. Dial Transplant 11: 871

153. Shinzato T, Sezaki R, Usuda M, Maeda K, Ohbayashi S, Toyota T (1982) Infusion-free hemodiafiltration: simultaneous hemofiltration and dialysis with no need for infusion fluid. Artif Organs 6: 453

154. Streicher E, Schneider H (1983) Stofftransport bei Hämodiafiltration. Nieren-Hochdruck-krankheiten 12: 339

155. Wizemann V, Rawer P, Schütterle G (1982) Ultrashort haemodiafiltration: long-term efficiency and haemodynamic tolerance. Proc Eur Dial Transplant Assoc 19: 175

156. Albertini B von, Shinaberger J, Gardner P, Miller J (1984) Performance characteristics of high-flux hemodiafiltration. Proc Eur Dial Transplant Assoc 21: 477

157. Dieker P (1982) Wirtschaftliche und organisatorische Konsequenzen der Einführung der simultanen Hämodialyse/Hämofiltration (Hämodiafiltration). In: Schütterle G, Wizemann V, Seyffart G (eds) Hemodiafiltration. Hygieneplan, Oberursel, p 146

158. Houda W, Kaden W (1980) Die simultane, getrennte Dialyse- und Ultrafiltrationsbehandlung bei chronischer Niereninsuffizienz. Z Urol Nephrol 73: 725

159. Schmidt R, Ivanovich P, Klinkmann H, Del Greco F (1980) Simultaneous hemodialysis and hemofiltration for chronic renal failure therapy (Abstract). Abstr Am Soc Artif Intern Organs 25: 63

160. Lewis AED, Goggin MH (1981) Two new techniques for regular dialysis, consecutive sequential ultrafiltration and hemodiafiltration (Abstract). Abstr Int Assoc Artif Organs 3: 45

161. Cioni L, Maccheroni M, Montali U, Palmarini D, Pilone N, Rindi P, Ronca C (1982) Emodiafiltrazione versus emofiltrazione. In: Emofiltrazione, aspetti technici e clinici, stato attuale e prospettive in Italia, p 57

162. Cioni L, Pilone N, Perossini M, Rindi P (1982) Two years experience with simultaneous hemofiltration/hemodialysis (HF/HD) (Abstract). Abstr Am Soc Artif Intern Organs 11: 45

163. Cioni L, Maccheroni M, Palmarini D, Rindi P, Pilone N (1983) The treatment of end-stage renal disease (ESRD) by hemodiafiltration (HD/HF) (Abstracts). Abstr Eur Dial Transplant Assoc 107

164. Ghezzi PM, Frigato G, Fantini GF, Dutto A, Meinero S, Cento G, Marazzi F, D'Andria V, Grivet V (1983) Theoretical model and first clinical results of the paired filtration-dialysis (PFD). Proc 10th ann meet europ soc artif organs, Bologna, Life Supp Syst 1 (Suppl 1): 271

165. Rindi P, Maccheroni M, Palmarini D, Pilone N, Cioni L (1983) High-performance hemofiltration (HF) and hemodiafiltration (HD/HF) (Abstract). Blood Purif 1: 54

166. Cioni L, Palmarini D, Pilone N, Rindi P (1984) Hemodiafiltration: 2 years experience (Abstract). Blood Purif 2: 47

167. Ghezzi PM, Marazzi F, Dutto A, Cento G, Meinero S, Nigrelli S, Rattalino G, Paglialunga A, Caneparoi G, Grivet V (1984) Extracorporeal blood purification in uremic patients by a separate convective-diffusive system (Abstract). Blood Purif 2: 51

168. Icardi A, Lamperi D, Cappelli G, Lamperi S (1984) Hemofiltration and biofiltration: a comparative study on the short-time effects (Abstract). Blood Purif 2: 52

169. Santoro A, Degli Esposti E, Sturani A, Ragiotto G, Spongano M, Cavalli F, Zuccala A, Chiari-
     ni C, Zucchelli P (1984) Trattamento a medio termine dell'uremia terminale con ultrafiltra-
     zione (Evaluation of biofiltration in chronic uremia). G Ital Nefrol 1: 143
170. Zucchelli P, Santoro A, Degli Esposti E, Sturani A (1984) Biofiltration (BF): a soft hemodiafil-
     tration (HDF) (Abstract). Blood Purif 2: 64
171. Leber H-W, Wizemann V, Rawer P (1981) Kurzzeitbehandlung dialysepflichtiger urämischer
     Patienten mittels simultaner Hämofiltration/Hämodialyse: Bericht über dreijährige Erfah-
     rungen. In: Dittrich P von, Seyffart G (eds) Aktuelle Probleme der Dialyseverfahren und der
     Niereninsuffizienz. Bindernagel, Friedberg, p 13
172. Rawer P, Wizemann V, Schütterle G (1982) Elimination of middle molecular compounds with
     hemodialysis, hemofiltration and hemodiafiltration. In: Schütterle G, Wizemann V, Seyffart G
     (eds) Hemodiafiltration. Hygieneplan, Oberursel, p 17
173. Wizemann A, Bernhardt O, Wizemann V (1980) Untersuchungen zum Einfluß der Serumos-
     molarität, des Wasserentzuges und des Blutdruckes auf den intraocularen Druck am Modell
     der Hämodialyse, Hämofiltration und simultanen Hämofiltration/Hämodialyse. Graefes
     Arch Clin Exp Ophthalmol 213: 43
174. Sprenger KBG, Bundschu D, Figueroa P, Franz HE (1981) Vergleich von Hämodiafiltration
     gegenüber Hämodialyse mit kontrollierter Ultrafiltration in einer ABA-Langzeitstudie. Nie-
     ren-Hochdruckkrk 10: 226
175. Vagge R, Cavatorta F, Solari P, Queirolo C (1984) Carnitine removal during haemodialytic
     treatment: comparison between conventional hemodialysis, haemofiltration and haemodiafil-
     tration (HDF). Blood Purif 2: 63
176. Wizemann V, Velcovsky HG, Bleyl H, Brüning S, Schütterle G (1985) Removal of hormones by
     hemofiltration and hemodialysis with a highly permeable polysulfone membrane. In: Strei-
     cher E, Seyffart G (eds) Highly permeable membranes. Contrib Nephrol 46: 61
177. Leber H-W, Wizemann V, Goubeaud G, Rawer P, Schütterle G (1977) Elimination nieder- und
     mittelmolekularer harnpflichtiger Substanzen bei Haemodialyse, Haemofiltration, Haemodia-
     filtration und Haemoperfusion. In: Dittrich P von, Kopp KF (eds) Aktuelle Probleme der
     Dialyseverfahren und der Niereninsuffizienz. Bindernagel, Friedberg, p 152
178. Wizemann V (1984) Hemodiafiltration – to be or not to be? Blood Purif 2: 76
179. Wizemann V, Rawer P, Schmidt H, Techert F, Schütterle G (1982) Efficiency of hemodialysis,
     hemofiltration, hemodiafiltration. In: Schütterle G, Wizemann V, Seyffart G (eds) Hemodiafil-
     tration. Hygieneplan, Oberursel, p 25
180. Jorstad S, Smeby LC, Wideroe T-E, Berg KJ (1979) Transport of uremic toxins through con-
     ventional hemodialysis membranes. Clin Nephrol 12: 168
181. Rabin EZ, Algom D, Freedman MH, Geunther L, Dardick I, Tattrie B (1981) Ribonuclease ac-
     tivity in renal failure. Nephron (BASEL) 27: 254
182. Falkenhagen D, Behm E, Böttcher M, Zinner G, Falkenhagen U, Ramlow W, Klinkmann H,
     Courtney JM (1985) Possibilities of reduction of complement activation in extracorporeal cir-
     culation (Abstract). Abstr symp on immune and metabolic aspects of therapeutic blood purifi-
     cation systems, Trondheim, Norway, p 21
183. Saito A, Chung TG, Kanazawa I, Oda O, Ohta K (1982) Middle and large molecule removal of
     protein-permeating hemodiafiltration. Proc Int Symp Hemoperfusion and Artif Organs 4: 42
184. Saito A, Ohta K, Chung TG, Oda O (1982) Clinical effects of larger molecules removal with
     protein-permeating hemodiafiltration (P-P HDF) (Abstract). Abstr Eur Dial Transplant Assoc
     123
185. Saito A, Ogawa H, Takagi T, Ohta K, Akasu H, Kawai S, Kubotsu A (1983) A new approach to
     glomerular filtration. Trans Am Soc Artif Intern Organs 29: 673
186. Saito A, Ohta K, Chung TG, Takagi T (1983) Clinical evaluation of protein-permeating hemo-
     diafiltration (Abstract). Blood Purif 1: 55
187. Saito A, Ohta K, Takay T, Chung TG (1983) One year experience of protein-permeating hemo-
     diafiltration. Artif Organs 7: 58
188. Saito A, Ogawa H, Chung TG, Takagi G (1984) Protein-permeating hemodiafiltration (Ab-
     stract). Blood Purif 2: 60
189. Leber H-W, Wizemann V (1982) Simultane Hämofiltration/Hämodialyse (SHFHD, Hämo-
     diafiltration): Ergebnisse und Indikationen. In: Streicher E, Schoeppe W (eds) Die adäquate
     Dialyse. Springer, Heidelberg Berlin New York, p 33
190. Vanholder R, Verbanck J, Schelstraete J, de Smeet R, Ringoir S (1982) Unipuncture simulta-

neous hemofiltration and dialysis. In: Schütterle G, Wizemann V, Seyffart G (eds) Hemodiafiltration. Hygieneplan, Oberursel, p 76

191. Wizemann V, Kramer W, Knopp G, Sychla M, Schmidt H, Rawer P, Schütterle G (1982) Cardiovascular function during hemodialysis, hemofiltration, hemodiafiltration. In: Schütterle G, Wizemann V, Seyffart G (eds) Hemodiafiltration. Hygieneplan, Oberursel, p 89

192. Mazzitello G, Candito C, Grandinetti F, Pugliesi G, Rondanini V (1984) Intolerance to hemodialysis and hemodiafiltration (Abstract). Blood Purif 2: 56

193. Wizemann V, Sychla M, Leber HW (1980) Simultaneous hemofiltration/hemodialysis versus hemofiltration and hemodialysis: hemodynamic parameters. Proc Eur Soc Artif Organs 7: 143

194. Wizemann V, Sychla M, Leber HW, Schütterle G (1982) Hemodynamics during five different techniques in the treatment of acute renal failure. In: Eliahou HE (ed) Acute renal failure. Proceedings of the Tel Aviv Satellite Symposion. Libbey, London, p 176

195. Schneider H, Liomin E, Streicher E (1985) Hemodynamic study of diffusive and convective procedures using a polysulfone membrane. In: Streicher E, Seyffart G (eds) Highly permeable membranes. Contrib Nephrol 46: 134

196. Jahn H, Bauler M, Schohn D (1985) Hemodynamic studies in chronic dialysis patients with a polysulfone hemodiafilter. In: Streicher E, Seyffart G (eds) Highly permeable membranes. Contrib Nephrol 46: 151

197. Schmidt M, Schoeppe W, Baldamus CA (1985) Hemodynamics during hemodialysis with dialyzers of high hydraulic permeability. In: Streicher E, Seyffart G (eds) Highly permeable membranes. Contrib Nephrol 46: 127

198. Shaldon S, Deschodt G, Branger B, Granolleras C, Baldamus CA, Koch KM, Dinarello CA (1985) Haemodialysis hypotension: the interleukin hypothesis restated. Proc Eur Dial Transplant Assoc 22: (in press)

199. Henderson L (1980) Symptomatic hypertension during hemodialysis. Kidney Int 17: 571

200. Shaldon S, Baldamus CA, Koch KM, Lysaght MJ (1983) Of sodium, symptomatology and syllogism. Blood Purif 1: 16

201. Gotch FA, Sargent JA (1983) Hemofiltration: an unnecessarily complex method to achieve hypotonic sodium removal and controlled ultrafiltration. Blood Purif 1: 9

202. Basile C, Di Maggio A, Longo S, Scatizzi A (1984) Sodium balance in hypertonic hemodiafiltration. Blood Purif 2: 70

203. Basile C, Aprile G, Gugliotta F, Di Maggio A, Pellegrino P, Longo S, Scatizzi A (1983) Role of osmolality in dialysis tolerance and vascular stability in hypertonic hemodiafiltration. Proc Pavia Workshop on dialysis tolerance and vascular stability. Int J Artif Organs (in press)

204. Wizemann V, Wizemann A (1984) Letter to the editor. Am J Nephrol 4: 134

205. Kramer W, Wizemann V, Kindler M, Thormann J, Grebe SF, Schütterle G, Lasch H-G, Schlepper M (1984) Influence of fluid removal rate on left ventricular performance and exercise tolerance in patients with coronary artery disease. Clin Nephrol 21: 280

206. Henderson LW, Koch KM, Dinarello CA, Shaldon S (1983) Hemodialysis hypotension: the interleukin hypothesis. Blood Purif 1: 3

207. Koch KM, Shaldon S, Baldamus CA, Lysaght MJ, Lonnemann G, Bingel M, Dinarello CA (1985) Convective mass transport in dialysis. Proc Eur Dial Transplant Assoc 22: (in press)

208. Wizemann V (1982) Erprobte Dialyseverfahren und ihre spezielle Indikation. Klinikarzt 11: 580

209. Schmidt R (1983) Untersuchungen zur Senkung der Frequenz akuter Komplikationen während der Hämodialyse. Thesis, Rostock, GDR

210. Klinkmann H, Ivanovich P (1984) Advantages and disadvantages of current dialysis techniques. In: Robinson RR (ed) Nephrology. Springer, New York Berlin Heidelberg Tokyo, p 1528

211. Fischbach M, Koehl C, Geisert J (1985) Hemodiafiltration – a superior method of blood purification in children? In: Streicher E, Seyffart G (eds) Highly permeable membranes. Contrib Nephrol 46: 162

212. Mion C, Oules R, Canaud B, Mourad G, Slingeneyer A, Branger B, Granolleras C, Al Sabadani B, Florence P, Chouzenoux R, Maurice F, Issautier R, Flavier JL, Polito C, Saunier F, Marty L, Fontanier P, Emond C, Ramtoolah H, Cornelissen F de, Huchard G, Fitte H, Boudet R (1984) Maintenance dialysis in the elderly. A review of 15 years experience in Languedoc-Roussillon. Proc Eur Dial Transplant Assoc 21: 490

213. Fischbach M, Attal Y, Geisert J (1984) Hemodiafiltration versus hemodialysis in children. A twelve months experience. Int J Pediatr Nephrol 5: 151

Comparative Economics of Hemofiltration Treatment

B. SCHÜNEMANN and V. BEHNCKE

Table of Contents

Introduction

The importance of hemofiltration (HF) as a safe and efficient method of treatment especially for critically ill patients, has been pointed out on numerous occasions. In addition, it proves to be of equal quality when compared with all conventional methods of treatment. One of the reasons which speaks against an increased application of HF routinely is that it is, as yet, a rather expensive method in comparison with hemodialysis (HD) and continuous ambulatory peritoneal dialysis (CAPD). The topic to be considered is a comparison of the various costs for the different methods of dialysis treatment, dealing not only with the direct costs but also with indirect or additional treatment costs. In illustrating such problems, it must then be possible to say how the total costs can be influenced by the increased application of one or more dialysis or other treatment methods.

An uniform and obligatory estimation of the costs is, however, not possible because, for example,

1) The cost prices of materials for each hospital are different, with sales prices and salaries showing considerable national differences.
2) Government regulations control the selection of the dialysis population, thereby influencing the market in one direction only.
3) National problems regarding supplies, are difficult to evaluate quantitatively,

e. g., HD places a large demand on water supplies and is rather costly in countries with a shortage of water, where HF would therefore be more economical.

4) Additional costs for medicines, hospitalization due to complications, taxi fares, and occupational rehabilitation, are difficult to quantitate comparably. (As far as occupational rehabilitation goes, many patients who would be able to work under certain conditions, do not find work because of the current unemployment situation.)

The following budget of expenses derives generally from a center with 60% HD patients and 40% HF patients. Ninety home-dialysis patients are on HD, HF, or CAPD treatment.

Direct Cost Analysis

A comparison of the costs for HF and HD in hospital and at home, as well as for CAPD, can be seen in Table 1 and Fig. 1. The overhead expenses including maintenance include the costs for items such as buildings and apparatus, their maintenance, disinfection, general hospital costs, electricity, water, material for laboratory investigations, ECG, and X-rays. The difference between DM 90 and DM 105 for in-hospital HD is due to additional expenses for disinfection, reverse osmosis, and repairs, as well as increased electricity and water consumption. Medical fees are included in the personnel costs for both hospital and home dialysis. This shows that one could economize most in the home-dialysis sector. For HF, less supervision is required, hence, lower personnel costs, i. e., DM 158 as against DM 168 for HD. The costs for dialysis material include those for dialyzers or filters, tubings, concentrates or substitution fluids, cannula for punctures, medicines, infusions, syringes, etc. Here we find the biggest differences between HF and HD or CAPD. This applies to both hospital and home treatments. Altogether, this amounts to DM 498 for hospital HF which proves to be the most expensive treatment method, followed by hospital HD (DM 418), home HF (DM 390), home HD (DM 281), and CAPD (DM 262).

Table 1. The per-treatment cost of different dialysis modalities

	Hospital dialysis (DM)		Home dialysis (DM)		
	HF	HD	HF	HD	CAPD[a]
Personnel	158	168	70	70	58
Overhead expenses and depreciation costs (including maintenance, etc.)	90	105	70	81	64
Dialysis material	250	145	250	130	140
Σ	498	418	390	281	262

[a] Per 2.3 days

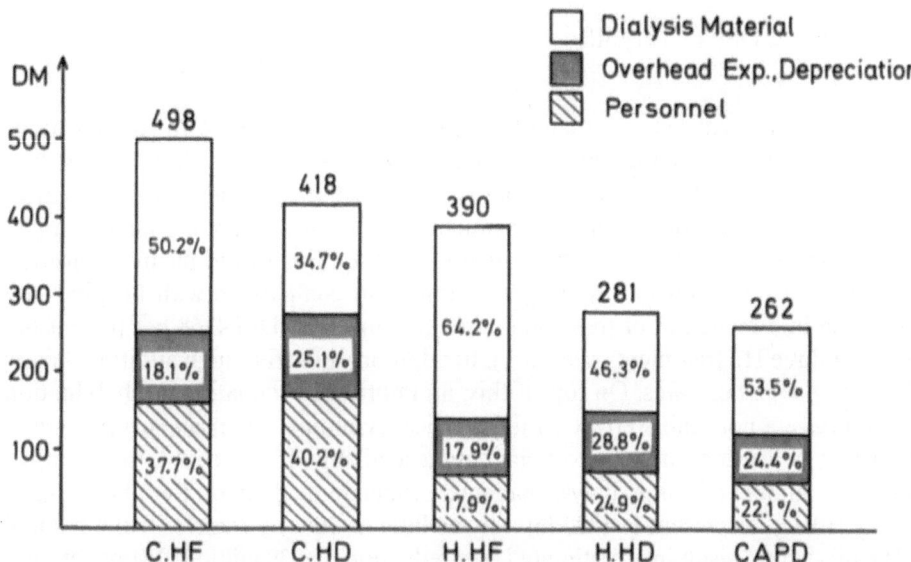

Fig. 1. The comparative per treatment costs for hospital hemofiltration *(C. HF)*, hospital hemodialysis *(C. HD)*, home hemofiltration *(H. HD)*, home hemodialysis *(H. HD)* and *CAPD*, including the percentages for dialysis material, overhead expenses, depreciation costs, maintenance, and personnel

Table 2. Comparative annual cost for dialysis equipment and material

	Relative cost
Standard hemodialysis	1.00
Bicarbonate hemodialysis	1.14
High-flux hemodialysis	1.38
Postdilution hemofiltration	1.85
Hemodiafiltration	2.04

For CAPD, we considered a treatment rate of 2.3 days which is equivalent to one HF/HD treatment.

The biggest cost differences between the various treatment methods apply to stocks for dialysis machines and other dialysis material as shown in Table 2. One can also see that hemodiafiltration (HDF) carries the highest costs for dialysis material, being reason enough for the hesitant advocation of this method.

An overall comparison of the costs, shows that home dialysis, in general, irrespective of the method, is the most reasonable. In addition, indirect costs such as those for taxi fares to and from hospital fall away, as has also been otherwise confirmed [1, 2]. Of course, transplantation is the most reasonable method as far as the costs go. A calculation made by D'APICE [3] shows that 60% of the costs for a standard HD treatment accumulate within the first year of treatment and 10% in every following year.

Indirect Cost Analysis

PLOUGH et al [4] have shown that a high percentage of patients with complications are found in hospital-based dialysis centers. As HF is supposed to be a safe method of treatment for patients with circulatory complications [5], these medical indications could be expanded for home treatment, i.e., the proportion of potential home-dialysis patients could be raised through home HF. This would mean a considerable overall reduction of DM 28 per treatment in comparison with hospital HD resulting in a reduction of treatment costs amounting to DM 4368 per patient per year (at three HF treatments per week). In addition, the rather high additional costs fall away, e.g., taxi fares. On top of this, an improved occupational rehabilitation would have a noticeable effect on the political economy. An exact survey cannot, however, be carried out as no official data is available. If one could, for example, raise the number of home-dialysis patients – which in the Federal Republic of Germany (FRG), at present is 1822 [6] – by as little as 10% by transfer from hospital HD, this would result in an estimated cost reduction of 4.39 million DM per annum (traveling costs of DM 20000 per patient per annum being included).

An improvement of the cost effectiveness of HF, particularly regarding personnel costs, compared with HD, can be reached with a shorter treatment time using high-flux filters. To add to this, the preparation phase of the modern HF machines is considerably shorter, as there is no disinfection and no hotrinsing phase, the functioning of the machines being relatively independent of a water installation. This makes

Table 3. Possible cost savings in hemofiltration

	Percentage
Self-produced replacement fluid	50–60
Reuse of hemofilter	50–60
Improvement of personnel effectiveness	30–40
Difference per treatment	30

Table 4. Comparative costs per treatment in hospital-based HD and HF with improved cost effectiveness

	Hemofiltration (DM)	Hemodialysis (DM)
Personnel	103	168
Overhead expenses and depreciation costs (including maintenance, etc.)	90	105
Dialysis material	150	112
Total	343	385
Difference	(11%)	

HF a fairly flexible method of treatment. It is possible to carry out three HF shifts with the same staff in the same time required for two HD shifts. This results in a saving of 30%–40% of the personnel costs.

The costs of dialysis material for HF in hospital and at home are comparatively high, being 50.2% and 64.2% of the total treatment costs respectively. One could, however, lower the costs for filters by 50%–60% with reusage, i.e., if they are used 4–5 times as is the case for dialyzers [7, 8]. In addition, it is possible to produce own substitution fluid on an off-line basis with special apparatus, e.g., Aquasart-Sartorius. Based on 3000 treatments per year, one could lower the costs for substitution fluid by a further 50%–60%. Table 3 shows an overall survey of possible realistic cost reductions. As is shown, the total potential cost reductions amount to 30% per treatment.

A calculation of the costs is shown in Table 4. One can see that the costs per HF treatment could be reduced to DM 343, which is 11% lower than the costs for HD. It was taken into account that the costs for dialyzers were likewise reduced because of reuse.

The main condition for this cost assessment, however, is the acceptance of HF as a routine method, which is then economical if enough patients are treated by this method.

Future Development

The development of reimbursed costs for HD over the past years is shown in Fig. 2. Although the personnel costs for dialysis treatment are continually increasing, there has been a significant drop in the HD costs over the years. This shows that the costs for dialysis material can be reduced. A similar policy is also to be expected with regard to HF. Costs for dialysis machines and filters could be reduced in the hospital-

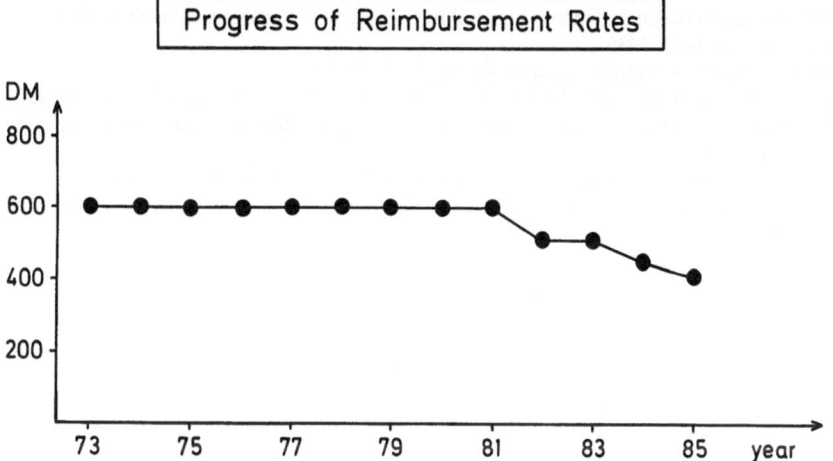

Fig. 2. Decrease of reimbursement rates for hemodialysis from 1973 to 1985

dialysis sector. On-line apparatus would allow a further drop in the costs for substitution fluid. Reusage could be further extended. Costs for machines could be lowered on the home-dialysis sector. Expensive high-flux filters are surely not necessary in every case, especially in home dialysis, as personnel costs are not of importance here.

Conclusion

A comparison of the direct costs per treatment shows HF as the most expensive and CAPD as the cheapest dialysis method. The difference is mainly due to material costs. Generally speaking, all home-dialysis methods are more reasonable as far as costs go. With HF the medical indications for home dialysis could also be extended to include dialysis patients with circulatory problems, thereby attaining a reduction of costs in contrast to hospital HD. With an improvement of personnel effectiveness, e. g., two HD shifts to three HF shifts simultaneously, reuse of filters, and self-produced substitution fluid, the HF costs can already be reduced by 30%, hospital HF then being 11% cheaper than hospital HD treatment. Future development with a reasonable market, i. e., sufficient HF treatments, will reduce prices for filters and machines and lead to a further reduction of costs for self-produced substitution fluid. HF, therefore, qualifies as a good and economical treatment method, making further cost reductions possible.

References

1. Clade H (1977) Finanzielle Grenzen des Dialyseprogramms. Dtsch Ärzteblatt 50: 2967–2972
2. Clade H (1977) Finanzielle Grenzen des Dialyseprogramms. Dtsch Ärzteblatt 51: 3021–3023
3. d'Apice AJF, Thomson NM, Heale WF, Kincaid-Smith PS (1983) Planning, developing and operating a dialysis programme. In: Drukker W, Parsons FM, Maher JF (eds) Replacement of renal function by dialysis, 2nd edn. Nijhoff, Boston, pp 820–829
4. Plough AL, Salem SR, Schwartz M, Weller JM, Ferguson WC (1984) Case mix in end-stage renal disease. Differences between patients in hospital-based and free-standing treatment facilities. N Engl J Med 310 (22): 1432–1436
5. Shaldon S (1981) Progress from haemodialysis. Nephron 27: 2–6
6. Kramer P, Broyer M, Brunner FP, Brynger H, Challah S, Oules R, Rizzoni G, Selwood NH, Wing AJ, Balas EA (1984) Combined report on regular dialysis and transplantation in Europe, XIV, 1983. Proc Eur Dial Transplant Assoc 21: 5–68
7. Foxen LG (1984) Is reuse cost effective? A case study. Dial Transplant 13 (5): 290–293
8. Ogden DA, Kopec G, Guy AD (1981) Cost effectiveness of multiple dialyzer use. Dial Transplant 10 (5): 407–411

The Future of Hemofiltration

L. W. HENDERSON

Table of Contents

Predilution hemofiltration (HF) was initiated as a test strategy to evaluate the pathophysiologic significance of "middle molecules" for the uremic patient [1, 2]. As such, the system was devised for use in the patient with stable end stage renal failure (ESRF). As originally applied, it was recognized to be at a disadvantage in the removal of low molecular weight solutes (< 350 daltons) when compared with hemodialysis (HD). Since then many changes have occurred in how convective mass transport is applied. Postdilution vs predilution [3] as a means of economizing on diluting fluid, hemodiafiltration (HDF) [4, 5, 6] which combines the best of both diffusion and convection, and continuous low efficiency HF for the treatment of acute renal failure (ARF) [7] are some of the creative applications to which this ultrafiltration methodology has been put. In placing this spectrum of techniques into the special perspective of "the future of hemofiltration" I wish to take a brief backward look in order to have you join me in extrapolating this line of development into the future.

Historical Perspective

It should be pointed out that the pioneering clinical work of Kolff [8] in applying his artificial kidney logically took him first to the application of this device in a young woman with chronic renal failure (CRF) ("malignant hypertension and shrunken kidneys"), not ARF, as has been erroneously reported [9]. Her survival of the artificial kidney treatment (for more than 4 weeks), if not her chronic uremia, was sufficiently encouraging to warrant the treatment of 15 more patients suffering from ARF. There was but a single survivor [8]. In spite of these dismal survival statistics, application of the technique continued, as it prolonged life. ARF was the disease entity to which this new device was applied until the early 1960s when BELDING SCRIBNER deliberately applied the artificial kidney to patients with CRF and plunged us into the era of maintenance dialysis [10].

Similarly, HF was first applied in a patient with CRF [11]. The recent upswing in application to treatment of patients with ARF, i. e., continuous arteriovenous hemo-filtration (CAVH), continues along the track of the historical development of HD. The late PETER KRAMER must be given full recognition for both identifying and pop-ularizing CAVH for this application [7]. His clinical reports of CAVH in Europe ini-tiated the logarithmic growth phase of this technique that we are presently experi-encing, both in Europe and North America. While description of the technique was initially made in the United States, [12, 13], the focus was more on the fluid removal aspects of the technique over the short term, rather than its continuous application to solute removal, as championed by Dr. Kramer.

HF and HD, during the recent past, have frequently been cast in adversarial roles, i. e., in a contest for which technique will eventually capture the market place for artificial kidneys. While this has made for some very lively discussions at nation-al and international meetings, I believe that this pedagogical device obscures the well-recognized goal of devising the very best treatment strategy possible for patient care. The new and persuasive evidence for the presence and pathophysiologic sig-nificance of intermediate molecular weight solutes (see chapter by HENDERSON and LEYPOLDT, this volume) coupled with the clear understanding that conventional small molecular weight uremic toxins are even more toxic, points us strongly to the logical conclusion that we must harness the capabilities of both techniques in order to provide the most efficient treatment. We must couple HF with its capability to re-move solutes that are just too big to move in satisfactory time-frame by diffusion with HD and its capability for swift small solute removal. Early studies of such cou-pling point towards a synergism between the two techniques in at least one rather complex dual membrane system [5]. The complexity of rigorously sifting out the re-spective contributions of diffusion and convection to the overall solute clearance pattern noted when both techniques are applied simultaneously [14] will probably not prove to be a worry for the clinician interested in maximizing the removal of ab-normal solutes of all molecular weights regardless of the underlying mechanisms. As such, creative application of this combination technique has already preceded the formal description of its kinetics. At present, two modes of application for HDF have been proposed. LEBER et al. [4] pioneered the simplest approach using a rou-tine dialysis membrane of high hydraulic permeability and conducting routine HD, but at a maximum ultrafiltration rate. Replacement of the plasma ultrafiltrate that is removed in excess of the required reduction in total body water necessary to restore dry weight is accomplished by simple "downstream" intravenous infusion. As such, a 6- to 10-liter convective solute removal is added to that accomplished by diffusion. The resulting solute removal pattern is more evenly balanced between large and small solutes. Minor variants of this approach have recently become popular in Ita-ly and Japan [15, 16]. We [5] and von ALBERTINI et al. [6] have favored a more com-plex approach in which two 1- to 1.5-m² membranes of high hydraulic permeability are used in series, as if doing routine HD (Fig. 1). A pressure gradient is generated from blood to bath in the first membrane and results in loss of filtrate which is swept to drain in the dialysate stream. A reversal of the pressure gradient in the sec-ond membrane seen by the blood results in an uptake of the freshly entering dialy-sate across the membrane. This replacement infusion must again be balanced with the loss of ultrafiltrate in a manner to accomplish the net loss of fluid required clin-

HEMODIAFILTRATION HYBRID SYSTEM

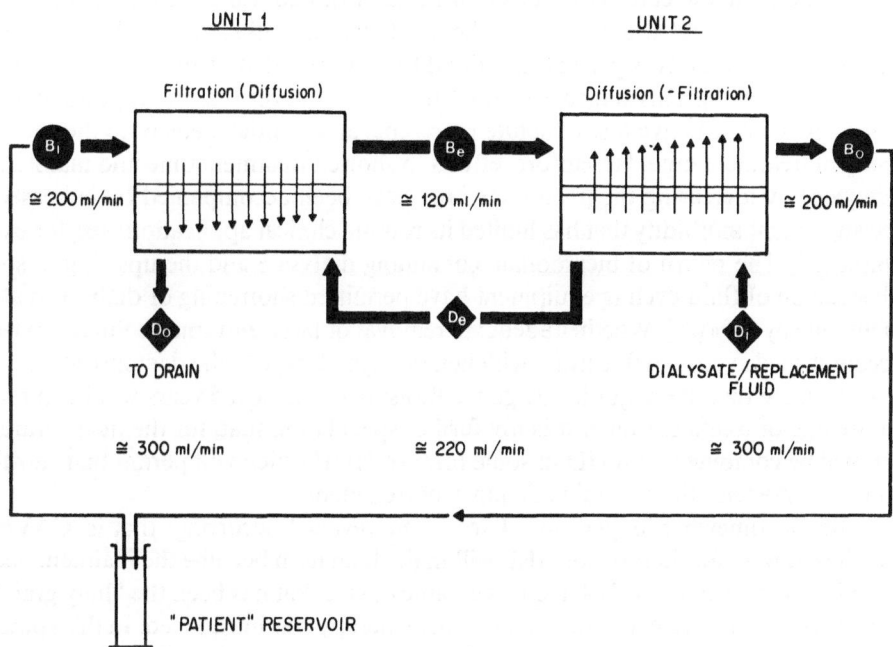

Fig. 1. Schematic diagram of a bench hemodiafiltration flow path. Blood enters unit 1 *(B_i)* at 200 ml/min where both ultrafiltration and diffusion occur. The reduced blood flow rate $(B_e = 120 \text{ ml/min})$ enters the second unit where back filtration reconstitutes the blood-flow rate returning to the patient $(B_o = 200 \text{ ml/min})$ and further diffusive solute loss takes place. Sterile pyrogen-free dialysate/reconstituting fluid flows in a countercurrent direction

ically for normalization of body water. VON ALBERTINI, in order to maximize efficiency, uses the highest possible blood flow rates that can be obtained from routine fistula access (500 + 50 ml/min) and with dialysate flow rates of 1000 ml/min. Internal filtration and replacement occurs at 112 ml/min. Removal of both urea and creatinine over the 6 h of treatment per week are equal to or greater than that offered by conventional 1.2 m² 12 h per week treatment, thus, assuring adequacy of treatment by analogy with solute removal patterns for adequate dialysis. In this way an exceedingly high and balanced clearance rate is achieved.

The fluid cycling hardware necessary to accomplish these goals is more complex than that used for routine dialysis, but quite comparable to that required for HF. Assurance of sterile pyrogen-free on-line production of replacement solution for this two-membrane HDF is a critical constituent for its success, but preliminary work suggests that this will be readily forthcoming [17, 18].

A very important result of the HF process is the identification of increased vascular stability with this technique when compared with HD [19, 20, 21, 22]. For reasons that are as yet unidentified, there is an appropriate release of norepinephrine with an attendant increase in total peripheral resistance that accompanies fluid removal with HF, which is lacking with HD [23, 24]. Contenders for the underlying mechanism are: A positive net sodium balance with HF, better biocompatibility (as assessed by complement activation) that accompanies use of the noncellulosic HF membranes, and the convective loos of a vascular destabilizing factor, i. e., blocker of norepinephrine release. I am sure other explanations will surface with time. This hemodynamic stability is preserved with HDF, as is reported by both LEBER [4] and VON ALBERTINI [6]. This unusual feature that, for whatever reason, appears to accompany the convective loss of solute represents an essential element to the shortening of treatment time. Heretofore, efforts to shorten treatment time and maintain adequacy by increasing the membrane area have been accompanied by increased intratreatment morbidity that has limited its routine clinical application; see, for example [25]. The return of bicarbonate containing dialysate and the upswing in sophistication of fluid cycling equipment have permitted shortening of dialysis treatment time by 25% [26]. Whether adequate removal of large and small solutes can be accomplished symptom free in 2 h with hemodialysis has yet to be demonstrated.

I speculate that the major investigative thrust over the next 5 years will be in the shortening of treatment time. It is my further speculation that, for the near future, HF will be combined with HD in some form of HDF which will permit that shortening of time and still maintain adequacy of treatment.

Taking a somewhat longer look, I see a role reversal occurring; that is, CAVH which is now a new therapy for ARF will in the long term become the maintenance technique for CRF as the 24-h a day wearable device that has been the "holy grail" of workers in this area ever since maintanance therapy was introduced. In this spirit, Fig. 2 shows LEWIS W. BLUEMLE'S concept of a "wristwatch dialyzer" put forward in the 1960s. To complete the speculation in this area, I see reprocessing of ultrafiltrate (i.e., adding a tubule) as the logical next step. Of the numerous possible options, I

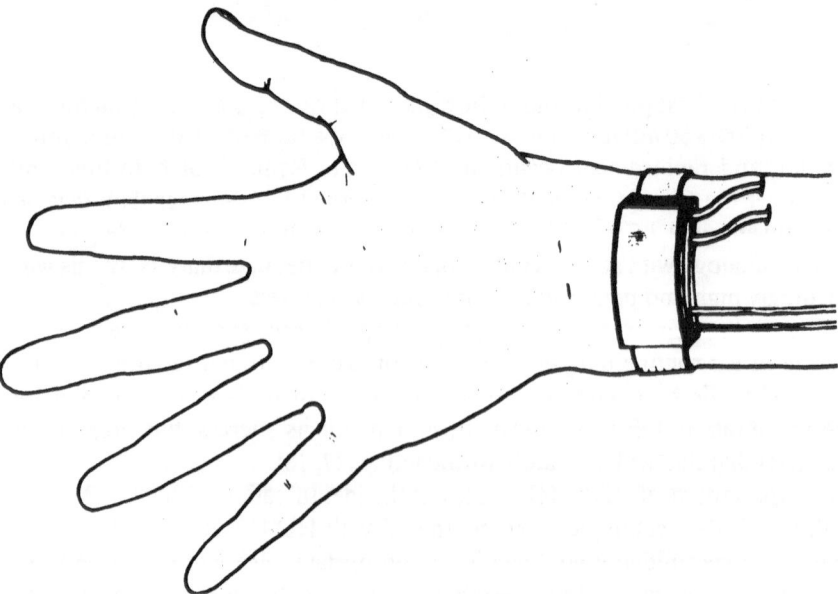

Fig. 2. The Bluemle "wristwatch dialyzer" as representative of our goal in 1965

GOAL

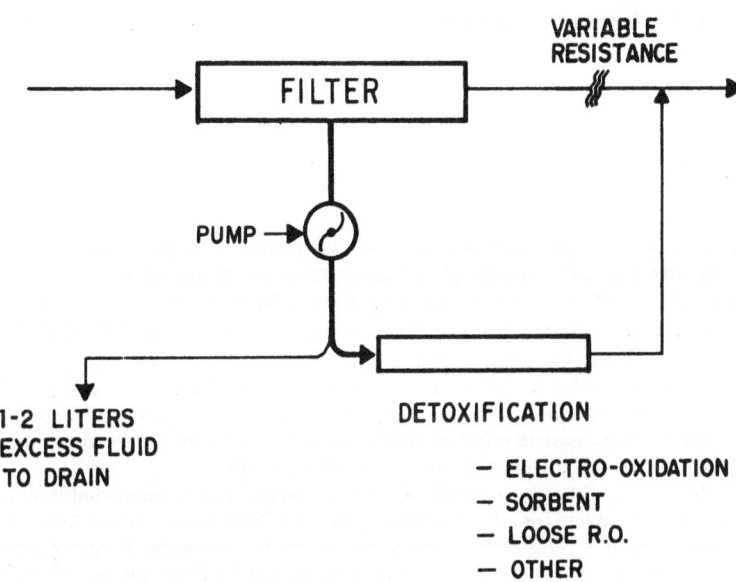

Fig. 3. An updated goal (from 1977) for a wearable artificial kidney

favor electrooxidation as a potentially compact system that could be battery powered and oxidize urea [26, 27] and possibly all of the organic constituents of the ultrafiltrate. This would mean reduction of carbohydrates and lipids to carbon dioxide and water with possibly a little inorganic phosphate remaining and the rendering of polypeptides to nitrogen gas with a little inorganic sulfate remaining. The inorganic "undetermined anions" might well yield to specific oral sorbents or selective trapping agents in the reprocessing path. Figure 3 is a diagram of such a circuit [1]. Excess total body water could be removed from the closed loop in an orderly manner through the day and discarded. The glucose and bicarbonate drain that this would impose could readily be offset orally. As the final role reversal, I see the patient with routine low catabolic rate ARF being treated with some variant of CAVH or peritoneal dialysis, but when high efficiency treatment is necessary (as for the high catabolic rate circumstances or to treat overdosages and poisoning), it will be with some variant of HDF.

A second but distinctly less likely scenario for the high efficiency treatment of ARF would be the utilization of pure HF with high blood flow rate (300–500 ml/min) in high flow predilution mode with membranes of sufficiently high hydraulic permeability (and/or area) to permit the system to operate in a blood-flow limited manner, i.e., the cross washing of every milliliter of blood traversing the blood path with sufficient diluting fluid to have unwanted solutes up to the molecular weight cutoff of the membrane asymptotically approaching zero concentration in the returning blood with clearance having little or no size discriminination. This would be expensive of diluting fluid and hence, to my mind, less desirable.

The future of HF in its pure form is then likely to reside with its continuous application to CRF as described in part by SHALDON [29], i.e., continuous ambulatory HF. In combination with dialysis, its contribution will be central to the design of any high efficiency membrane-based device for short-term intermittent treatment of renal failure.

References

1. Henderson LW (1977) Development of a convective blood cleansing technique. Proceedings of the 10th Annual Contractors Conference, Bethesda, Maryland, p 130
2. Henderson LW (1981) The beginning of hemofiltration. In: Beryne GM, Giovannetti S, Thomas S (eds) Contributions to nephrology series, vol 32. Shaefer K, Koch KM, Quellhorst E, von Herrath D (eds) Symposium on hemofiltration volume. Karger, Basel, p 1
3. Henderson LW (1979) Pre- vs. postdilution hemofiltration. Clin Nephrol 11: 120
4. Leber HW, Wizemann V, Goubeaud G, Rawer P, Schutterle G (1978) Simultaneous hemofiltration/hemodialysis: an effective alternative to hemofiltration and conventional hemodialysis in the treatment of uremic patients. Clin Nephrol 9: 115
5. Cheung AK, Kato Y, Leypoldt JK, Henderson LW (1982) Hemodiafiltration using a hybrid membrane system for self-generation of diluting fluid. Trans Am Soc Artif Intern Organs 28: 61
6. von Albertini B, Miller JH, Gardner PW, Norris KC, Roberts CE, Shinaberger JH (1984) High flux hemodiafiltration. Abstract, American Society for Nephrology, 17th annual meeting, p 76
7. Kramer P (ed) (1982) Arterio-venous hemofiltration, Vandenhoeck and Ruprecht, Göttingen
8. Kolff WJ (1965) First clinical experience with the artificial kidney. Ann Intern Med 62: 608
9. McBride PT (1979) Genesis of the artificial kidney, chap 3. Travenol Labs, Deerfield, Illinois, USA, p 9
10. Quinton WE, Dillard DH, Cole JJ, Scribner BH (1962) Eight months experience with silastic-teflon bypass cannulas. Trans Am Soc Artif Intern Organs 8: 236
11. Henderson LW, Besarab A, Michaels A, Bluemle LW Jr (1967) Blood purification by ultrafiltration and fluid replacement (diafiltration). Trans Am Soc Artif Intern Organs 12: 216
12. Silverstein ME, Ford CA, Lysaght MJ, Henderson LW (1974) Treatment of severe fluid overload by ultrafiltration. N Engl J Med 291: 747
13. Paganini EP, Nakamoto S (1980) Continuous slow flow ultrafiltration in oliguric acute renal failure. Trans Am Soc Artif Intern Organs 26: 203
14. Leypoldt JK, Frigon RP, Henderson LW (1985) Characterization of solutes transport in membrane ultrafiltration. J Membrane Sci (in review)
15. Maeda K, Shinzato T, Sezaki R, Yamada K, Saito A, Ohta K (1984) Decrease sieving coefficient for middle molecule during hemofiltration and infusion free hemodiafiltration. Blood Purif 2: 54 (Abstract)
16. Icardi A, Lamperi B, Cappelli G, Lamperi S (1984) Hemofiltration and biofiltration: a comparative study on the short term effects. Blood Purif 2: 52 (Abstract)
17. Henderson LW, Beans E (1978) Successful production of sterile pyrogen free electrolyte solution by ultrafiltration. Kidney Int 14: 522
18. Henderson LW, Sanfelippo ML, Beans E (1978) "On line" preparation of sterile pyrogen free electrolyte solution. Trans Am Soc Artif Intern Organs 24: 465
19. Baldamus CA (1983) Clinical value and technical feasibility of long term hemofiltration. Assaio J 6: 192
20. Bosch JP, von Albertini B, Geronemus R, Glabman S, Goldstein MH, Kahn T, Kupfer S (1979) Comparison of hemofiltration and ultrafiltration plus hemodialysis to conventional hemodialysis. Annual Progress report to the Artificial Kidney Chronic Uremia Program, National Institute of Arthritis, Metabolic and Digestive Diseases, 15 March 1979
21. Henderson LW (1980) Symptomatic hypotension during hemodialysis. Kidney Int 17: 571
22. Quellhorst EA, Schuenemann B, Hildebrand U (1983) Morbidity and mortality in long term hemofiltration. Asaio J 6: 185

23. Baldamus CA, Ernst W, Fassbinder W, Koch KM (1980) Differing haemodynamics stability due to differing sympathetic response: comparison of ultrafiltration, haemodialysis and haemofiltration. Proc Eur Dial Transplant Assoc 17: 205
24. Quellhorst E, Schuenemann B, Hildebrand U, Falda Z (1980) Response of the vascular system to different modifications of haemofiltration and haemodialysis. Proc Eur Dial Transplant Assoc 17: 197
25. Graefe U, Milutinovich J, Follette WC, Vizzo JE, Babb AL, Scribner BH (1978) Less dialysis induced morbidity and vascular instability with bicarbonate and dialysate. Ann Intern Med 88: 332
26. Schuenemann B, Quellhorst E, Kaiser H, Richter G, Mundt K, Weidlich E, Loeffler G, Zachariae M and Schunk O (1982) Regeneration of filtrate and dialysis fluid by electro-oxidation and absorption. Trans Am Soc Artif Intern Organs 28: 49
27. Wright JC (1982) Electrochemical dialysate regeneration: the electrooxidation of urea at the ruthenium titanium oxide electrode. Ph D Dissertation, Stanford University
28. Shaldon S, Beau MC, Deschodt G, Lysaght MJ, Ramperez P, Mion C (1980) Continuous ambulatory hemofiltration. Trans Am Soc Artif Intern Organs 26: 210

Subject Index

Numbers printed in italics refer to pages upon which the keyword is dealt with more extensively